VOLUME 1

RADIOGRAPHIC ANATOMY, POSITIONING, & PROCEDURES WORKBOOK

*This workbook is dedicated to the most important person in my life,
my wife, Sharon Hayes. Her love and support for me have created all the happiness
in my life. She was the motivation that inspired me to become
a radiologic technology educator, and she is the reason I still pursue goals;
therefore, this publication is for her.*

VOLUME 1

RADIOGRAPHIC ANATOMY, POSITIONING, & PROCEDURES WORKBOOK

Third Edition

Steven G. Hayes, Sr., BSRT, MEd, RT(R)

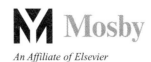

An Affiliate of Elsevier

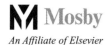
An Affiliate of Elsevier

11830 Westline Industrial Drive
St. Louis, Missouri 63146

RADIOGRAPHIC ANATOMY, POSITIONING, AND PROCEDURES WORKBOOK   0-323-01480-1
Copyright © 2003, Mosby, Inc. All rights reserved.

NOTICE

Previous editions copyrighted 1996, 1999

International Standard Book Number 0-323-01480-1

Acquisitions Editor: Jeanne Wilke
Editorial Assistant: Paige Mosher
Project Manager: Joy Moore
Senior Designer: Mark A. Oberkrom

Printed in the United States of America

Last digit is the print number: 9   8   7   6   5   4   3

Preface

This two-volume workbook has been developed to accompany *Mosby's Radiographic Instructional Series (MRIS): Anatomy, Positioning, and Procedures* multimedia and *Merrill's Atlas of Radiographic Positions and Radiologic Procedures* (commonly referred to as *Merrill's Atlas* or just, *Merrill's*). The chapters in this workbook are presented in the same order as the 27 units in *Mosby's Radiographic Instructional Series: Anatomy, Positioning, and Procedures* multimedia and the first 27 chapters of *Merrill's Atlas of Radiographic Positions and Radiologic Procedures.* However, the material presented in this workbook can function as a useful review for any anatomy and positioning course or as a review for the certification exam. The exercises found in this workbook are designed to give you a thorough review of osteology, anatomy, physiology, arthrology, and radiographic examinations.

The following features were revised or newly added to the second edition.

- Updated and standardized anatomy terminology to reflect the usage in *Merrill's Atlas* as well as the most current anatomy texts and *Nomina Anatomica*
- New questions on computed radiography (CR), including the slight positioning changes and the kVp setting changes necessary for CR
- New exercise sections on radiographic quality in Chapter 1, identifying projections of the vertebral column in Chapter 8, and review of essential mammographic projections in Chapter 24
- New chapter review self-tests for Chapters 20 through 23
- More film evaluations, offering additional opportunities to evaluate images for proper positioning
- More positioning questions to complement the workbook's strong anatomy review
- Reformatted exercises for ease of writing in answers while working through the MRIS multimedia tutorials

The following features have been revised or newly added to the third edition.

- More than 60 new pictures, radiographic images, and illustrations
- New matching exercises for pathology terms in 12 chapters that have essential projections
- New exercises for identifying projections of the upper limb in Chapter 4, for identifying projections of the shoulder girdle in Chapter 5, and for identifying mammographic projections in Chapter 24
- New review exercises for the tangential projection for the intertubercular groove in Chapter 5 and for the verticosubmental projection for the cranium in Chapter 20

- New review exercises for the completely revised Chapter 13, "Trauma Radiography"
- Improved sequencing of exercise items with the text of *Merrill's Atlas of Radiographic Positions and Radiologic Procedures*
- Numerous exercises updated to reflect related changes found in the current edition of *Merrill's Atlas of Radiographic Positions and Radiologic Procedures*
- Chapter 24, Mammography, expanded to seven separate exercises from its original three exercises

All chapters that have essential projections are divided into two sections: (1) an anatomy section and (2) a positioning section.

- The anatomy sections consist of various exercises such as labeling and identification diagrams, short-answer and multiple-choice questions, matching exercises, and crossword puzzles.
- The positioning sections include short-answer and multiple-choice questions, true-false statements, fill-in-the-blank statements, matching exercises, identification exercises, and radiographic comparisons of standard radiographic projections.
- At the end of each chapter is a collection of multiple-choice questions that reviews the entire chapter.
- Answers for all exercises are provided at the end of each volume.

Some of the radiographic projections included and described in *Merrill's Atlas* are for reference purposes only and are no longer routinely performed in radiologic imaging facilities. Therefore, we have chosen to focus on essential terminology, anatomy, and positioning information for the projections identified as necessary for entry-level competency as determined by a survey of radiologic technology programs in the United States and Canada. For more information on the survey consult the Preface contained in *Merrill's Atlas.*

Some chapters of *Merrill's Atlas* (Volumes 1 and 2) have limited radiographic applications or consist of radiographic procedures only rarely performed today because of technological advances in adjunct medical imagery modalities (e.g., computed tomography, magnetic resonance imaging, and diagnostic ultrasound). Because those chapters do not include radiographic examinations deemed essential for entry-level competency, this workbook provides only cursory coverage for those chapters.

To use this workbook most effectively you should first study the appropriate anatomic and radiographic sections from *Merrill's Atlas* and the multimedia series. Then complete the exercises that relate to the chapter of interest.

Steven G. Hayes, Sr.

Acknowledgments

My appreciation is extended to those who were instrumental in the development of this workbook. The first, of course, is my wife Sharon. The simple dedication in the front of this workbook does not adequately express my appreciation for all her support and assistance with this publication and with every goal I have ever pursued. For more than 30 years, she has given me more than I can ever return in kind.

The difficulties of a major writing project are, sometimes, not fully realized by an author on initially accepting the task. Support from family members can often affect how successful an author is in completing a publication. I am fortunate to have the complete support of my family. For that reason, I need to recognize my two children, who allowed me to temporarily withdraw my presence from their activities. My son, Steven G. Hayes, Jr., ASRT, RT(R) (ARRT), is very supportive of everything I do, especially with the development of this workbook. Because he is an experienced radiologic educator and technologist, his knowledge of radiographic positioning was very beneficial to me in obtaining some of the radiographic images I needed and with assisting in the development of the text. I value his support and advice. I also want to thank my daughter, Tonya, for her understanding when I was excusing myself from family activities so I could sustain my production schedule. To both, I apologize for depriving them of my time during the development of this workbook.

Another radiologic educator, Jackie Miller, BSRT, RT(R) (ARRT), has been a close friend and colleague of mine longer than either of us can remember. I know no one who has more common sense than Jackie. Other than my wife, he probably knows me better than does anyone else. I appreciate his assistance with obtaining some of the radiographs used in this workbook and the long-term encouragement he has given me in all my endeavors.

I also want to recognize my Mosby editors, Jeanne Wilke, Lisa Potts, and Carole Glauser. Jeanne is the acquisitions editor who first proposed this workbook project to me. I appreciate the confidence she had in me from the very onset. Lisa, an accomplished developmental editor, was very important in assisting me throughout the entire development of the first edition of this workbook. She was always available to answer every question I had and provided useful advice that made my work so much easier. Thank you, Lisa. For the preparation of the second edition, I thank Carole Glauser for coordinating the many activities that transform a manuscript into the finished publication.

I also thank Philip W. Ballinger, MS, RT, FAERS, and Eugene Frank, MA, RT(R), FASRT, co-authors for *Merrill's Atlas of Radiographic Positions and Radiologic Procedures,* ninth edition. Philip was quick to answer my technical questions concerning *Merrill's Atlas* and offered significant suggestions. For the preparation of the second edition, in addition to Philip, I thank Eugene for his replies to the countless e-mail messages I sent him almost nightly for months as the revision neared its completion.

For the preparation of the second edition, in addition to the preceding, I sincerely appreciate the comments and suggestions from students, educators, and reviewers. Their collective input helped make this workbook a better learning aid.

For the preparation of the third edition I want to specifically thank Eugene Frank, MA, RT(R), FASRT, author of *Merrill's Atlas of Radiographic Positions and Radiologic Procedures,* tenth edition. In addition to some face-to-face meetings, almost daily we sent e-mail messages between us to ensure that our publications are the highest quality possible and that essential information is identical in both our publications. He is a constant source of technical expertise for me, and his suggestions immensely helped me throughout the writing of this edition. Additionally, my sincere appreciation is extended to Jeanne Wilke, Executive Editor, for her continual support and management strategies in all aspects of the production of this workbook. One valuable service Jeanne provided me was ensuring that I always had very competent editorial assistants and developmental editors throughout the development of this edition. Specifically, Jennifer Genett and Rebecca Swisher, Developmental Editors, and Melissa Kuster and Paige Mosher, Editorial Assistants, provided important services during this revision project. Jennifer was in on the initial planning stages, Melissa helped with the illustrations and figures, and Paige and Rebecca coordinated all the end activities that culminate with the final printed product. To those four ladies I offer my sincere appreciation for their constant efforts to keep this edition moving along by taking care of so many tasks that authors are unable to do for themselves.

I have been lucky to have the love and support of many wonderful people. Those I have just mentioned are the ones who really are responsible for this workbook.

Steven G. Hayes, Sr.

Contents

VOLUME 1

RADIOGRAPHIC ANATOMY, POSITIONING, & PROCEDURES WORKBOOK

CHAPTER 1

Preliminary Steps in Radiography

Review

Instructions: Many important factors must be considered every time a radiograph is obtained. This exercise provides a comprehensive review of those important areas. Items require you to fill in missing words, select answers from a list, provide a short answer, or choose true or false (provide an explanation for any statement you believe to be false).

1. Define the following radiographic terms:

    a. Optical density: _____

    _____

    _____

    b. Contrast: _____

    _____

    _____

    c. Recorded detail: _____

    _____

    _____

    d. Shape distortion: _____

    _____

    _____

2. From the following list, circle the three primary factors that can be used to control radiographic density.
    a. Time, in second(s)
    b. Milliamperage (mA)
    c. Kilovoltage peak (kVp)
    d. Central ray–film alignment
    e. Object-to-image receptor distance (OID)
    f. Combination of milliamperage and time (mAs)

3. Fig. 1-1 shows two images with different radiographic density. Compare these images and identify each according to its density. (The choices are insufficient density and proper density.)

    a. Image A: _____

    b. Image B: _____

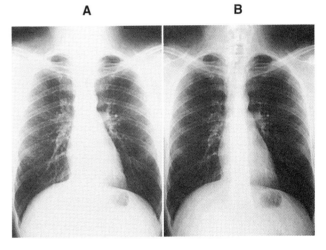

Fig. 1-1 Two images showing different radiographic density.

4. What exposure factor controls radiographic contrast?

    _____

5. Fig. 1-2 shows two images with different radiographic contrast. Compare the images and identify each according to its contrast. (The choices are short scale [high contrast] and long scale [low contrast].)

   a. Image A: _____

   b. Image B: _____

7. Fig. 1-3 shows two images with different levels of recorded detail. Compare the images and identify each according to its recorded detail. (The choices are sharp image and unsharp image.)

   a. Image A: _____

   b. Image B: _____

A   **B**

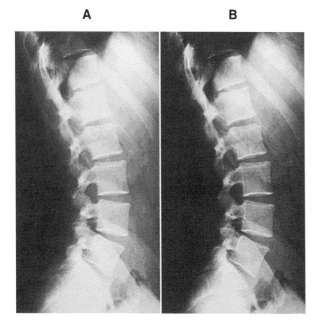

Figure 1-2 Two images showing different scales of radiographic contrast.

A   **B**

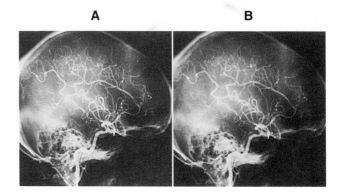

Figure 1-3 Two images showing different levels of recorded detail.

6. From the following list, circle the six factors that control recorded detail.

   a. Film
   b. Screen
   c. Motion
   d. Distance
   e. Exposure
   f. Geometry
   g. Focal spot size
   h. Milliamperage (mA)
   i. Kilovoltage peak (kVp)

8. From the following list, circle the two factors that control radiographic magnification.

   a. Time, in second(s)
   b. Milliamperage (mA)
   c. Kilovoltage peak (kVp)
   d. Object-to-image receptor distance (OID)
   e. Source-to-image receptor distance (SID)

9. True or False. All radiographs yield some degree of magnification.

10. Fig. 1-4 shows two images with different degrees of magnification. Assuming that both patients are average-size adults, which image—A or B—shows the most magnification?

A   **B**

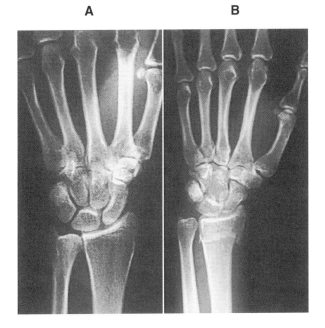

Figure 1-4 Two images showing different levels of magnification.

11. From the following list, circle the five factors that control or affect shape distortion.
    a. Alignment
    b. Angulation
    c. Central ray
    d. Image receptor
    e. Anatomical part
    f. Object-to-image receptor distance (OID)
    g. Source-to-image receptor distance (SID)

12. Describe how a posteroanterior (PA) projection radiograph of the chest should be displayed on a viewing device.

13. Fig. 1-5 shows two images of a PA projection of a chest.
    Which image—A or B—is correctly displayed?

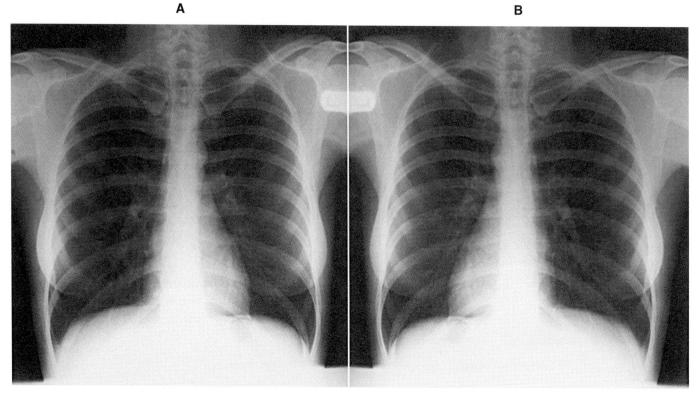

A   **B**

Figure 1-5 Two images of a chest.

14. Describe how lateral projection radiographs should be dis-
    played.

15. Fig. 1-6 shows two lateral projection chest radiographs. Which image—A or B—is correctly displayed as a left lateral chest radiograph?

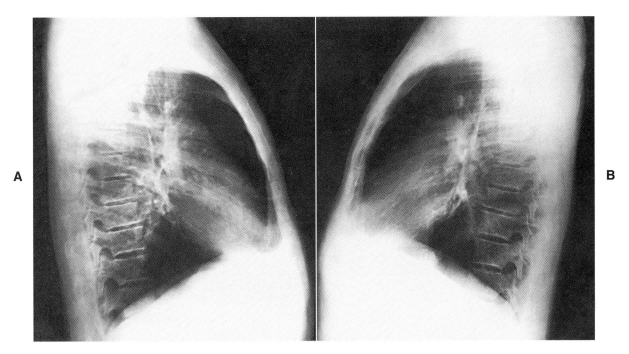

A

B

Figure 1-6 Two lateral projection radiographs of a chest.

16. Describe how hand and foot radiographs should be displayed.

17. Fig. 1-7 shows two images of a PA left hand radiograph.
    Which image—A or B—is correctly displayed?

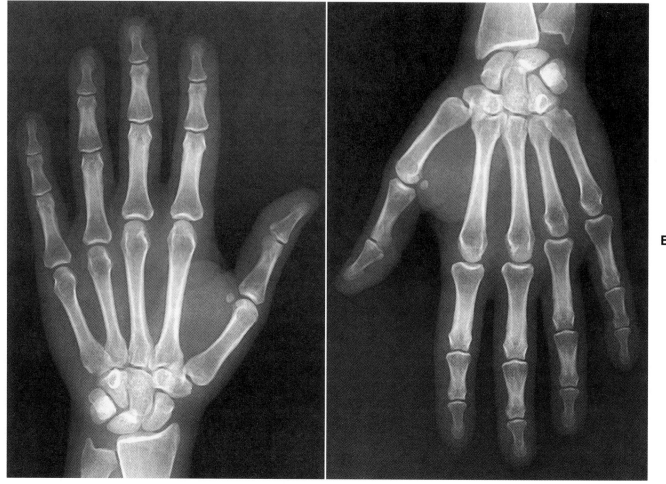

A

B

Figure 1-7 Two images of a hand.

18. Fig. 1-8 shows two images of an anteroposterior (AP) right knee. Which image —A or B—is correctly displayed?

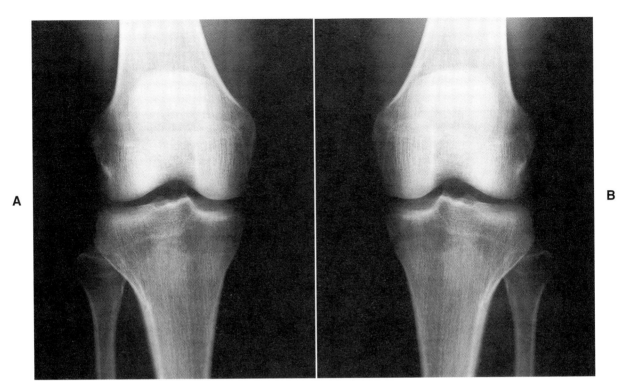

A   B

Figure 1-8 Two images of a knee.

19. Describe the two most common ways that lateral decubitus radiographs are displayed.

20. Fig. 1-9 shows two AP chest radiographs with the patient in a lateral decubitus position. The patient has fluid present in the right lung. Correctly identify each image as either left lateral decubitus or right lateral decubitus.

    a. Image A: _____

    b. Image B: _____

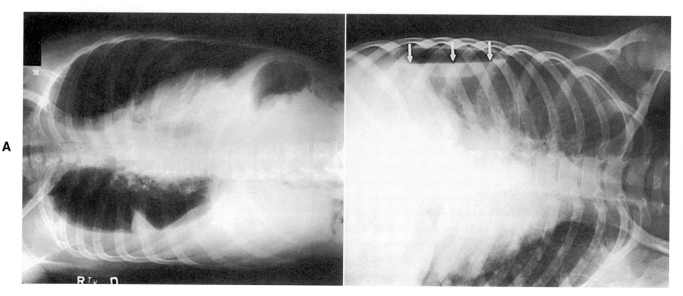

A   B

Figure 1-9 Two AP chest radiographs, lateral decubitus position.

21. When the radiologist is unable to see the patient, who is responsible for ensuring that an adequate clinical history accompanies the radiographs?

_____

22. What is the easiest and most convenient method to prevent the spread of microorganisms?

_____

23. According to the Centers for Disease Control, all human blood and certain bodily fluids should be treated as if they contain _____ _____.

24. What protective apparel should radiographers wear if the possibility of touching blood exists?

_____

25. What procedure should be followed to properly dispose of used hypodermic needles?

26. Define the following terms:

   a. Disinfectant: _____

   _____

   _____

   b. Antiseptic: _____

   _____

   _____

   c. Sterilization: _____

   _____

   _____

   d. Disinfection: _____

   _____

   _____

27. Which term—antiseptic or disinfectant—classifies isopropyl alcohol?

28. What information should be included in a procedures (or protocol) book that identifies each examination performed in the radiography department?

29. List the three ways a patient's colon may be cleansed for an abdominal examination.

30. Identify the three types of muscular tissue and state the type of motion (voluntary or involuntary) associated with each.

31. The rhythmic motion of smooth muscle structures is called

_____

32. What exposure factor is used to control involuntary motion?

_____

33. What body system controls the movement of voluntary muscles?

_____

34. From the following list, circle the five ways voluntary motion can be controlled by a radiographer.

    a. Increase mAs
    b. Decrease mAs
    c. Apply immobilization
    d. Give clear instructions
    e. Adjust support devices
    f. Increase exposure time
    g. Decrease exposure time
    h. Provide patient comfort
    i. Use slower film–screen system
    j. Use mammography film for extremities

35. Why is it necessary to ensure that any folds in cloth gowns are straightened out before making the radiographic exposure?

36. What devices must be removed from the patient within the area of interest when the skull is examined?

37. Before beginning a radiographic examination, what should the radiographer do to gain the cooperation of a coherent patient?

38. What is the minimum number of personnel that should be used to transfer a helpless patient from a gurney to the radiographic table?

39. What are the two phases of respiration?

_____

40. What respiration phase is requested when the goal is to expand lung fields to the maximum extent possible?

_____

41. What respiration procedure provides for lung motion but not rib motion?

_____

42. Match the patient conditions in Column A with the appropriate radiation exposure compensation necessary to provide a diagnostic image listed in Column B.

    Column A

    ___ 1. Ascites

    ___ 2. Edema

    ___ 3. Old age

    ___ 4. Atrophy

    ___ 5. Emaciation

    ___ 6. Pneumonia

    ___ 7. Emphysema

    ___ 8. Enlarged heart

    ___ 9. Pneumothorax

    ___ 10. Hydrocephalus

    ___ 11. Pleural effusion

    ___ 12. Degenerative arthritis

    Column B

    a. Requires a decrease in radiation exposure

    b. Requires an increase in radiation exposure

43. From the following list, circle the four items of identification information that should be on every radiograph.

    a. Patient's name
    b. Patient's diagnosis
    c. Date of examination
    d. Institutional identity
    e. Patient's marital status
    f. Side marker (right or left)
    g. Requesting physician's name

44. In addition to the standard required information, what additional information is needed for each of the following examinations?

    a. Linear tomography: _____

    b. Excretory urography: _____

45. For each projection in Column A, select from Column B the *best* choice for how side markers should be used for that particular projection.

Column A	Column B
____ 1. PA hand	a. The R marker is typically used
____ 2. PA chest	
____ 3. AP forearm	b. The L marker is typically used
____ 4. Lateral skull	c. Use the appropriate R or L marker
____ 5. PA of the skull	
____ 6. AP cervical spine	d. Always mark the side closest to the IR
____ 7. Lateral lumbar spine	e. Always mark the side farthest from the IR
____ 8. Lateral decubitus chest	f. Always mark the side up (opposite the side laid on)
____ 9. AP oblique lumbar spine	g. Use both the R and L markers to identify the two sides
____ 10. Bilateral AP knees (side-by-side on one IR)	

46. What adjustment can be made by the radiographer to compensate for an increase in OID?

47. List four reasons why it would become necessary to angle the central ray.

48. How is radiographic contrast affected when the radiation beam is restricted to only the area under examination? Explain why.

49. List the three guidelines for determining when gonadal shielding should be used.

50. For computed radiography, what is the purpose for the imaging plate?

Self-Test: Preliminary Steps in Radiography

Instructions: Answer the following questions by selecting the best choice.

1. Which factor controls radiographic contrast?
   a. Exposure time(s)
   b. Milliamperage (mA)
   c. Kilovoltage peak (kVp)

2. Which radiographic term refers to the degree of blackness between two adjacent areas on a radiograph?
   a. Density
   b. Contrast
   c. Magnification
   d. Recorded detail

3. Which of the following factors controls shape distortion?
   a. Alignment
   b. Milliamperage (mA)
   c. Milliamperage-time (mAs)
   d. Source-to-image receptor distance (SID)

4. How should a left lateral projection radiograph of the chest be displayed on a viewbox?
   a. As though the patient were standing in front of and facing to the left of the viewer
   b. As though the patient were standing in the normal anatomical position, face-to-face with the viewer
   c. So that the side of the patient where the x-ray beam enters is the side of the image closer to the viewbox
   d. So that the side of the patient closer to the IR during the procedure is the side of the image closer to the viewbox

5. How should a PA projection radiograph of the chest be displayed on a viewbox?
   a. As viewed from the perspective of the x-ray tube
   b. So that the side of the patient closer to the IR during the procedure is the side of the image closer to the viewbox
   c. As though the patient were standing in front of the viewer, with the patient's right side nearer the viewer's right side and the patient's left side nearer the viewer's left side
   d. As though the patient were standing in front of the viewer, with the patient's right side nearer the viewer's left side and the patient's left side nearer the viewer's right side

6. A PA projection radiograph of the hand should be displayed:
   a. From the perspective of the x-ray tube and with the fingers pointing upward
   b. From the perspective of the x-ray tube and with the fingers pointing downward
   c. With the patient in the anatomical position and with the fingers pointing upward
   d. With the patient in the anatomical position and with the fingers pointing downward

7. Who is responsible for obtaining a necessary clinical history when the radiologist is unable to see the patient?
   a. Radiographer
   b. Radiology nurse
   c. Chief technologist
   d. Department receptionist

8. To properly dispose of a hypodermic needle, it should be:
   a. Bent
   b. Recapped
   c. Broken to prevent its reuse
   d. Placed in a puncture-proof container

9. What is the medical property classification of isopropyl alcohol?
   a. Sterilizer
   b. Antiseptic
   c. Germicide
   d. Disinfectant

10. Within the operating room, who should remove sterile items that are in the way of the radiographer?
    a. Surgeon
    b. Radiographer
    c. Anesthesiologist
    d. Circulating nurse

11. To prepare the patient for a radiographic examination of the abdomen, what are the three methods used for cleansing the patient's bowel?
    a. Laxatives, enemas, and exercise
    b. Limited diet, enemas, and exercise
    c. Limited diet, laxatives, and enemas
    d. Limited diet, laxatives, and exercise

12. Which type of muscle tissue produces peristalsis?
    a. Cardiac
    b. Striated
    c. Smooth

13. Which type of muscle tissue comprises skeletal muscle?
    a. Cardiac
    b. Striated
    c. Smooth

14. Which pathologic condition requires a decrease in exposure factors from the routine procedure?
    a. Edema
    b. Pneumonia
    c. Emphysema
    d. Pleural effusion

15. Which change in exposure factors should be used to control voluntary motion that is a result of the patient's age or mental illness?
    a. Increase the milliamperage
    b. Decrease the milliamperage
    c. Increase the exposure time
    d. Decrease the exposure time

16. Which procedure best reduces the possibility of patient-controlled motion?
    a. Increase the milliamperage
    b. Increase the exposure time
    c. Give understandable instructions to the patient
    d. Use par-speed film with detail-intensifying screens

17. Which side marker placement rule applies when performing an AP oblique of the cervical spine?
    a. The R marker is typically used.
    b. The L marker is typically used.
    c. Always mark the side closest to the IR.
    d. Always mark the side farthest from the IR.

18. Which piece of information is not required as part of the identification of radiographs?
    a. Name of the patient
    b. Date of the examination
    c. Name of the radiographer
    d. Name of the medical facility

19. Why is it desirable to collimate to the area of interest?
    a. Lengthens the scale of contrast
    b. Reduces the required milliamperage
    c. Reduces the amount of scatter radiation produced
    d. Compensates for an increase in object-to-image receptor distance (OID)

20. How is a radiographic image affected when the radiation beam is restricted to the area under examination only?
    a. Improved recorded detail and increased radiographic density
    b. Improved recorded detail and increased radiographic contrast
    c. Reduction in part magnification and increased radiographic density
    d. Reduction in part magnification and increased radiographic contrast

21. Which of the following is not a consideration for determining when to use gonadal shielding?
    a. The patient has a reasonable reproductive potential.
    b. The purpose of the examination will be compromised.
    c. The patient is aware of the application of the gonadal shield.
    d. The gonads lie within or close (about 5 cm) to the primary x-ray field.

22. Which change will most improve recorded detail when the sternum is imaged?
    a. Increasing the OID
    b. Decreasing the SID
    c. Decreasing the source-to-object distance
    d. Collimating from a 35 × 43 cm field size to the area of interest only

23. For which examination is the use of gonadal shielding most important for the patient of childbearing age?
    a. Wrist
    b. Skull
    c. Chest
    d. Lumbar-sacral

24. Which computed radiography accessory houses the image storage phosphors that acquire the latent image?
    a. Image reader
    b. Control panel
    c. Imaging plate
    d. Video monitor

25. For computed radiography, what is the purpose of using laser film?
    a. Aids in patient positioning
    b. Measures radiation output from the tube
    c. Prints a permanent image of the examined body part
    d. Protects the video monitor screen from overexposure

CHAPTER 2

Radiation Protection

Review

Instructions: This exercise is a comprehensive review of radiation protection. Items require you to fill in missing words, select the correct answer, provide a short answer, or choose true or false (provide an explanation for any statement you believe to be false).

1. From the following list, circle the three early effects of high-dose radiation exposure.
   a. Cancer
   b. Lethality
   c. Leukemia
   d. Skin erythema
   e. Genetic effects
   f. Hematologic depression

2. From the following list, circle the two natural categories for late effects of radiation exposure.
   a. Genetic
   b. Somatic
   c. Pathogenic
   d. Hematologic

3. True or False. Significant evidence exists to prove that late genetic effects of radiation exposure on humans do occur within the diagnostic range of radiation energies.

4. True or False. Producing a measurable hematologic depression with any radiation exposure is possible.

5. Why is the life span–shortening effect that results from nonspecific premature aging no longer prevalent among radiographic workers today?

6. Which radiation-induced malignant disease—cancer or leukemia—is more readily observed in a heavily irradiated population?

7. What are the dose–response relationships for early and late effects of radiation exposure?
   a. Early effects and late effects have a threshold.
   b. Early effects have a threshold, but late effects have no threshold.
   c. Early effects have no threshold, but late effects have a threshold.
   d. Early effects and late effects have no threshold.

8. List conventional unit terms and SI unit terms for the following radiation quantities.

Quantity	Conventional Unit Term	SI Unit Term
a. Exposure:	_____	_____
b. Absorbed dose:	_____	_____
c. Dose equivalent:	_____	_____
d. Activity:	_____	_____

9. Complete the following conversion table.

	rems	mrems	sieverts (Sv)	millisieverts (mSv)
a.	1 _____	_____	_____	_____
b.	_____	500 _____	_____	_____
c.	_____	_____	0.10 _____	_____
d.	_____	_____	_____	250 _____

10. Which source causes most of the occupational exposure received by radiographers?

    a. Radionuclides
    b. X-ray tube/primary beam
    c. Scattered radiation from the patient

11. What is the current whole-body dose limit recommendation for radiographers?

    a. 5 Sv (500 rems)
    b. 50 Sv (5000 rems)
    c. 5 mSv (500 mrems)
    d. 50 mSv (5000 mrems, or 5 rems)

12. What is the current annual dose limit recommendation for the general public?

    a. 1 Sv (100 rems)
    b. 10 Sv (1000 rems)
    c. 1 mSv (100 mrems)
    d. 10 mSv (1000 mrems, or 1 rem)

13. How is it possible for the skin of a mammography technologist to reach its dose limit without exceeding the whole-body limit for the person?

    a. Tube filtration for mammography tubes is higher than tube filtration for diagnostic units.
    b. Milliamperage levels used for mammography are greater than those used for other diagnostic procedures.
    c. Radiation energy levels used for mammography are not as penetrating as those used for other diagnostic procedures.

14. Circle the three terms from the following list that refer to the dose received by patients during diagnostic radiographic examinations.

    a. Fetal dose
    b. Organ dose
    c. Primary dose
    d. Terrestrial dose
    e. Occupational dose
    f. Entrance skin exposure

15. Which of the following type of patient dose can be directly measured by thermoluminescent dosimeters?

    a. Fetal dose
    b. Organ dose
    c. Entrance skin exposure

16. Which gender has the higher gonadal dose for abdominal radiography?

    a. Male
    b. Female

17. What is the purpose of adding filtration to the x-ray tube?

    a. Increase the radiation output from the tube
    b. Enable the use of higher levels of exposure factors
    c. Reduce the amount of low-energy radiation that enters the patient

18. How many millimeters of aluminum filtration must be added to an x-ray tube that is capable of producing x-rays with energies above 70-kilovoltage peak (kVp)?

    a. 1.5
    b. 2.5
    c. 3.5

19. State the relationship between x-ray tube filtration and patient dose.

20. State the relationship between collimation and patient dose.

21. State the relationship between kilovoltage peak and patient dose.

22. List the three guidelines for determining when gonadal shielding should be used.

23. When compared with a conventional calcium tungstate screen-film combination, rare earth screen-film combinations _____ (increase or decrease) the patient dose.

24. Assume that a radiograph of acceptable radiographic density is produced using 30 milliampere-seconds (mAs) and 70 kVp. Exposure factors are adjusted as necessary, and a subsequent radiograph of equal density is produced using 80 kVp. Why does the second radiographic procedure offer a lower patient dose?

25. Define the following terms:

    a. Primary barrier: _____

    _____

    _____

    b. Secondary barrier: _____

    _____

    _____

26. Identify the following structures as either primary or secondary barriers:

    a. Floors: _____

    b. Walls: _____

    c. Ceilings: _____

    d. Control booth barriers: _____

27. Define the following terms:

    a. Controlled area: _____

    _____

    _____

    b. Uncontrolled area: _____

    _____

    _____

28. Which area—controlled or uncontrolled—is permitted the higher dose limit recommendation?

29. Define the following terms:

    a. Use factor: _____

    _____

    _____

    b. Occupancy factor: _____

    _____

    _____

30. List the three cardinal aspects of radiation protection.

33. List three types of personnel monitoring devices.

31. List three steps the radiographer can take to minimize occupational exposure during fluoroscopic procedures.

34. Where should the radiographer wear a film badge during fluoroscopic procedures?

32. For how many minutes should the fluoroscopic reset timer be set for fluoroscopic procedures?

_____

35. By approximately what percentage is the gonadal dose reduced to an irradiated area that is protected by a contact gonadal shield?

_____

Self-Test: Radiation Protection

Instructions: Answer the following questions by selecting the best choice.

1. Which type of radiation injury causes radiation-induced malignant disease?
   a. Late genetic effect
   b. Late somatic effect
   c. Early genetic effect
   d. Early somatic effect

2. Which radiation injuries have not been detected in humans?
   a. Solid tumor neoplasias
   b. Late genetic effect injuries
   c. Late somatic effect injuries
   d. Early somatic effect injuries

3. Which phrase best describes radiation-induced cataracts?
   a. Low-dose, late effect injury
   b. Low-dose, early effect injury
   c. High-dose, late effect injury
   d. High-dose, early effect injury

4. How many rads equal 1 gray (Gy)?
   a. 1
   b. 10
   c. 100
   d. 1000

5. How many sieverts (Sv) equal 1 rem?
   a. 0.01
   b. 0.10
   c. 10
   d. 100

6. What is the basic difference between the rem and other radiation units?
   a. The rem is the SI unit for radiation dose.
   b. The rem is used only for radiation protection purposes.
   c. The rem is used to indicate the activity level of radionuclides.
   d. The rem is used to indicate the exposure rate for a given exposure.

7. The radiation intensity of a given exposure of x-rays is measured in:
   a. Rads (or Gy)
   b. Rems (or Sv)
   c. Curies (or Becquerels [Bq])
   d. Milliroentgens (or coulombs [C]/kg)

8. Which radiation unit refers to the amount of occupational exposure received by radiographers?
   a. Millirads (or mGy)
   b. Milliroentgens (or C/kg)
   c. Millicuries (or mBq)
   d. Millirems (or mSv)

9. Which radiation unit refers to the amount of radiation received by a patient during an examination?
   a. Millirads (or mGy)
   b. Milliroentgens (or C/kg)
   c. Millicuries (or mBq)
   d. Millirems (or mSv)

10. Which condition is considered an early effect of radiation exposure?
    a. Cancer
    b. Leukemia
    c. Cataracts
    d. Skin erythema

11. Which condition is considered a late effect of radiation exposure?
    a. Lethality
    b. Leukemia
    c. Skin erythema
    d. Hematologic depression

12. Which late effect of radiation exposure no longer exists today because of improved radiation protection practices?
    a. Cancer
    b. Leukemia
    c. Solid tumor neoplasia
    d. Reduced life expectancy

13. Which dose–response model best represents the basis for radiation protection guidelines?
    a. Linear, threshold
    b. Linear, nonthreshold
    c. Nonlinear, threshold
    d. Nonlinear, nonthreshold

14. Which radiation injury exhibits a threshold type of dose–response relationship?
    a. Cancer
    b. Leukemia
    c. Skin erythema
    d. Solid tumor neoplasia

15. With reference to dose–response relationships, what does the threshold indicate?
    a. Dose level below which no response will occur
    b. Dose level below which all exposures pose a significant threat
    c. Dose level above which no response will occur
    d. Dose level above which no early somatic effects are observed

16. Which area of the body can best withstand the effects of radiation exposure?
    a. Skin
    b. Hands
    c. Forearms
    d. Lenses of the eyes

17. According to NCRP Report No. 91 (1987), what is the current cumulative dose equivalent for occupational exposures?
    a. 10 Sv (1000 rems) times the age of the radiographer
    b. 50 Sv (5000 rems) times the age of the radiographer
    c. 10 mSv (1 rem) times the age of the radiographer
    d. 50 mSv (5 rems) times the age of the radiographer

18. What is the only diagnostic radiography examination in which exposure to the radiographer's skin can reach its limit before the whole-body limit is reached?
    a. Fluoroscopy
    b. Mammography
    c. Mobile radiography
    d. Surgical radiography

19. Which device is used most often to measure entrance skin exposure (ESE)?
    a. Ion chamber
    b. Densitometer
    c. Geiger counter
    d. Thermoluminescent dosimeters (TLD)

20. Which radiographic examination produces the least ESE?
    a. Skull
    b. Chest
    c. Retrograde urography
    d. Thoracic vertebral column

21. Which radiographic examination produces the greatest mean marrow dose?
    a. Skull
    b. Chest
    c. Humerus
    d. Lumbar vertebral column

22. Which radiographic examination produces the greatest fetal dose?
    a. Skull
    b. Chest
    c. Gallbladder
    d. Lumbar vertebral column

23. Which radiographic examination produces the greatest exposure to the radiographer?
    a. Skull
    b. Fluoroscopy
    c. Excretory urography
    d. Lumbar vertebral column

24. Where should the radiographer wear a TLD during fluoroscopic procedures?
    a. Under the lead apron, at the level of the waist
    b. Under the lead apron, at the level of the collar
    c. Outside the lead apron, at the level of the waist
    d. Outside the lead apron, at the level of the collar

25. Where should a pregnant radiographer wear a "baby badge" (fetal monitor) during fluoroscopic procedures?
    a. Under the lead apron, at the level of the waist
    b. Under the lead apron, at the level of the collar
    c. Outside the lead apron, at the level of the waist
    d. Outside the lead apron, at the level of the collar

CHAPTER 3

General Anatomy and Radiographic Positioning Terminology

Review

Instructions: No one can succeed in a profession without first mastering its terminology. This exercise reviews the terminology unique to radiography. Items require you to identify illustrations, fill in missing words, provide a short answer, match columns, select answers from a list, or complete a crossword puzzle.

1. Define the following terms:

   a. Anatomy: _____

   _____

   _____

   _____

   b. Physiology: _____

   _____

   _____

   _____

   c. Osteology: _____

   _____

   _____

   _____

2. Describe the anatomic position.

3. List the four fundamental planes of the body.

4. Any plane passing vertically through the body from front to back and dividing the body into right and left segments is called a(n) _____ plane.

5. Any plane passing vertically through the body from side to side and dividing the body into anterior and posterior segments is called a(n) _____ plane.

6. The plane that passes vertically through the midline of the body from side to side and divides the body into equal anterior and posterior segments is called the _____ plane.

7. The plane passing through the midline of the body and dividing it into equal right and left halves is known as the _____ plane.

8. A plane that passes crosswise through the body and divides the body into superior and inferior segments is a(n) _____ plane.

9. Identify the four body planes shown in Fig. 3-1.

A. _____

B. _____

C. _____

D. _____

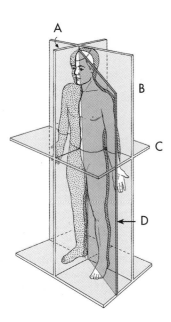

Figure 3-1 Planes of the body.

10. List the two major cavities of the torso.

11. Match the structures (Column a) with the body cavities in which they are found (Column b).

Column A	Column B
_____ 1. Liver	a. Thoracic
_____ 2. Lungs	b. Abdominal
_____ 3. Heart	c. Pelvic
_____ 4. Uterus	
_____ 5. Spleen	
_____ 6. Rectum	
_____ 7. Ureters	
_____ 8. Trachea	
_____ 9. Ovaries	
_____ 10. Stomach	
_____ 11. Pancreas	
_____ 12. Intestines	
_____ 13. Esophagus	
_____ 14. Gallbladder	
_____ 15. Peritoneum	
_____ 16. Pericardium	
_____ 17. Urinary bladder	

12. Identify each body cavity shown in Fig. 3-2.

    A. _____

    B. _____

    C. _____

    D. _____

    E. _____

13. Identify the four quadrants of the body shown in Fig. 3-3.

    A. _____

    B. _____

    C. _____

    D. _____

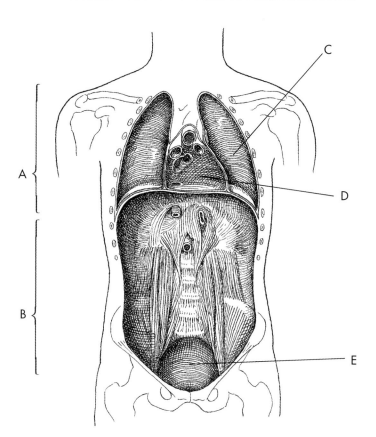

Figure 3-2 Anterior view of the torso.

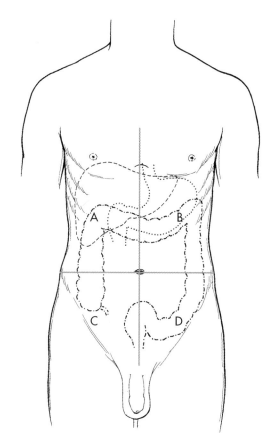

Figure 3-3 Clinical divisions of the four quadrants of the abdomen.

14. Identify the nine regions of the abdomen shown in Fig. 3-4.

A. _____

B. _____

C. _____

D. _____

E. _____

F. _____

G. _____

H. _____

I. _____

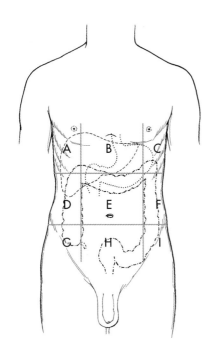

Figure 3-4 Anatomic divisions of the nine regions of the abdomen.

15. Match the vertebrae (Column A) with the appropriate external landmark present at the same body level (Column B).

Column A	Column B
____ 1. C1	a. Gonion
____ 2. C2, C3	b. Mastoid tip
____ 3. C3, C4	c. Hyoid bone
____ 4. C5	d. Thyroid cartilage
____ 5. C7, T1	e. Vertebra prominens
____ 6. T1	f. Inferior costal margin
____ 7. T2, T3	g. Level of sternal angle
____ 8. T4, T5	h. Level of jugular notch
____ 9. T7	i. Level of xiphoid process
____ 10. T9, T10	j. Level of inferior angles of scapulae
____ 11. L2, L3	k. Level of anterior superior iliac spines
____ 12. L4, L5	l. Level of most superior aspect of crests of ilia
____ 13. S1, S2	m. Level of symphysis pubis and greater trochanters
____ 14. Coccyx	n. Approximately 2 inches (5 cm) above level of jugular notch

16. Identify the surface landmarks of the head and neck shown in Fig. 3-5.

    A. _____

    B. _____

    C. _____

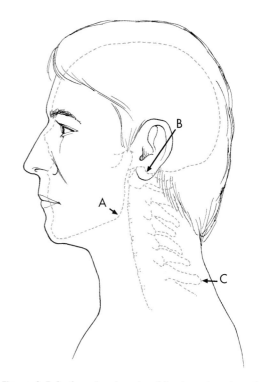

Figure 3-5 Surface landmarks of the head and neck.

17. Identify the vertebral level or surface landmark (or both) for each marked location shown in Fig. 3-6.

    A. _____

    B. _____

    C. _____

    D. _____

    E. _____

    F. _____

    G. _____

    H. _____

    I. _____

    J. _____

18. List the four major types of body habitus.

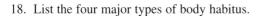

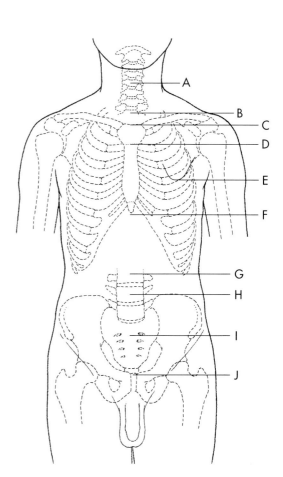

Figure 3-6 Surface landmarks of the torso.

19. Identify the body habitus illustrated in Figs. 3-7 through 3-10.

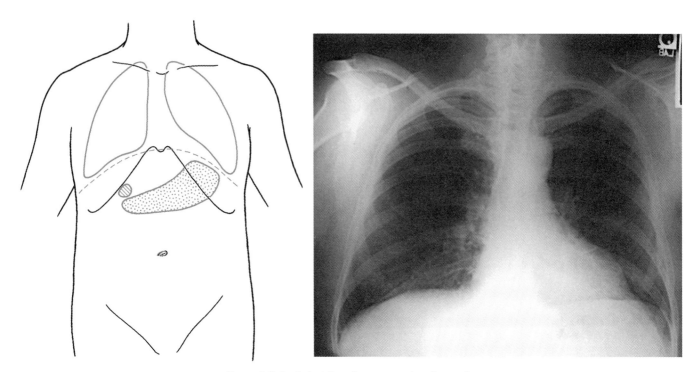

Figure 3-7 Body habitus diagram and radiograph.

a. Fig. 3-7: _____

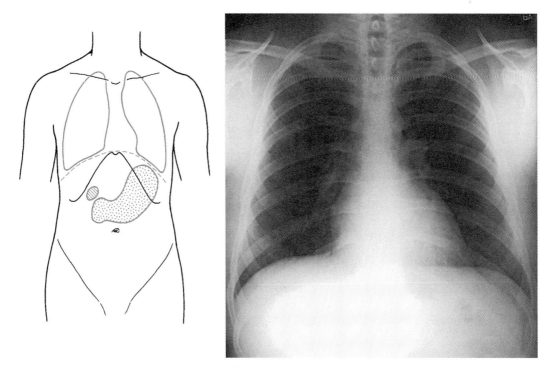

Figure 3-8 Body habitus diagram and radiograph.

b. Fig. 3-8: _____

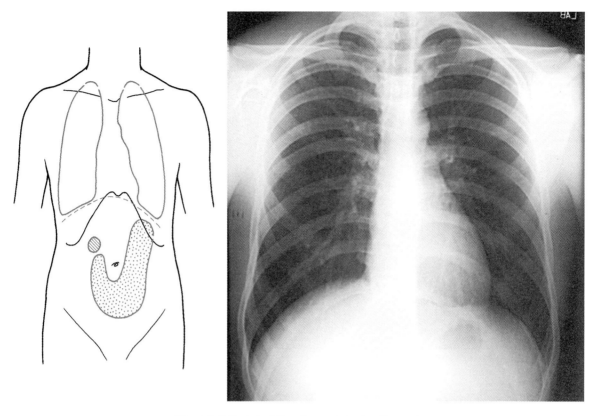

Figure 3-9 Body habitus diagram and radiograph.

c. Fig. 3-9: _____

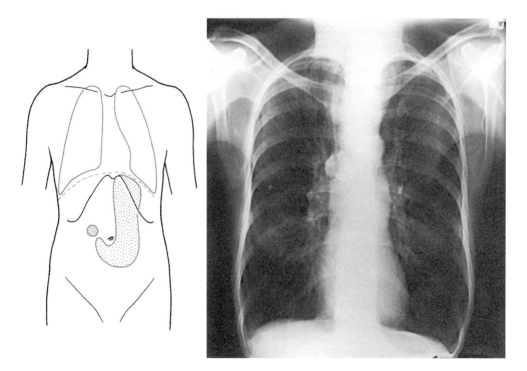

Figure 3-10 Body habitus diagram and radiograph.

d. Fig. 3-10: _____

20. How many bones comprise the typical adult skeleton?

_____

21. List the two main skeletal groups that make up the bony framework of the body.

22. From the following list, circle the four main parts of the appendicular skeleton.

    a. Ribs
    b. Pelvic girdle
    c. Shoulder girdle
    d. Vertebral column
    e. Upper limbs (extremities)
    f. Lower limbs (extremities)

23. From the following list, circle the four main parts of the axial skeleton.

    a. Ribs
    b. Skull
    c. Sternum
    d. Vertebral column
    e. Upper limbs (extremities)
    f. Lower limbs (extremities)

24. Match the definitions in Column A with the terms in Column B.

    Column A

    ___ 1. Outer layer of bony tissue

    ___ 2. Inner trabeculated portion of the bone

    ___ 3. Central cylindrical canal of long bones

    ___ 4. Tough, fibrous membrane that covers the bone. (except where bone is covered by articular cartilage)

    Column B

    a. Periosteum

    b. Spongy bone

    c. Compact bone

    d. Medullary cavity

25. From the following list, circle the four classifications (by shape) of bones.

    a. Flat
    b. Long
    c. Short
    d. Small
    e. Cranial
    f. Irregular
    g. Appendicular

26. Match the bones in Column A with the classifications in Column B.

    Column A

    ___ 1. Tibia

    ___ 2. Lunate

    ___ 3. Radius

    ___ 4. Patella

    ___ 5. Sacrum

    ___ 6. Maxilla

    ___ 7. Scapula

    ___ 8. Capitate

    ___ 9. Sternum

    ___ 10. Humerus

    ___ 11. Occipital

    ___ 12. Mandible

    ___ 13. Vertebrae

    ___ 14. Calcaneus

    ___ 15. Trapezium

    Column B

    a. Flat

    b. Long

    c. Short

    d. Irregular

27. Define the following bone classifications:

a. Long: _____

_____

_____

b. Short: _____

_____

_____

c. Flat: _____

_____

_____

d. Irregular: _____

_____

_____

e. Sesamoid: _____

_____

_____

_____

28. List the three functional classifications of articulations.

29. Match the functional classifications of articulations in Column A with the types of movements in Column B.

Column A	Column B
____ 1. Diarthroses	a. Immovable
____ 2. Synarthroses	b. Freely movable
____ 3. Amphiarthroses	c. Limited or slight movement

30. List the three structural classifications of articulations.

31. Match the structural classifications of articulations in Column A with the functional classifications in Column B.

Column A	Column B
____ 1. Fibrous	a. Diarthroses
____ 2. Synovial	b. Synarthroses
____ 3. Cartilaginous	c. Amphiarthroses

32. Identify the following articulations according to their functional and structural classifications:

	Functional Classification	Structural Classification
a. Knee:	_____	_____
b. Cranial sutures:	_____	_____
c. Symphysis pubis:	_____	_____

33. Match the definitions in Column A with the articulation terms in Column B.

Column A

_____ 1. Fibrous envelope that encloses a synovial joint

_____ 2. Joint in which two bones are joined by hyaline cartilage

_____ 3. Lubricant and nutrient compound found within synovial joints

_____ 4. Joining together of two midline bones in the body by a plate of fibrocartilage

_____ 5. Fluid-containing sacs that are interposed between sliding surfaces to reduce friction

_____ 6. Fibrocartilaginous disk pad located between the ends of bones in some synovial joints

Column B

a. Bursae

b. Meniscus

c. Symphysis

d. Synovial fluid

e. Synchondrosis

f. Articular capsule

34. Match each type of synovial joint in Column A with the kinds of movement that are applicable from Column B. Some synovial joints may have more than one selection from Column B. Some selections from Column B may be used more than once.

Column A

_____ 1. Gliding (plane)

_____ 2. Hinge (ginglymus)

_____ 3. Pivot (trochoid)

_____ 4. Ellipsoid (condyloid)

_____ 5. Saddle (sellar)

_____ 6. Ball and socket (spheroid)

Column B

a. Sliding

b. Gliding

c. Flexion

d. Extension

e. Rotation

f. Abduction

g. Adduction

h. Circumduction

35. Match the articulations in Column A with the corresponding synovial-type joint in Column B.

Column A

_____ 1. Hip

_____ 2. Knee

_____ 3. Elbow

_____ 4. Wrist

_____ 5. Shoulder

_____ 6. C1 and C2

_____ 7. Intertarsal

_____ 8. Interphalangeal

_____ 9. Metacarpophalangeal

_____ 10. Carpometacarpal joint of the thumb

Column B

a. Saddle (sellar)

b. Gliding (plane)

c. Pivot (trochoidal)

d. Hinge (ginglymus)

e. Ellipsoid (condyloid)

f. Ball and socket (spheroidal)

36. Match the process or projection terms in Column A with the definitions in Column B.

Column A	Column B
___ 1. Head	a. Sharp process
___ 2. Horn	b. Bony projection
___ 3. Crest	c. Beaklike process
___ 4. Facet	d. Ridgelike process
___ 5. Spine	e. Club-shaped process
___ 6. Styloid	f. Hook-shaped process
___ 7. Tubercle	g. Long, pointed process
___ 8. Condyle	h. Projection above a condyle
___ 9. Hamulus	i. Hornlike process on a bone
___ 10. Coracoid	j. Expanded end of a long bone
___ 11. Malleolus	k. Small, rounded, elevated process
___ 12. Trochanter	
___ 13. Tuberosity	l. Large, rounded, elevated process
___ 14. Epicondyle	m. Rounded process at an articular extremity
___ 15. Protuberance	
	n. Small, smooth-surfaced process for articulation
	o. Large, rounded, elevated process located at the junction of the neck and shaft of the femur

37. Match the terms for depressions in Column A with the definitions in Column B.

Column A	Column B
___ 1. Fossa	a. Cleft or groove
___ 2. Sinus	b. Pit, fovea, or hollow
___ 3. Sulcus	c. Shallow, linear depression
___ 4. Groove	d. Recess, groove, cavity, or hollow space
___ 5. Fissure	
___ 6. Foramen	e. Furrow, trench, or fissurelike depression
	f. Hole in a bone for transmission of blood vessels and nerves

38. **Instructions:** Use the following clues to complete the crossword puzzle. All answers refer to anatomic terms for processes or depressions.

ACROSS

3. Hook-shaped process
6. Furrow, trench, or fissurelike depression
8. Long, pointed process
9. Large process located at junction of neck and shaft of femur
11. Rounded process at an articular extremity
12. Large, rounded, elevated process
17. Expanded end of long bone
18. Hole in bone for the transmission of blood vessels and nerves
20. Ridgelike process
21. Shallow, linear depression
22. Cleft or groove
23. Projection above a condyle

DOWN

1. Pit, fovea, or hollow
2. Club-shaped process
4. Sharp process
5. Bony projection
7. Small, smooth-surfaced process for articulation
10. Indentation into the border of a bone
13. Small, rounded, elevated process
14. Beaklike process
15. Less prominent ridge than a crest
16. Tubelike passageway
19. Recess, groove, cavity, or hollow space

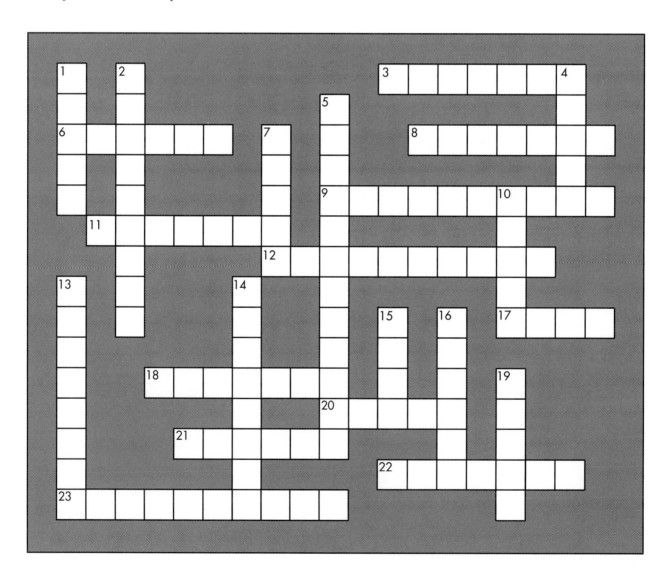

39. Match the body parts in Column A with the definitions in Column B. Some definitions may be used more than once.

Column A

___ 1. Deep

___ 2. Distal

___ 3. Lateral

___ 4. Dorsal

___ 5. Medial

___ 6. Central

___ 7. Ventral

___ 8. Caudad

___ 9. Palmar

___ 10. Plantar

___ 11. Inferior

___ 12. Internal

___ 13. Dorsum

___ 14. Visceral

___ 15. Anterior

___ 16. External

___ 17. Superior

___ 18. Proximal

___ 19. Cephalad

___ 20. Posterior

___ 21. Ipsilateral

___ 22. Peripheral

___ 23. Superficial

___ 24. Contralateral

Column B

a. Refers to the sole of the foot

b. Refers to the palm of the hand

c. Refers to the covering of an organ

d. Refers to parts far from the surface

e. Refers to a part near the skin or surface

f. Refers to nearer the feet or situated below

g. Refers to nearer the head or situated above

h. Refers to parts toward the head of the body

i. Refers to a part on the same side of the body

j. Refers to the back part of the body or an organ

k. Refers to parts away from the head of the body

l. Refers to the middle area or main part of an organ

m. Refers to a part within or on the inside of an organ

n. Refers to a part or parts on the opposite side of the body

o. Refers to a part outside of an organ or on the outside of the body

p. Refers to parts at or near the surface, edge, or outside of a body part

q. Refers to the forward or front part of the body or to the forward part of an organ

r. Refers to parts toward the median plane of the body or toward the middle of a body part

s. Refers to parts nearest the point of attachment, point of reference, origin, or beginning

t. Refers to parts farthest from the point of attachment, point of reference, origin, or beginning

u. Refers to the top or anterior surface of the foot, or to the back or posterior surface of the hand

v. Refers to parts away from the median plane of the body or away from the middle of a part to the right or the left

40. **Instructions:** Use the following clues to complete the crossword puzzle. All answers refer to body part terminology.

ACROSS

1. Away from the head of the body
5. Near the skin or surface
7. Sole of the foot
9. Toward the head of the body
10. Within or on the inside of an organ
11. Nearest the point of attachment or origin
14. Away from the median plane to the right or left
15. Outside an organ or the body
16. Pertaining to caudad
17. Opposite of superior

DOWN

2. Posterior side
3. Opposite of lateral
4. Far from the surface
5. Opposite of inferior
6. Farthest from the point of reference or origin
7. At or near the edge of a body part
8. Front part of the body
9. On the opposite side of the body
10. On the same side of the body
12. Back part of the body or an organ
13. Middle or main part of an organ

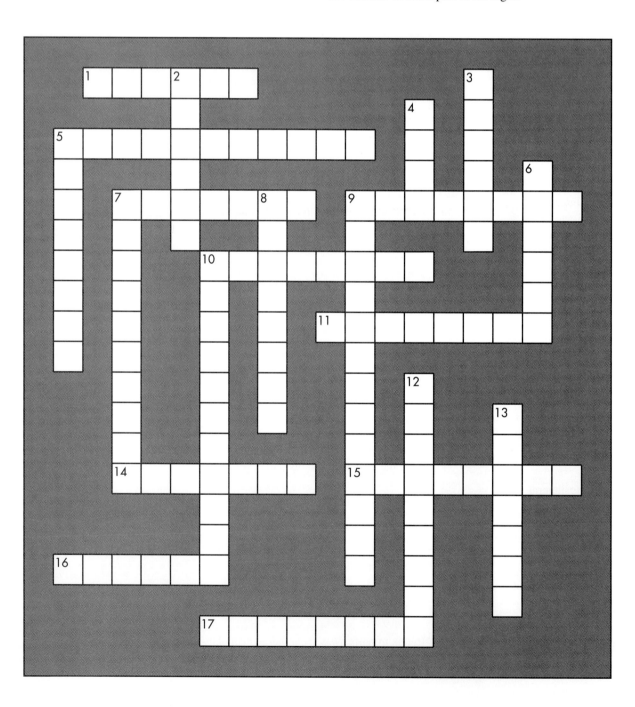

41. Define the following positioning terms:

    a. Projection: _____

    _____

    _____

    b. Position: _____

    _____

    _____

    c. View: _____

    _____

    _____

    d. Method: _____

    _____

    _____

    _____

42. Classify each of the following terms by writing *P* in the space provided if the term refers to a projection, *B* if the term refers to a body position, or *R* if the term refers to a radiographic position.

    ____ a. AP   ____ i. Dorsoplantar

    ____ b. Supine   ____ j. Left lateral

    ____ c. Upright   ____ k. Transthoracic

    ____ d. AP axial   ____ l. Trendelenburg

    ____ e. Lordotic   ____ m. Parietoacanthial

    ____ f. Recumbent   ____ n. Right anterior oblique

    ____ g. Tangential   ____ o. Right lateral decubitus

    ____ h. AP oblique

43. Match the descriptions in Column A with the projection terms in Column B.

Column A	Column B
____ 1. Central ray is angled longitudinally with the long axis of the body	a. AP
	b. PA
____ 2. Central ray enters the anterior body surface and exits the posterior body surface	c. Axial
____ 3. Central ray enters the posterior body surface and exits the anterior body surface	d. Lateral
	e. Oblique
____ 4. Central ray enters the side or lateral aspect of the body or body part and exits the other side	f. Tangential
____ 5. Central ray enters the body or body part from a side angle into the anterior or posterior surface of the body	
____ 6. Central ray is directed toward the outer margin of a curved body to profile a body part and project it free of superimposition	

44. Identify the projections illustrated in Figs. 3-11 through 3-16.

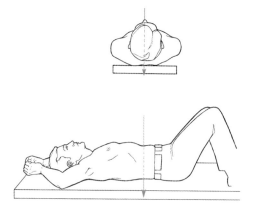

Figure 3-11 Diagram showing the path of an x-ray beam.

a. Fig. 3-11: _____

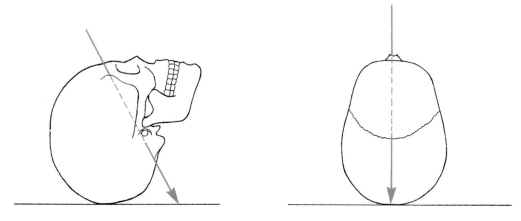

Figure 3-12 Diagram showing the path of an x-ray beam.

b. Fig. 3-12: _____

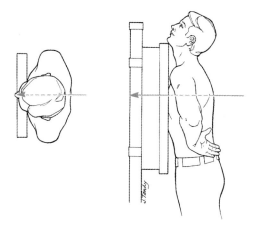

Figure 3-13 Diagram showing the path of an x-ray beam.

c. Fig. 3-13: _____

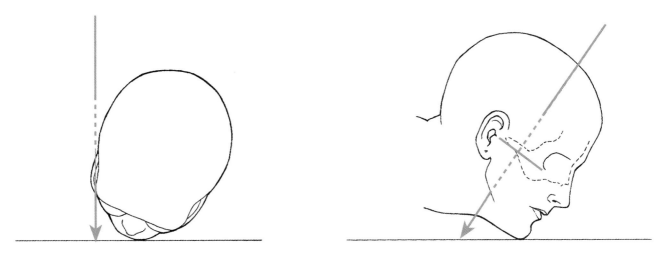

Figure 3-14 Diagram showing the path of an x-ray beam.

d. Fig. 3-14: _____

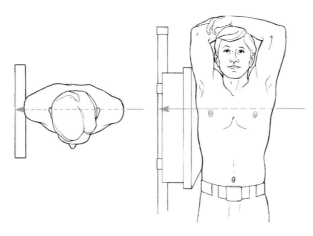

Figure 3-15 Diagram showing the path of an x-ray beam.

e. Fig. 3-15: _____

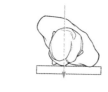

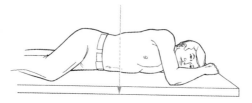

Figure 3-16 Diagram showing the path of an x-ray beam.

f.   Fig. 3-16: _____

45. Match the position descriptions in Column A with the terms in Column B.

Column A

_____ 1.   Lying face down

_____ 2.   Lying on the back

_____ 3.   Lying down in any position

_____ 4.   Erect or marked by a vertical position

_____ 5.   Lying supine with the head lower than the feet

_____ 6.   Lying supine with the head higher than the feet

Column B

a. Upright position

b. Fowler's position

c. Recumbent position

d. Trendelenburg's position

e. Prone (ventral recumbent) position

f. Supine (dorsal recumbent) position

46. Identify the body positions illustrated in Figs. 3-17 through 3-19.

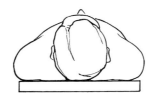

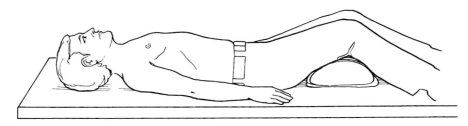

Figure 3-17 A body position.

a. Fig. 3-17: _____

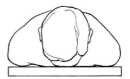

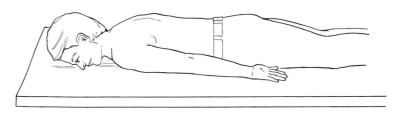

Figure 3-18 A body position.

b. Fig. 3-18: _____

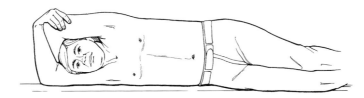

Figure 3-19 A body position.

c. Fig. 3-19: _____

47. Identify the radiographic positions illustrated in Figs. 3-20 through 3-28.

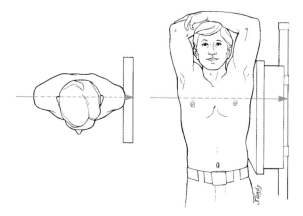

Figure 3-20 A radiographic position.

a. Fig. 3-20: _____

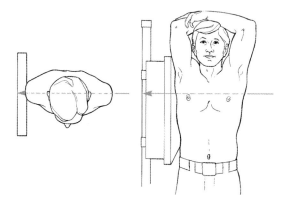

Figure 3-21 A radiographic position.

b. Fig. 3-21: _____   _____

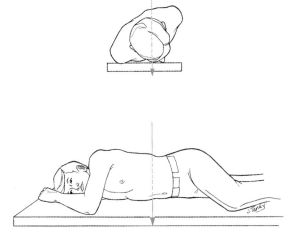

Figure 3-22 A radiographic position.

c. Fig. 3-22: _____

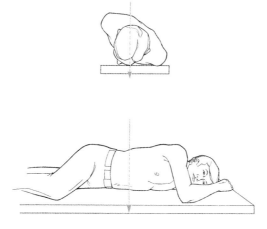

Figure 3-23 A radiographic position.

d. Fig. 3-23: _____

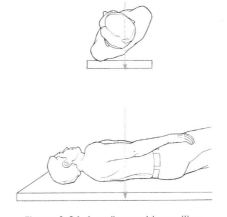

Figure 3-24 A radiographic position.

e. Fig. 3-24: _____

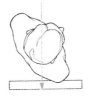

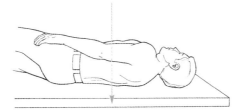

Figure 3-25 A radiographic position.

f. Fig. 3-25: _____

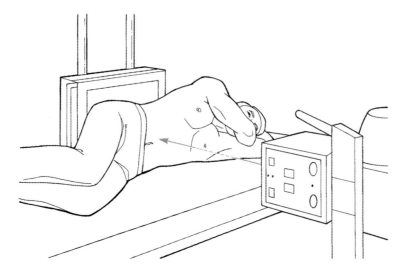

Figure 3-26 A radiographic position.

g. Fig. 3-26: _____

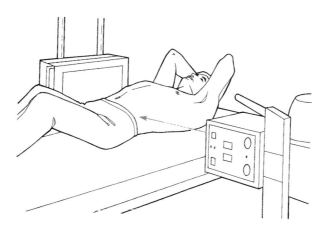

Figure 3-27 A radiographic position.

h. Fig. 3-27: _____

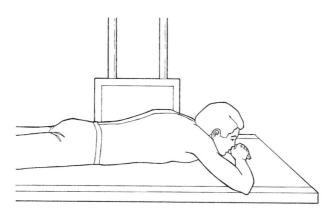

Figure 3-28 A radiographic position.

i. Fig. 3-28: _____

48. Match the body movements in Column A with the definitions in Column B.

Column A

____ 1. Tilt

____ 2. Rotate

____ 3. Flexion

____ 4. Pronate

____ 5. Eversion

____ 6. Supinate

____ 7. Deviation

____ 8. Extension

____ 9. Inversion

____ 10. Abduction

____ 11. Adduction

____ 12. Hyperflexion

____ 13. Circumduction

____ 14. Hyperextension

Column B

a. To turn around an axis

b. Straightening of a joint

c. Circular movement of a limb

d. Forced or excessive straightening of a joint

e. Forced or excessive flexion of a joint or part

f. A turning away from the regular standard or course

g. To turn the forearm so that the palm of the hand faces forward

h. To turn the forearm so that the palm of the hand faces backward

i. Movement of a part toward the central axis of a body or body part

j. Movement of the foot when it is turned inward at the ankle joint

k. Movement of the foot when it is turned outward at the ankle joint

l. Movement of a part away from the central axis of a body or body part

m. Bending movement of a joint whereby the angle between contiguous bones is diminished

n. Movement of a part so that the sagittal (longitudinal) plane is angled so that it is not parallel with the long axis of the body

49. Identify the body movements illustrated in Figs. 3-29 through 3-34.

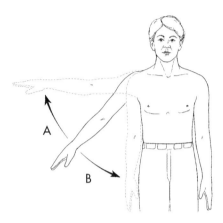

Figure 3-29 Two types of body movements.

a. Fig. 3-29: A. _____

           B. _____

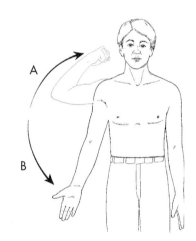

Figure 3-30 Two types of body movements.

b. Fig. 3-30: A. _____

           B. _____

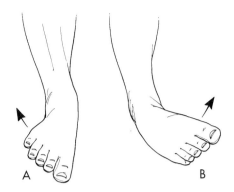

Figure 3-31 Two types of body movements.

c. Fig. 3-31: A. _____

            B. _____

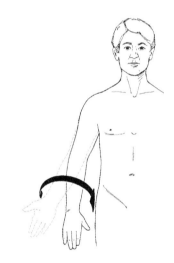

Figure 3-32 One type of body movement.

d. Fig. 3-32: _____

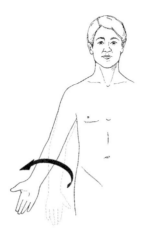

Figure 3-33 One type of body movement.

e. Fig. 3-33: _____

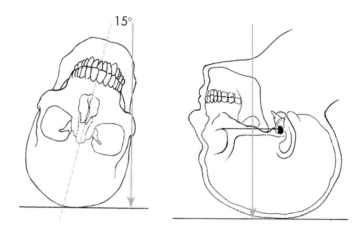

Figure 3-34 One type of body movement.

f. Fig. 3-34: _____

50. Provide the plural form for each of the following medical terms:

a. Ala: _____   f. Diverticulum: _____

b. Alveolus: _____   g. Ganglion: _____

c. Appendix: _____   h. Ilium: _____

d. Calculus: _____   i. Lamina: _____

e. Diagnosis: _____   j. Metastasis: _____

Self-Test: General Anatomy and Radiographic Positioning Terminology

Instructions: Answer the following questions by selecting the best choice.

1. Which term refers to the study of the function of the body organs?
   a. Anatomy
   b. Osteology
   c. Physiology

2. Which are the four fundamental body planes?
   a. Sagittal, coronal, horizontal, and oblique
   b. Sagittal, coronal, midaxillary, and transverse
   c. Midsagittal, midcoronal, horizontal, and oblique
   d. Midsagittal, midcoronal, midaxillary, and transverse

3. Which plane divides the body into equal right and left halves?
   a. Oblique
   b. Horizontal
   c. Midsagittal
   d. Midcoronal

4. Which are the two great cavities of the torso?
   a. Pelvic and pleural
   b. Pelvic and abdominal
   c. Thoracic and pleural
   d. Thoracic and abdominal

5. Which body structure is located within the thoracic cavity?
   a. Liver
   b. Heart
   c. Gallbladder
   d. Urinary bladder

6. In which quadrant of the abdomen is the appendix located?
   a. Right upper quadrant
   b. Right lower quadrant
   c. Left upper quadrant
   d. Left lower quadrant

7. Which region of the abdomen is located below the umbilical region?
   a. Epigastrium
   b. Hypogastrium
   c. Left hypochondrium
   d. Right hypochondrium

8. Which vertebra is located at the level of the xiphoid process?
   a. C7
   b. T7
   c. T10
   d. L3

9. Which body habitus represents a person of large, massive stature in whom the stomach is located high and nearly horizontal within the abdomen?
   a. Sthenic
   b. Asthenic
   c. Hyposthenic
   d. Hypersthenic

10. Excluding small sesamoid and accessory bones in the skull, how many bones comprise the skeleton?
    a. 202
    b. 206
    c. 210
    d. 215

11. Which structure belongs to the axial skeleton?
    a. Skull
    b. Lower limb
    c. Upper limb
    d. Pelvic girdle

12. Which bone has a medullary cavity?
    a. Tibia
    b. Sacrum
    c. Parietal
    d. Sternum

13. Bones are classified according to their:
    a. Size
    b. Shape
    c. Function
    d. Origination

14. Which bone classifications are vertebrae?
    a. Flat
    b. Long
    c. Short
    d. Irregular

15. Which bone classification is the trapezium?
    a. Flat
    b. Long
    c. Short
    d. Irregular

16. Which bone classification consists largely of compact cortex tissue in the form of two plates that enclose a layer of diploë?

    a. Flat
    b. Long
    c. Short
    d. Irregular

17. Which term specifically refers to the study of the joints?

    a. Anatomy
    b. Osteology
    c. Arthrology
    d. Physiology

18. Which functional classification of articulations refers to joints that have only limited or slight movement?

    a. Diarthroses
    b. Synarthroses
    c. Amphiarthroses

19. Which functional classification of articulations are synovial joints?

    a. Diarthroses
    b. Synarthroses
    c. Amphiarthroses

20. Which structural classification of articulations are cranial sutures?

    a. Fibrous
    b. Synovial
    c. Cartilaginous

21. Which type of movement occurs in a ginglymus joint?

    a. Rotational
    b. Gliding or sliding
    c. Flexion and extension
    d. Abduction and adduction

22. Which of the following joints is an example of a condyloid joint?

    a. Hip
    b. Intercarpal
    c. Interphalangeal
    d. Metacarpophalangeal

23. Which term refers to a long, pointed process?

    a. Crest
    b. Styloid
    c. Condyle
    d. Tuberosity

24. Which term for a depression refers to a hole in a bone through which blood vessels and nerves pass?

    a. Sinus
    b. Sulcus
    c. Groove
    d. Foramen

25. Which term refers to a fracture in which a broken bone projects though the skin?

    a. Open
    b. Closed
    c. Displaced
    d. Nondisplaced

26. Which term refers to a body part on the opposite side of the body?

    a. Lateral
    b. Posterior
    c. Ipsilateral
    d. Contralateral

27. Which term refers to the path of the central x-ray?

    a. View
    b. Method
    c. Position
    d. Projection

28. Which term refers to a general body position?

    a. Axial
    b. Recumbent
    c. Tangential
    d. Left anterior oblique (LAO)

29. Which term refers to the movement of a body part away from the central axis of the body?

    a. Flexion
    b. Inversion
    c. Abduction
    d. Adduction

30. Which term is the plural form for diagnosis?

    a. Diagnosix
    b. Diagnoses
    c. Diagnosae
    d. Diagnosum

CHAPTER 4

Upper Limb

SECTION 1

Osteology and Arthrology of the Upper Limb

Exercise 1

Instructions: Label the diagram of a hand shown in Fig. 4-1 by writing *D* on each distal phalanx, *M* on each middle phalanx, and *P* on each proximal phalanx. Label each metacarpal by writing its identification number (1 through 5) on the appropriate bone.

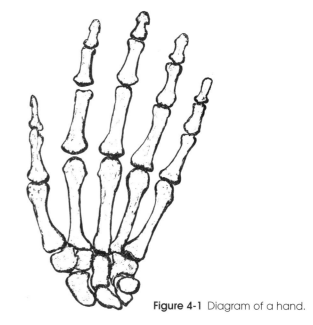

Figure 4-1 Diagram of a hand.

Exercise 2

Instructions: Identify each lettered bone or articulation shown in Fig. 4-2.

A. _____

B. _____

C. _____

D. _____

E. _____

F. _____

G. _____

H. _____

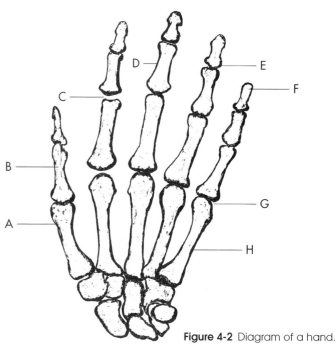

Figure 4-2 Diagram of a hand.

Exercise 3

Instructions: Identify each lettered carpal bone in the proximal row shown in Fig. 4-3.

A. _____

B. _____

C. _____

D. _____

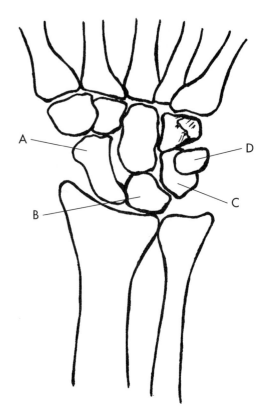

Figure 4-3 Diagram of a wrist.

Exercise 4

Instructions: Identify each lettered carpal bone in the distal row shown in Fig. 4-4.

A. _____

B. _____

C. _____

D. _____

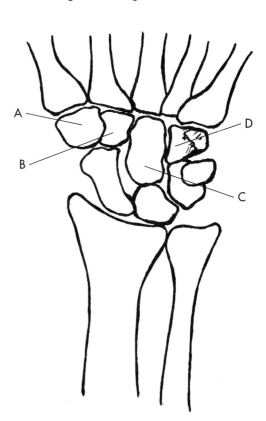

Figure 4-4 Diagram of a wrist.

Exercise 5

Instructions: Identify each lettered bone shown in Fig. 4-5.

A. _____   D. _____

B. _____   E. _____

C. _____   F. _____

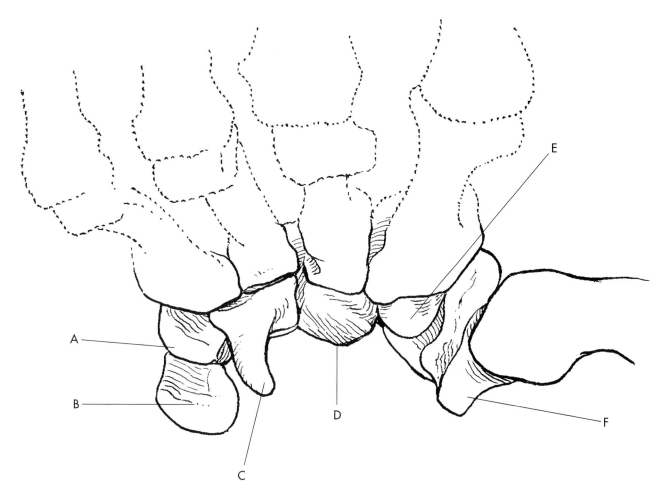

Figure 4-5 Inferosuperior aspect of the carpal sulcus.

Exercise 6

Instructions: Use the following clues to complete the crossword puzzle. All answers refer to the bones and joints of the hand and wrist.

ACROSS

2. Next to trapezium
7. Thumb joint
9. Finger bones
10. Largest carpal bone
11. Opposite of proximal
13. Joint proximal to the hand
14. One finger bone
16. Synonym for joint
17. Carpal bone classification
18. Number of carpal bones
19. Opposite of distal

DOWN

1. Where bones articulate
3. Lateral carpal in the distal row
4. Long bones in the hand
5. Wrist bones
6. Medial carpal in the distal row
8. Distal from the wrist
9. Smallest carpal bone
11. Metacarpal shaft
12. Hamate's other name
15. Between scaphoid and triquetrum

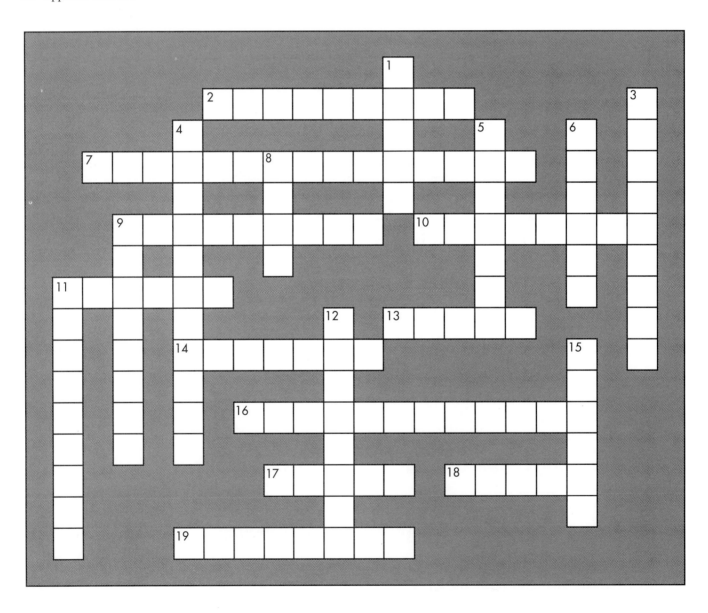

Exercise 7

Instructions: Identify each lettered structure shown in Fig. 4-6.

A. _____

B. _____

C. _____

D. _____

E. _____

F. _____

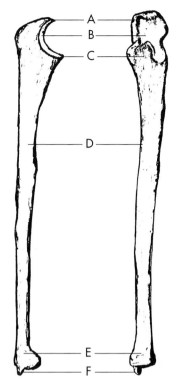

Figure 4-6 Two views of the ulna.

Exercise 8

Instructions: Identify each lettered structure shown in Fig. 4-7.

A. _____

B. _____

C. _____

D. _____

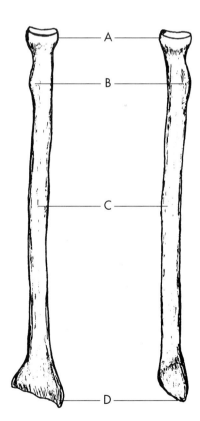

Figure 4-7 Two views of the radius.

Exercise 9

Instructions: Identify each lettered articulation in Fig. 4-8.

A. _____

B. _____

C. _____

D. _____

E. _____

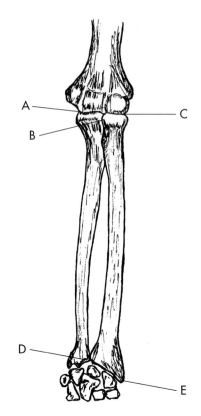

Figure 4-8 The forearm.

Exercise 10

Instructions: Identify each lettered structure in Fig. 4-9.

A. _____

B. _____

C. _____

D. _____

E. _____

F. _____

G. _____

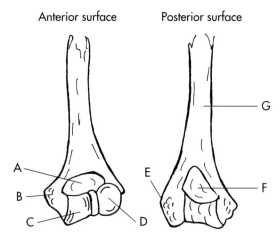

Figure 4-9 Distal end of the humerus.

Exercise 11

Instructions: Identify each lettered structure in Fig. 4-10.

A. _____

B. _____

C. _____

D. _____

E. _____

F. _____

G. _____

H. _____

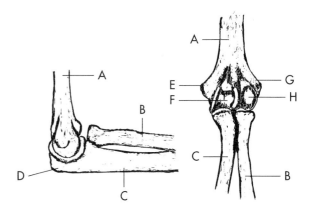

Figure 4-10 Two views of the elbow.

Exercise 12

Instructions: Identify each lettered structure illustrated in Fig. 4-11.

A. _____

B. _____

C. _____

D. _____

E. _____

F. _____

G. _____

H. _____

I. _____

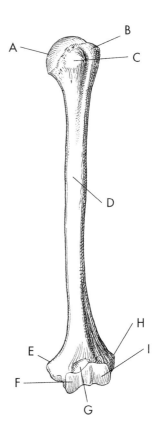

Figure 4-11 Anterior aspect of the humerus.

Exercise 13

Instructions: Match the structures located on the distal portion of the humerus in Column A with the descriptions in Column B. Not all descriptions may apply to the listed structures.

Column A

____ 1. Trochlea

____ 2. Capitulum

____ 3. Coronoid fossa

____ 4. Olecranon fossa

____ 5. Medial epicondyle

Column B

a. A round, marblelike structure

b. Bony prominence; easily palpated

c. A spool-like structure

d. Depression; located on the anterior surface

e. Depression; located on the posterior surface

f. Lateral to the humeral head

Exercise 14

Instructions: Listed following are structures found on the radius, ulna, or humerus. In the space provided, write *P* if the structure is proximal or *D* if the structure is distal on the bone.

____ 1. Trochlea

____ 2. Capitulum

____ 3. Ulnar head

____ 4. Radial head

____ 5. Humeral head

____ 6. Radial tubercle

____ 7. Coronoid fossa

____ 8. Trochlear notch

____ 9. Greater tubercle

____ 10. Olecranon fossa

____ 11. Coronoid process

____ 12. Olecranon process

____ 13. Medial epicondyle

____ 14. Ulnar styloid process

____ 15. Radial styloid process

Exercise 15

Instructions: Listed following are structures found on the radius, the ulna, or the humerus. In the space provided, write *R* for radius, *U* for ulna, or *H* for humerus to indicate on which bone the part is located. Some structures may be found on more than one bone.

_____ 1. Head

_____ 2. Trochlea

_____ 3. Capitulum

_____ 4. Radial notch

_____ 5. Radial fossa

_____ 6. Coronoid fossa

_____ 7. Styloid process

_____ 8. Olecranon fossa

_____ 9. Trochlear notch

_____ 10. Greater tubercle

_____ 11. Radial tuberosity

_____ 12. Coronoid process

_____ 13. Olecranon process

_____ 14. Medial epicondyle

_____ 15. Lateral epicondyle

Exercise 16

Instructions: Match the articulations in Column A with the types of movement listed in Column B. More than one choice from Column B may be used for some articulations.

Column A	Column B
_____ 1. Intercarpal	a. Gliding
_____ 2. Radiocarpal	b. Flexion
_____ 3. Interphalangeal	c. Extension
_____ 4. Metacarpophalangeal	d. Abduction
_____ 5. Distal radioulnar	e. Adduction
_____ 6. Proximal radioulnar	f. Circumduction
_____ 7. Elbow joint (humeroulnar and humeroradial)	g. Rotational (around a single axis)

Exercise 17

Instructions: Use the following clues to complete the crossword puzzle. All answers refer to the humerus, radius, and ulna.

ACROSS

3. Most lateral tubercle
5. Lateral bone of forearm
6. Medial from the capitulum
10. Process and fossa
11. Medial bone of forearm
13. Greater and lesser _____
14. Distal radial process
15. Distal forearm articulation

DOWN

1. Most proximal ulnar process
2. Joint between humerus and forearm
4. On each side of humerus
7. Humeral shaft
8. Upper arm bone
9. Articulates with radial head
12. Articulates with scapula

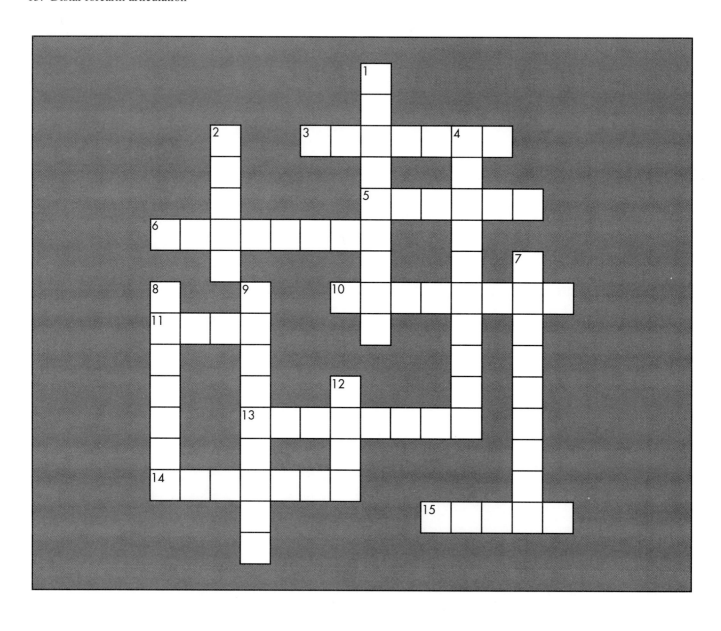

Exercise 18

Match the pathology terms in Column A with the appropriate definition in Column B. Not all choices from Column B should be selected.

Column A

_____1. Gout

_____2. Fracture

_____3. Bone cyst

_____4. Dislocation

_____5. Joint effusion

_____6. Osteomyelitis

_____7. Osteoarthritis

_____8. Enchondroma

_____9. Osteosarcoma

_____10. Ewing's sarcoma

_____11. Colle's fracture

_____12. Smith's fracture

_____13. Boxer's fracture

_____14. Bennett's fracture

_____15. Torus or Buckle fracture

Column B

a. Loss of bone density

b. Disruption in the continuity of bone

c. Benign tumor consisting of cartilage

d. Fracture at the base of the first metacarpal

e. Fracture at the base of the fifth metacarpal

f. Displacement of a bone from the joint space

g. Malignant tumor arising from cartilage cells

h. Fluid-filled cyst with a wall of fibrous tissue

i. Impacted fracture with bulging of the periosteum

j. Inflammation of bone due to a pyogenic infection

k. Chronic, systemic, inflammatory collagen disease

l. Malignant tumor of bone arising in medullary tissue

m. Hereditary form of arthritis where uric acid is deposited in joints

n. Malignant, primary tumor of bone with bone or cartilage formation

o. Fracture of the distal radius and ulnar styloid with anterior displacement

p. Fracture of the distal radius and ulnar styloid with posterior displacement

q. Accumulation of fluid in the joint associated with an underlying condition

r. Form of arthritis marked by progressive cartilage deterioration in synovial joints and vertebrae

Exercise 19

Instructions: This exercise is a comprehensive review of the osteology and arthrology of the upper limb. Provide a short answer or select the correct answer for each question.

1. List the names of the three groups of bones that comprise the hand and wrist and indicate the quantity of bones in that group in each upper limb.

2. Which bone classification are the metacarpals?
   a. Flat
   b. Long
   c. Short
   d. Irregular

3. Which bone classification are the carpal bones?
   a. Flat
   b. Long
   c. Short
   d. Irregular

4. Which bones articulate with the head of metacarpal bones?
   a. Carpals
   b. Distal phalanges
   c. Proximal phalanges

5. What group of bones articulates with the base of metacarpal bones?

6. What part of a metacarpal bone—base or head—forms part of each metacarpophalangeal joint?

7. Which of the following types of upper limb joints are formed in part by the bases of the metacarpals?
   a. Interphalangeal
   b. Carpometacarpal
   c. Metacarpophalangeal

8. How are the metacarpals identified?
   a. Letters A to E from medial (little finger side) to lateral (thumb side)
   b. Letters A to E from lateral (thumb side) to medial (little finger side)
   c. Numbered 1 through 5 from lateral (thumb side) to medial (little finger side)
   d. Numbered 1 through 5 from medial (little finger side) to lateral (thumb side)

9. What is the most distal portion of each metacarpal?
   a. Head
   b. Base
   c. Tubercle

10. How many proximal, middle, and distal phalanges are found in one hand?

    a. Proximal: _____

    b. Middle: _____

    c. Distal: _____

11. Which kinds of movements do the interphalangeal joints allow?
    a. Gliding and sliding
    b. Flexion and extension
    c. Rotational movements around a single axis

12. Which joint is the most distal joint in the upper limb?
    a. Carpometacarpal
    b. Distal interphalangeal
    c. Metacarpophalangeal
    d. Proximal interphalangeal

13. Identify each carpal bone by listing its name first, followed by any additional names it may have. Indicate whether each bone is proximal or distal by writing *P* for proximal or *D* for distal in the parentheses found after each blank.

    a. _____ (   )

    b. _____ (   )

    c. _____ (   )

    d. _____ (   )

    e. _____ (   )

    f. _____ (   )

    g. _____ (   )

    h. _____ (   )

14. What other name refers to the radiocarpal joint?

19. On which end of the ulna—proximal or distal—is the olecranon process located?

15. List the names of the two bones that comprise the forearm and indicate which bone is lateral and which bone is medial.

20. Which two bony processes are located on the proximal end of the ulna?

    a. Ulnar head and styloid process
    b. Ulnar head and coronoid process
    c. Olecranon process and styloid process
    d. Olecranon process and coronoid process

21. Which of the following is located on the proximal ulna?

    a. Ulnar notch
    b. Humeral notch
    c. Trochlear notch

16. On which end of the radius—proximal or distal—is the styloid process located?

22. On which bone is the trochlear notch located?

    a. Ulna
    b. Radius
    c. Humerus

23. Which joint do the radial notch of the ulna and the head of the radius form?

    a. Humeroulnar
    b. Humeroradial
    c. Distal radioulnar
    d. Proximal radioulnar

17. On which end of the radius—proximal or distal—is the radial head located?

24. Which joint do the head of the ulna and the ulnar notch of the radius form?

    a. Humeroulnar
    b. Humeroradial
    c. Distal radioulnar
    d. Proximal radioulnar

18. On which end of the ulna—proximal or distal—is the styloid process located?

25. With which of the following structures of the distal humerus does the radial head articulate?

    a. Trochlea
    b. Capitulum
    c. Lateral epicondyle
    d. Medial epicondyle

26. With which of the following structures of the distal humerus does the trochlear notch articulate?

    a. Trochlea
    b. Capitulum
    c. Lateral epicondyle
    d. Medial epicondyle

27. From the following list, circle the three articulations that form the complete elbow joint.

    a. Radiocarpal
    b. Humeroulnar
    c. Humeroradial
    d. Scapulohumeral
    e. Distal radioulnar
    f. Proximal radioulnar

28. With reference to the capitulum, where is the trochlea located?

    a. Lateral
    b. Medial
    c. Distal
    d. Proximal

29. Write the name of each articulation of the humerus.

30. Write the name of each fossa found on the distal humerus and indicate on which surface each is located.

SECTION 2

Positioning of the Upper Limb

Exercise 1: Positioning for the Fingers

Instructions: A typical radiographic series to demonstrate fingers usually includes a posteroanterior (PA) projection, PA oblique projection, and lateral projection. This exercise pertains to those projections. Identify structures, fill in missing words, or provide a short answer for each question.

1. Identify each lettered bone or joint shown in Fig. 4-12.

   A. _____

   B. _____

   C. _____

   D. _____

   E. _____

   F. _____

   G. _____

2. The radiograph shown in Fig. 4-12 demonstrates a

   _____ (PA or lateral) projection.

3. When performing the radiograph illustrated in Fig. 4-12, toward which joint should the central ray be directed?
   a. Metacarpophalangeal
   b. Distal interphalangeal
   c. Proximal interphalangeal

4. How should the hand be placed for the PA projection of the fingers?
   a. Prone
   b. Lateral
   c. Supine
   d. Internal rotation

5. Compare Fig. 4-12 with Fig. 4-13. Describe how the patient's position as shown in Fig. 4-12 was adjusted to produce the image shown in Fig. 4-13.

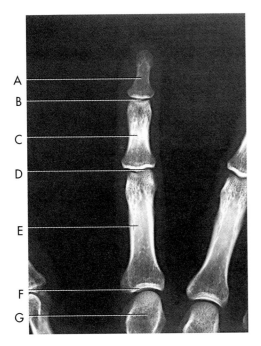

Figure 4-12 Second digit (index finger).

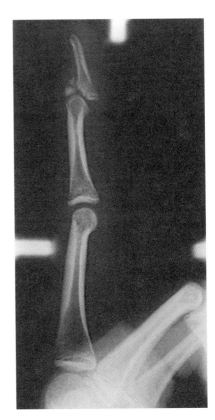

Figure 4-13 Second digit.

6. On which hand surface should the hand be rested when performing the lateral projection radiograph of the fourth or fifth digit?
   a. Medial (ulnar)
   b. Lateral (radial)
   c. Anterior (palmar)
   d. Posterior (ventral)

7. For lateral projections of the third or fourth digit, why should the affected digit be positioned so that its long axis is parallel with the image receptor?

8. How many degrees from the PA position should a finger be rotated for PA oblique projection?

9. For the PA oblique projection of the second digit, what is the advantage of rotating the second digit medially compared with the advantage of rotating the digit laterally?

10. For the PA oblique projection of the third digit, what is the advantage of placing the patient's fingers on a 45-degree foam wedge?

Exercise 2: Positioning for the Thumb

Instructions: This exercise pertains to projections of the thumb. Identify structures, fill in missing words, choose the correct answer, or provide a short answer for each question.

1. Anteroposterior (AP) projections of the thumb require that the patient's hand be rotated into extreme

   _____   _____.

2. The central ray should be directed perpendicular to the first

   _____ joint.

3. In what position should the thumb be placed when the hand is pronated with fingers extended?

4. Which projection of the thumb produces the greatest object-to-image receptor distance (OID)?
   a. AP projection
   b. PA projection
   c. Lateral projection
   d. Oblique projection

5. Which carpal bone should be included in all radiographs of the thumb?
   a. Scaphoid
   b. Trapezoid
   c. Trapezium

6. Identify each lettered structure or joint shown in Fig. 4-14.

A. _____

B. _____

C. _____

D. _____

E. _____

F. _____

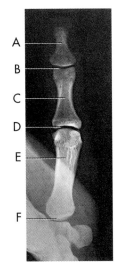

Figure 4-14 AP thumb.

Exercise 3: Positioning for the Hand

Instructions: This exercise pertains to radiographic positions for the hand. Identify structures, fill in missing words, provide a short answer, or choose an answer from a list for each question.

1. Which surface of the hand—palmar or dorsal—should be in contact with the image receptor (IR) for the PA projection?

2. The central ray should be directed perpendicular to the

   third _____ joint.

3. Which two groups of joints of the hand and digits should be demonstrated open on the radiograph of the PA projection of the hand?
   a. Intercarpal and interphalangeal
   b. Intercarpal and carpophalangeal
   c. Metacarpophalangeal and interphalangeal
   d. Metacarpophalangeal and carpophalangeal

4. Identify each lettered bone or joint shown in Fig. 4-15.

A. _____

B. _____

C. _____

D. _____

E. _____

F. _____

G. _____

H. _____

I. _____

J. _____

K. _____

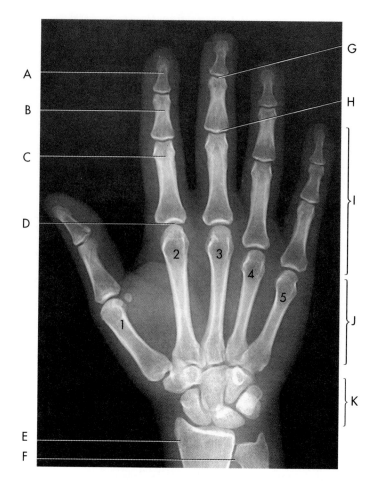

Figure 4-15 PA hand.

5. Figs. 4-16 and 4-17 illustrate two different ways to position the hand for PA oblique projections. Which figure represents the position that best demonstrates interphalangeal joints? Explain why.

6. Examine the radiographs shown in Figs. 4-18 and 4-19. What difference in positioning most likely caused the difference in appearance of these two images?

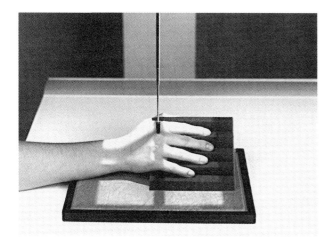

Figure 4-16 PA oblique hand.

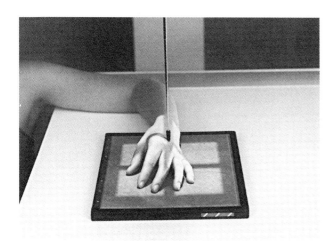

Figure 4-17 PA oblique hand.

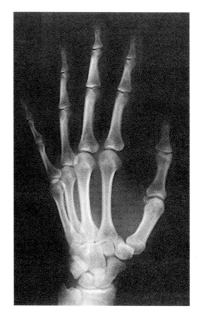

Figure 4-18 PA oblique hand.

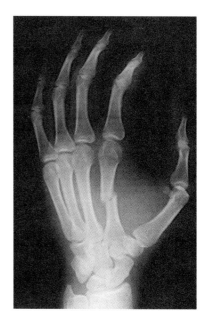

Figure 4-19 PA oblique hand.

7. For lateral projections, toward which joint should the central ray be directed?

   a. First metacarpophalangeal
   b. Second metacarpophalangeal
   c. First proximal interphalangeal
   d. Second proximal interphalangeal

8. Which projection of the hand should demonstrate superimposed phalanges?

   a. PA
   b. PA oblique
   c. Lateral

9. Fig. 4-20 shows a lateral projection radiograph of the hand. In this image, which group of bones is of primary interest?

   a. Carpals
   b. Phalanges
   c. Metacarpals

10. Identify each lettered individual bone or group of bones in Fig. 4-21.

    A. _____

    B. _____

    C. _____

    D. _____

    E. _____

    F. _____

    G. _____

    H. _____

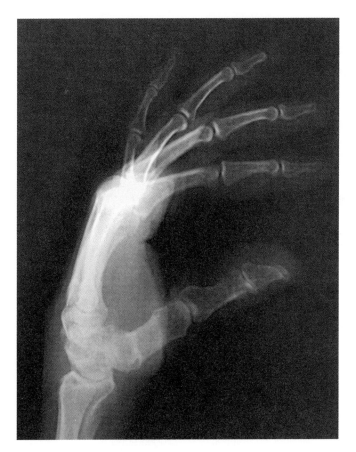

Figure 4-20 Fan lateral hand.

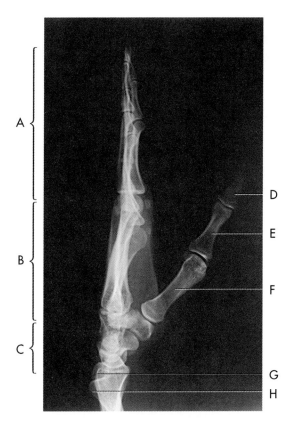

Figure 4-21 Lateral hand.

Exercise 4: Positioning for the Wrist

Instructions: This exercise pertains to radiographic positions for the wrist. Identify structures, fill in missing words, provide a short answer, and select answers from a list for each question.

1. Which surface of the wrist—anterior or posterior—should be in contact with the IR for PA projection radiographs?

2. Why should the hand and digits be slightly flexed for the PA projection of the wrist?

3. When performing the PA projection radiograph, the central ray should be directed perpendicularly, entering in the

   _____ area.

4. Identify each lettered carpal bone shown in Fig. 4-22.

   A. _____

   B. _____

   C. _____

   D. _____

   E. _____

   F. _____

   G. _____

   H. _____

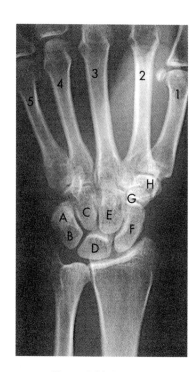

Figure 4-22 PA wrist.

5. For the lateral projection of the wrist, how should the elbow be positioned?
   a. Fully extended
   b. Flexed 45 degrees
   c. Flexed 90 degrees

6. For the lateral projection of the wrist, which surface of the wrist should be in contact with the IR?
   a. Medial
   b. Lateral
   c. Anterior
   d. Posterior

7. Identify each lettered structure in Fig. 4-23.

A. _____

B. _____

C. _____

D. _____

E. _____

F. _____

G. _____

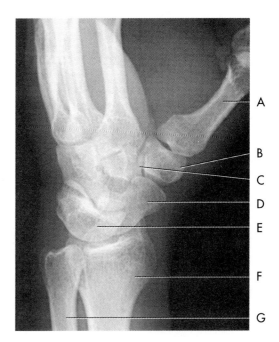

Figure 4-23 Lateral wrist.

8. Referring again to Fig. 4-23, what other bones in addition to the metacarpals and the carpals should be superimposed for this projection?

_____

9. Which surface of the wrist—anterior or posterior—should be in contact with the IR when beginning to position for PA oblique projections?

_____

10. How much should the wrist be rotated for PA oblique projections?

a. 25 degrees
b. 35 degrees
c. 45 degrees

11. For the PA oblique projection when the scaphoid is of primary interest, the scaphoid can sometimes be better demonstrated if the patient flexes the wrist toward the

_____.

12. Identify each lettered structure shown in Fig. 4-24.

A. _____

B. _____

C. _____

D. _____

E. _____

F. _____

G. _____

Figure 4-24 PA oblique wrist.

Questions 13 through 15 pertain to the *PA projection of the wrist in ulnar deviation.* Examine Fig. 4-25 as you answer the questions.

Questions 16 through 20 pertain to the *PA axial projection, Stecher method.* Examine Figure 4-26 as you answer the following questions.

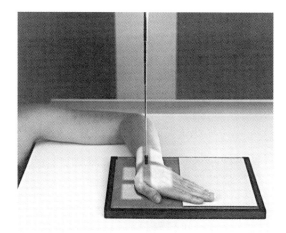

Figure 4-25 PA wrist in ulnar deviation.

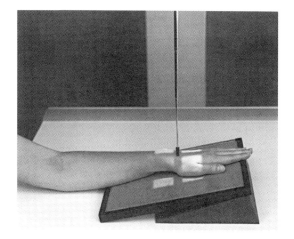

Figure 4-26 PA axial wrist, Stecher method.

13. Which bone is of primary interest with this projection?

    a. Ulna

    b. Lunate

    c. Radius

    d. Scaphoid

14. How should the central ray be directed to the wrist?

    a. Perpendicular

    b. 5 degrees distally

    c. 5 degrees proximally

15. To better delineate a fracture line with a PA projection of the wrist in ulnar deviation, how many degrees and in which direction may the central ray be directed?

    a. 10 to 15 degrees medially or laterally

    b. 20 to 25 degrees medially or laterally

    c. 10 to 15 degrees proximally or distally

    d. 20 to 25 degrees proximally or distally

16. Which surface of the wrist—anterior or posterior—should be in contact with the IR?

17. Which carpal bone is of primary interest with this position?

    a. Lunate

    b. Capitate

    c. Scaphoid

18. How far from horizontal should the IR be inclined toward the elbow?

    a. 10 degrees

    b. 20 degrees

    c. 30 degrees

19. When using a wedge to elevate the IR (as in question 18), how should the central ray be directed toward the wrist?

    a. Perpendicular
    b. At a 10-degree angle toward the elbow
    c. At a 20-degree angle toward the elbow
    d. At a 30-degree angle toward the elbow

20. If no wedge is used to angle the IR, how should the central ray be directed toward the wrist?

    a. Perpendicularly
    b. At a 10-degree angle toward the elbow
    c. At a 20-degree angle toward the elbow
    d. At a 30-degree angle toward the elbow

Items 21 through 25 pertain to the *tangential projection for the carpal canal.*

21. With the patient seated at the end of the table, how should the affected forearm be positioned with reference to the long axis of the table?

22. How should the wrist be placed into position—hyperextended or hyperflexed?

23. With reference to the plane of the IR, how should the long axis of the hand be positioned?

    a. Angled
    b. Vertical
    c. Parallel

24. With reference to the long axis of the hand, how much should the central ray be angled?

    a. 5 to 10 degrees
    b. 15 to 20 degrees
    c. 25 to 30 degrees

25. Identify each lettered structure shown in Fig. 4-27.

    A. _____

    B. _____

    C. _____

    D. _____

    E. _____

    F. _____

    G. _____

    H. _____

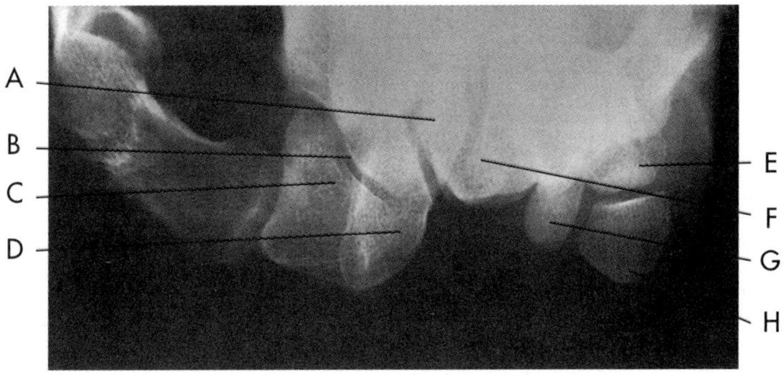

Figure 4-27 Tangential (inferosuperior) carpal canal.

Exercise 5: Positioning for the Forearm

Instructions: This exercise pertains to the two radiographic positions for the forearm, the AP projection and the lateral projection. Identify structures, provide a short answer, select the answer from a list, or choose true or false (explaining any statement you believe to be false) for each question.

1. When positioning for the AP projection, select an IR long enough to include the entire forearm from the _____ of the ulna to the _____ of the radius.
   a. head; head
   b. head; styloid process
   c. olecranon process; head
   d. olecranon process; styloid process

2. For the AP projection of the forearm, how should the elbow be positioned?
   a. Fully extended
   b. Flexed 45 degrees
   c. Flexed 90 degrees

3. True or False. The hand should be pronated for the AP projection.

4. True or False. The central ray should be directed perpendicular to the forearm for the AP projection.

5. Identify each lettered structure shown in Fig. 4-28.

   A. _____

   B. _____

   C. _____

   D. _____

   E. _____

   F. _____

   G. _____

   H. _____

   I. _____

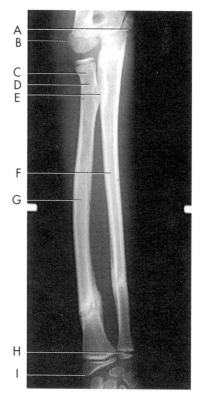

Figure 4-28 AP forearm.

6. For the lateral projection of the forearm, how should the elbow be positioned?
   a. Fully extended
   b. Flexed 45 degrees
   c. Flexed 90 degrees
   d. Rotated medially 45 degrees

7. For the lateral projection, how should the coronal plane through the humeral epicondyles be placed with reference to the IR?

   a. Parallel

   b. Perpendicular

   c. Rotated medially 45 degrees

8. True or False. The hand should be supinated for the lateral projection.

9. True or False. The central ray should be directed perpendicularly to the forearm for the lateral projection.

10. Identify each lettered structure shown in Fig. 4-29.

   A. _____

   B. _____

   C. _____

   D. _____

   E. _____

   F. _____

   G. _____

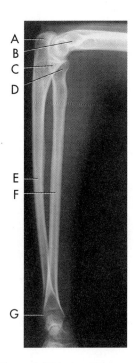

Figure 4-29 Lateral forearm.

Exercise 6: Positioning for the Elbow

Instructions: This exercise pertains to radiographic positions for the elbow. Identify structures, provide a short answer, match columns, or select answers from a list for each question.

1. For the AP projection of the elbow, the hand should be

   _____. (pronated or supinated).

2. For the AP projection, why should the hand be positioned with the palm facing up?

3. For the AP projection, how should the coronal plane through the humeral epicondyles be placed with reference to the IR?

   a. Parallel

   b. Perpendicular

   c. Rotated medially 45 degrees

4. For the AP projection, how should the central ray be directed?

   a. Perpendicular

   b. Angled caudally

   c. Angled cephalically

5. Identify each lettered structure shown in the AP projection of an elbow in Fig. 4-30.

A. _____

B. _____

C. _____

D. _____

E. _____

F. _____

G. _____

H. _____ (tuberosity)

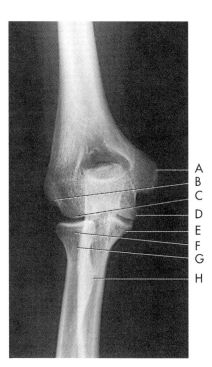

Figure 4-30 AP elbow.

6. For the lateral projection, how should the coronal plane through the humeral epicondyles be placed with reference to the IR?

a. Parallel
b. Perpendicular
c. Rotated medially 45 degrees

7. For the lateral projection of the elbow, how should the hand be adjusted?

a. Pronated
b. Supinated
c. Lateral with the thumb side up
d. Lateral with the thumb side down

8. How many degrees of flexion of the elbow are necessary for the lateral projection?

9. How should the humeral epicondyles appear in the image of the lateral projection of the elbow?

10. Identify each lettered structure shown in Fig. 4-31.

A. _____

B. _____

C. _____

D. _____

E. _____

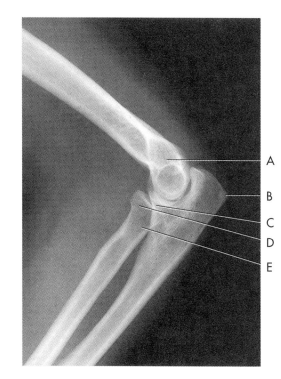

Figure 4-31 Lateral elbow.

11. How much medial rotation of the elbow is needed to position it for AP oblique projections?

    a. 25 degrees
    b. 35 degrees
    c. 45 degrees
    d. 55 degrees

12. For AP oblique projections, how should the central ray be directed?

    a. Perpendicularly
    b. Angled laterally
    c. Angled medially

13. Which AP oblique projection positioning movement—medial rotation or lateral rotation—requires the hand to be pronated?

14. Identify each lettered structure shown in Fig. 4-32.

    A. _____

    B. _____

    C. _____

    D. _____

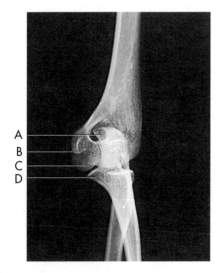

Figure 4-32 AP oblique elbow (medial rotation).

15. Identify each lettered structure in Fig. 4-33.

    A. _____

    B. _____

    C. _____

    D. _____

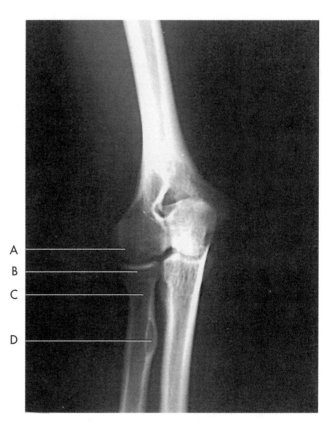

Figure 4-33 AP oblique elbow (lateral rotation).

16. Again examining Figs. 4-32 and 4-33, identify which image best demonstrates the following structures.

    ____ a. Open elbow joint

    ____ b. Coronoid process in profile

    ____ c. Radial head projected free of the ulna

    ____ d. Elongated medial humeral epicondyle

    ____ e. Ulna superimposed by the radial head and neck

17. Figs. 4-34 and 4-35 are AP projection radiographs of the elbow with the elbow partially flexed. Examine the images and answer the questions that follow.

    a. Which image demonstrates an AP distal projection of the humerus?

    _____

    b. Which image demonstrates an AP proximal projection of the forearm?

    _____

    c. Which image demonstrates a radiograph of the elbow joint partially opened?

    _____

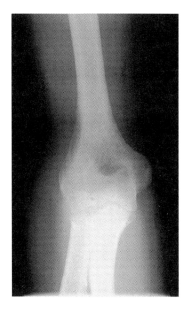

Figure 4-34 AP elbow, partial flexion.

    d. For the AP distal humerus projection (partially flexed elbow), what part of the upper limb should be parallel and in contact with the IR?

    _____

    e. In the AP distal humerus projection (partially flexed elbow) radiograph, what part of the upper limb will appear greatly foreshortened in the image?

    _____

    f. For the AP proximal forearm projection (partially flexed elbow), what part of the upper limb should be parallel and in contact with the IR?

    _____

    g. In the AP proximal forearm projection (partially flexed elbow) radiograph, what part of the upper limb will appear greatly foreshortened in the image?

    _____

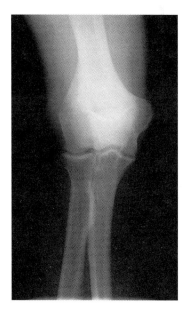

Figure 4-35 AP elbow, partial flexion.

18. Match the projections of the elbow in Column A with the evaluation criteria in Column B. Not all evaluation criteria may apply to the listed projections.

Column A

_____ 1. AP projection

_____ 2. Lateral projection

_____ 3. AP lateral oblique projection

_____ 4. AP medial oblique projection

_____ 5. AP proximal forearm projection (partially flexed elbow)

Column B

a. Distal humerus will be foreshortened.

b. Coronoid process should be seen in profile.

c. Olecranon process should be seen in profile.

d. Proximal forearm will be greatly foreshortened.

e. Radial head should be projected free of the ulna.

f. Humeral epicondyles should not be rotated or superimposed.

Exercise 7: Positioning for the Humerus

Instructions: This exercise pertains to the positioning of the humerus for AP and lateral projections. Identify structures, fill in missing words, provide a short answer, or select answers from a list.

Questions 1 through 7 pertain to the *AP projection.*

1. Describe how the image receptor should be positioned with reference to the patient.

2. Which part(s) of the humerus should be palpated and correctly placed to ensure that the humerus is correctly positioned for AP projections?

   a. Head
   b. Epicondyles
   c. Lesser tubercle
   d. Greater tubercle

3. How should a coronal plane passing through the humeral epicondyles be positioned with reference to the plane of the IR?

   a. Parallel
   b. Perpendicular
   c. Rotated laterally 45 degrees
   d. Rotated medially 45 degrees

4. How should the hand be placed?

5. For the AP projection with the patient supine, why is it sometimes necessary to elevate the unaffected shoulder on a firm support?

6. From the following list, circle the three evaluation criteria that indicate the humerus was correctly positioned for the AP projection.

   a. Epicondyles are superimposed.
   b. Epicondyles are maximally seen and not rotated.
   c. Greater tubercle is superimposed over the humeral head.
   d. Humeral head and greater tubercle are both seen in profile.
   e. Lesser tubercle is seen in profile and toward the glenoid fossa.
   f. Outline of the lesser tubercle is located between the humeral head and the greater tubercle.

7. Identify each lettered structure shown in Fig. 4-36.

A. _____

B. _____

C. _____

D. _____

E. _____

F. _____

G. _____

H. _____

I. _____

J. _____

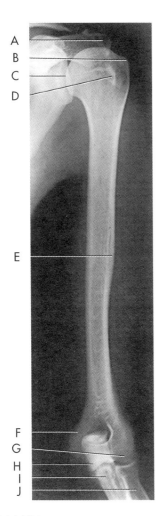

Figure 4-36 Upright AP humerus.

Questions 8 through 15 pertain to the *lateral projection.*

8. Describe how the image receptor should be positioned with reference to the patient.

9. Unless contraindicated by a possible fracture, describe how the upper limb should be maneuvered with the patient sitting or standing.

10. When performing the lateral projection, with reference to the plane of the IR, ensure that a coronal plane passing through the humeral epicondyles is

    _____ (parallel or perpendicular).

11. How does the divergence of the beam affect the demonstration of the elbow joint in the lateral projection radiograph?

12. The superimposition of what structures confirms that a true lateral image was produced?

13. For the lateral projection with the patient in the lateral recumbent position and an IR placed between the arm and the thorax, which portion of the humerus is missing from the radiograph?

14. From the following list, circle the three evaluation criteria that indicate the humerus was in a true lateral position when properly imaged for the lateral projection.

   a. The epicondyles are superimposed.
   b. The epicondyles are maximally seen and not rotated.
   c. The greater tubercle is superimposed over the humeral head.
   d. The humeral head and greater tubercle are both seen in profile.
   e. The lesser tubercle is seen in profile and toward the glenoid fossa.
   f. The outline of the lesser tubercle is located between the humeral head and the greater tubercle.

15. Identify each lettered structure shown in Fig. 4-37.

   A. _____

   B. _____

   C. _____

   D. _____

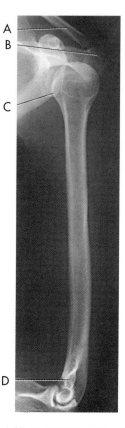

Figure 4-37 Upright lateral humerus.

Exercise 8: Positioning of the Upper Limb

Instructions: This exercise is a comprehensive review of the standard projections that demonstrate structures of the upper limb. Provide a short answer for each item.

1. Where is the centering point for the central ray for the AP projection of the thumb?

2. Which projection of the thumb requires the patient to rotate the hand into extreme internal rotation?

3. Where is the centering point for the central ray for the PA projection of the third digit of the hand?

4. Explain why the hand should be rotated into extreme internal rotation until the lateral surface of the index finger is in contact with the IR, rather than positioning that finger with its medial (ulnar) surface toward the IR, for the lateral projection of the index finger (second digit).

5. Name the three bones that should be completely seen in the image of the AP projection of the thumb.

6. Excluding the thumb, name the two digits of the hand that should rest directly on the IR for the lateral projection of individual digits.

7. Describe how and where the central ray should be directed for the PA projection of the hand.

8. What surface of the hand should be in contact with the IR for the PA projection of the hand?

9. From the prone position, how many degrees should the hand be rotated for the PA oblique projection? For the lateral projection?

10. To best demonstrate all digits, how should the thumb and index finger be positioned with respect to the IR for the PA oblique projection of the hand?

11. Which bones of the hand are of primary interest if the fingertips are allowed to rest on the IR for the PA oblique projection of the hand?

12. What group of bones of the hand is best demonstrated with the fan lateral projection of the hand?

13. For the PA projection of the wrist, why should the hand be slightly arched by flexing the fingers?

14. Describe how and where the central ray should be directed for the PA projection of the wrist.

15. In addition to the eight carpal bones, what other bones should be seen in the image of the PA projection of the wrist?

16. How many degrees from the prone position should the wrist be rotated for the PA oblique projection of the wrist?

17. Which projection of the wrist requires the superimposition of the radial and ulnar styloid processes?

18. Which surface of the wrist should be in contact with the IR for the lateral projection of the wrist?

19. In which projection of the wrist should the metacarpals appear superimposed in the image?

20. For the PA oblique projection of the wrist, which side of the wrist should be elevated from the IR?

21. What two carpal bones on the lateral side of the wrist should be clearly demonstrated in the image of the PA oblique projection of the wrist?

22. What carpal bone is best demonstrated with the ulnar deviation position of the wrist?

23. How does the placement of the IR for the PA axial projection of the scaphoid (Stecher method) differ from IR placement for PA projections of the wrist?

24. How does the forearm appear if the hand is pronated when performing the AP projection of the forearm?

25. To prevent radial crossover, how should the hand be positioned for the AP projection of the forearm?

26. What structure on the distal end of the ulna should be seen in the image of the AP projection of the forearm?

27. How should the humeral epicondyles appear in the image of the lateral projection of the forearm?

28. How should the hand be positioned for the lateral projection of the forearm?

29. What would most likely cause the bones of the forearm to appear rotated in the image of the AP projection of the elbow?

30. Why should the patient lean laterally for the AP projection of the elbow?

31. What structures of the proximal radius are seen slightly superimposed over the proximal ulna in the AP projection of the elbow?

32. How should the hand be positioned for the lateral projection of the elbow? Explain why.

33. What oblique projection of the elbow best demonstrates the coronoid process in profile?

34. How should the forearm and elbow be rotated to best demonstrate the radial head free of superimposition from the ulna?

35. How many AP projections are necessary to best demonstrate the elbow without distortion when an injury prevents full extension of the elbow?

36. Explain how the humerus and the forearm are positioned differently for each AP projection of the elbow when the elbow is in partial flexion.

37. With reference to the patient, where should the top border of the IR be positioned to ensure its proper placement for the AP projection of the humerus?

38. What humeral processes should be palpated to ensure proper alignment when the humerus is being positioned?

39. Which projection for the humerus requires the patient's hand to be supinated?

40. Describe how to best position the IR for the lateral projection of the humerus if the AP projection radiograph clearly shows a fracture 2 inches (5 cm) superior to the elbow.

Exercise 9: Identifying Projections of the Upper Limb

Instructions: This exercise uses photographs that show patients being positioned for various projections of the upper limb. Examine each photograph and identify the projection by name and the part of the upper limb that is being demonstrated.

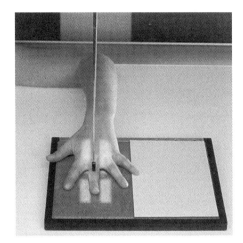

Figure 4-38

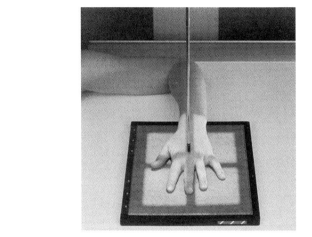

Figure 4-40

1. Fig. 4-38: _____

3. Fig. 4-40: _____

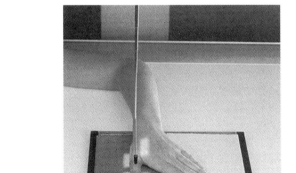

Figure 4-39

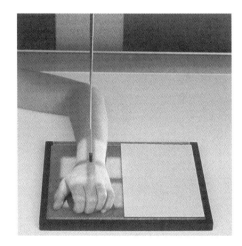

Figure 4-41

2. Fig. 4-39: _____

4. Fig. 4-41: _____

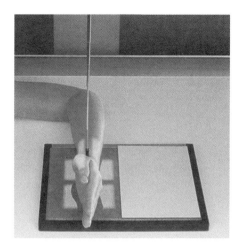

Figure 4-42

5. Fig. 4-42: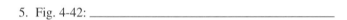

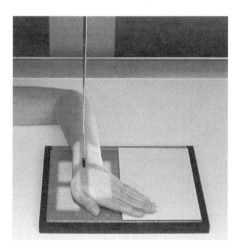

Figure 4-43

6. Fig. 4-43: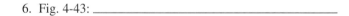

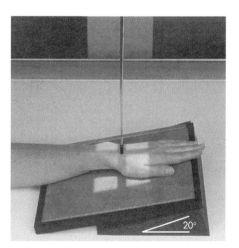

Figure 4-44

7. Fig. 4-44: _____

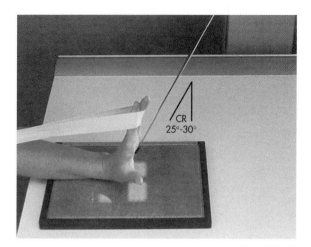

Figure 4-45

8. Fig. 4-45: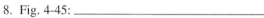

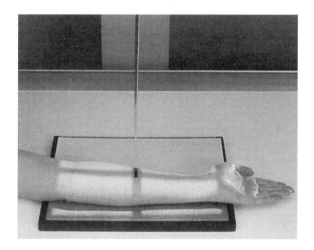

Figure 4-46

9. Fig. 4-46: _____

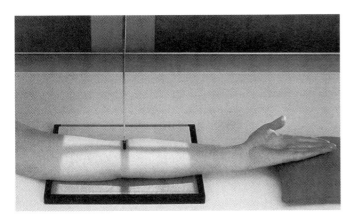

Figure 4-47

10. Fig. 4-47: _____

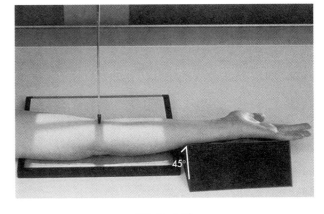

Figure 4-49

12. Fig. 4-49: _____

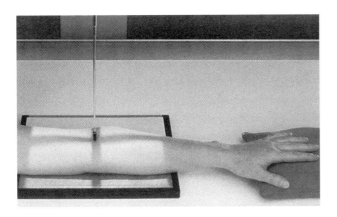

Figure 4-48

11. Fig. 4-48: _____

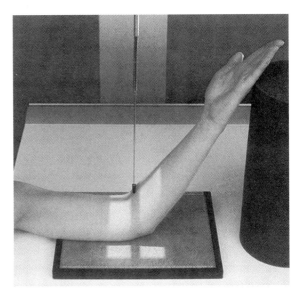

Figure 4-50

13. Fig. 4-50: _____

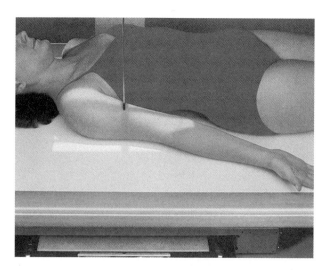

Figure 4-51

14. Fig. 4-51: _____

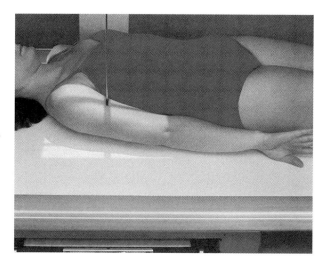

Figure 4-52

15. Fig. 4-52: _____

Exercise 10: Evaluating Radiographs of the Upper Limb

Instructions: This exercise consists of radiographs of the upper extremity to give you practice evaluating extremity positioning. These images are not from *Merrill's Atlas of Radiographic Positions and Radiologic Procedures.* Each radiograph shows at least one positioning error. Examine each image and answer the questions that follow by providing a short answer or choosing the correct answer from a list.

1. Fig. 4-53 shows a PA finger projection of inferior quality. Examine the image and state why it does not meet the evaluation criteria for this projection.

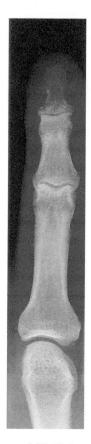

Figure 4-53 PA finger.

2. Fig. 4-54 shows an AP projection radiograph of the thumb. Examine the image and state why it does not meet the evaluation criteria for this projection.

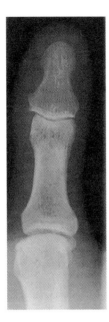

Figure 4-54 AP thumb.

3. Fig. 4-55 shows an AP projection radiograph with the forearm incorrectly positioned. State the positioning error that occurred in this image.

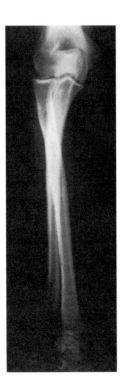

Figure 4-55 AP forearm with improper positioning.

4. Fig. 4-56 shows an attempted lateral projection radiograph with the forearm incorrectly positioned. From the following list, select the positioning error that most likely occurred in this image.
   a. The hand was pronated.
   b. The hand was supinated.
   c. The upper arm was not parallel and in contact with the IR and table.

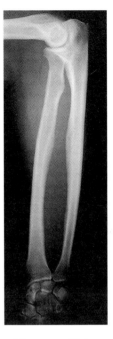

Figure 4-56 Lateral forearm with improper positioning.

Fig. 4-57 shows a lateral projection radiograph with the elbow incorrectly positioned. Examine the image and answer the questions that follow.

Fig. 4-58 is another lateral view with the elbow incorrectly positioned. Examine the image and answer the questions that follow.

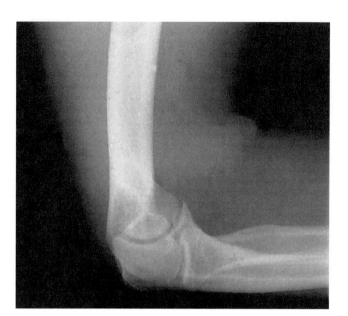

Figure 4-57 Lateral elbow with improper positioning.

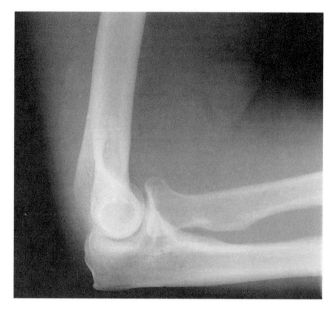

Figure 4-58 Lateral elbow with improper positioning.

5. Which part of the image indicates that the elbow was incorrectly positioned for this view?

   a. The radial head is seen in profile.
   b. The radial tuberosity is facing anteriorly.
   c. The humeral epicondyles are not superimposed.

6. Which positioning error most likely caused the elbow to appear as it does in this image?

   a. The hand was pronated, causing radial crossover of the ulna.
   b. The upper arm was not parallel and in contact with the IR and table.
   c. The central ray was angled longitudinally with the long axis of the forearm.

7. Which part of the image indicates that the elbow was incorrectly positioned for this view?

   a. The olecranon process is seen in profile.
   b. The radial tuberosity does not face anteriorly.
   c. The humeral epicondyles are not superimposed.

8. Which positioning error most likely caused the elbow to appear as it does in this image?

   a. The hand was supinated.
   b. The hand was medially rotated.
   c. The upper arm was not parallel and in contact with the IR and table.

Self-Test: Osteology, Arthrology, and Positioning of the Upper Limb

Instructions: Answer the following questions by selecting the best choice.

1. How many interphalangeal joints are found in one upper limb?
   a. 8
   b. 9
   c. 10
   d. 14

2. Each proximal phalanx articulates with a:
   a. Metacarpal
   b. Carpal bone
   c. Distal phalanx
   d. Carpometacarpal joint

3. Which bones comprise the palm of the hand?
   a. Carpals
   b. Phalanges
   c. Metatarsals
   d. Metacarpals

4. Which joint is formed by the articulation of the proximal end of the middle phalanx with the distal end of the proximal phalanx of the ring finger?
   a. The distal interphalangeal joint of the third digit
   b. The distal interphalangeal joint of the fourth digit
   c. The proximal interphalangeal joint of the third digit
   d. The proximal interphalangeal joint of the fourth digit

5. Which joint is formed by the articulation of the distal end of the middle phalanx with the proximal end of the distal phalanx of the index finger?
   a. The distal interphalangeal joint of the first digit
   b. The distal interphalangeal joint of the second digit
   c. The proximal interphalangeal joint of the first digit
   d. The proximal interphalangeal joint of the second digit

6. Which joint is a hinge-type joint?
   a. Interphalangeal
   b. Scapulohumeral
   c. Carpometacarpal
   d. Metacarpophalangeal

7. How many metacarpal bones are found in one upper limb?
   a. 2
   b. 5
   c. 8
   d. 14

8. Which of the following articulates with the bases of metacarpal bones?
   a. Carpals
   b. Phalanges
   c. Forearm
   d. Metacarpophalangeal joints

9. Which joint of the hand is formed by the articulation of the head of a metacarpal with a digit?
   a. Carpometacarpal
   b. Metacarpophalangeal
   c. Distal interphalangeal
   d. Proximal interphalangeal

10. Which joints of the hand are formed by the articulation of the bases of the metacarpals with the bones of the wrist?
    a. Radiocarpal
    b. Interphalangeals
    c. Carpometacarpals
    d. Metacarpophalangeals

11. Which joint is a condyloid joint?
    a. Interphalangeal
    b. Scapulohumeral
    c. Carpometacarpal
    d. Metacarpophalangeal

12. Which articulation of the upper limb is a saddle joint that allows the thumb to oppose the fingers?
    a. Radiocarpal
    b. Distal radioulnar
    c. Proximal radioulnar
    d. First carpometacarpal

13. Which bones are located in the proximal row of the wrist?
    a. Scaphoid, lunate, capitate, and hamate
    b. Scaphoid, lunate, pisiform, and triquetrum
    c. Trapezium, trapezoid, capitate, and hamate
    d. Trapezium, trapezoid, pisiform, and triquetrum

14. Which bones are located in the distal row of the wrist?
    a. Hamate, capitate, lunate, and scaphoid
    b. Hamate, capitate, trapezium, and trapezoid
    c. Pisiform, triquetrum, lunate, and scaphoid
    d. Pisiform, triquetrum, trapezium, and trapezoid

15. Where in the wrist is the scaphoid located?
    a. Medial side of the distal row
    b. Medial side of the proximal row
    c. Lateral side of the distal row
    d. Lateral side of the proximal row

16. Where in the wrist is the trapezium located?

    a. Medial side of the distal row
    b. Medial side of the proximal row
    c. Lateral side of the distal row
    d. Lateral side of the proximal row

17. Where in the wrist is the hamate located?

    a. Medial side of the distal row
    b. Medial side of the proximal row
    c. Lateral side of the distal row
    d. Lateral side of the proximal row

18. What other name refers to the carpal bone known as the hamate?

    a. Unciform
    b. Capitatum
    c. Cuneiform
    d. Os magnum

19. What other name refers to the carpal bone known as the capitate?

    a. Pisiform
    b. Unciform
    c. Scaphoid
    d. Os magnum

20. What other name refers to the carpal bone known as the triquetrum?

    a. Navicular
    b. Cuneiform
    c. Lesser multangular
    d. Greater multangular

21. What other name refers to the carpal bone known as the trapezium?

    a. Trapezoid
    b. Semilunar
    c. Lesser multangular
    d. Greater multangular

22. What other name refers to the carpal bone known as the trapezoid?

    a. Pisiform
    b. Unciform
    c. Lesser multangular
    d. Greater multangular

23. Which carpal bone has only one name?

    a. Hamate
    b. Capitate
    c. Pisiform
    d. Scaphoid

24. Which bone classification are carpal bones?

    a. Flat
    b. Long
    c. Short
    d. Irregular

25. Which bones are classified as short bones?

    a. Carpals
    b. Vertebrae
    c. Phalanges
    d. Metacarpals

26. Which joint is the most distal articulation of the wrist?

    a. Intercarpal
    b. Radiocarpal
    c. Carpometacarpal
    d. Metacarpophalangeal

27. Which joint is the most proximal articulation of the wrist?

    a. Intercarpal
    b. Radiocarpal
    c. Carpometacarpal
    d. Metacarpophalangeal

28. Which two carpal bones are the most lateral bones of the wrist?

    a. Lunate and trapezoid
    b. Lunate and trapezium
    c. Scaphoid and trapezoid
    d. Scaphoid and trapezium

29. Between which two bones is the lunate situated?

    a. Trapezoid and scaphoid
    b. Trapezoid and trapezium
    c. Triquetrum and scaphoid
    d. Triquetrum and trapezium

30. What other name refers to the carpal bone known as the scaphoid?

    a. Unciform
    b. Navicular
    c. Semilunar
    d. Capitatum

31. Which carpal bone does not articulate with the radius?

    a. Lunate
    b. Capitate
    c. Scaphoid
    d. Triquetrum

32. Which bony structures are located on the proximal end of the ulna?
    a. Radial notch, styloid process, and ulnar head
    b. Radial head, olecranon process, and ulnar head
    c. Radial head, styloid process, and coronoid process
    d. Radial notch, olecranon process, and coronoid process

33. Which bony structures are located on the distal end of the ulna?
    a. Ulnar head and styloid process
    b. Ulnar head and olecranon process
    c. Coronoid process and styloid process
    d. Coronoid process and olecranon process

34. Which bony structure is located on the distal end of the radius?
    a. Head
    b. Neck
    c. Tubercle
    d. Styloid process

35. Which bony structures are located on the proximal radius?
    a. Head and tubercle
    b. Head and styloid process
    c. Olecranon process and tubercle
    d. Olecranon process and styloid process

36. Which bones comprise the forearm?
    a. Radius and ulna
    b. Radius and carpals
    c. Humerus and ulna
    d. Humerus and carpals

37. Which structure is located on the lateral aspect of the distal forearm?
    a. Ulnar head
    b. Radial head
    c. Ulnar styloid process
    d. Radial styloid process

38. Which large bony process is easily located by touching on the posterior aspect of the proximal forearm?
    a. Styloid process
    b. Radial tuberosity
    c. Coronoid process
    d. Olecranon process

39. Which structure is located on the medial side of the distal forearm?
    a. Coronoid process
    b. Olecranon process
    c. Ulnar styloid process
    d. Radial styloid process

40. Which two structures unite to form the trochlear notch?
    a. Radial notch and styloid process
    b. Radial notch and olecranon process
    c. Coronoid process and styloid process
    d. Coronoid process and olecranon process

41. Where is the trochlear notch located?
    a. Distal ulna
    b. Distal radius
    c. Proximal ulna
    d. Proximal radius

42. Which two structures articulate to form the proximal radioulnar joint?
    a. Head of the ulna and radial notch of the ulna
    b. Head of the ulna and ulnar notch of the radius
    c. Head of the radius and radial notch of the ulna
    d. Head of the radius and ulnar notch of the radius

43. Which two structures articulate to form the distal radioulnar joint?
    a. Head of the ulna and radial notch of the ulna
    b. Head of the ulna and ulnar notch of the radius
    c. Head of the radius and radial notch of the ulna
    d. Head of the radius and ulnar notch of the radius

44. Which articulation do the trochlea and the trochlear notch form?
    a. Humeroulnar
    b. Humeroradial
    c. Distal radioulnar
    d. Proximal radioulnar

45. Which structure articulates with the capitulum?
    a. Ulnar head
    b. Radial head
    c. Glenoid fossa
    d. Humeral head

46. Which structure articulates with the capitulum?
    a. Distal ulna
    b. Distal radius
    c. Proximal ulna
    d. Proximal radius

47. Which structure articulates with the trochlea?
    a. Distal ulna
    b. Distal radius
    c. Proximal ulna
    d. Proximal radius

48. Which structure articulates with the trochlear notch?

    a. Trochlea
    b. Capitulum
    c. Distal ulna
    d. Distal radius

49. Which joint classification is the elbow?

    a. Diarthrodial
    b. Synarthrodial
    c. Amphiarthrodial

50. In which joint is the capitulum located?

    a. Hip
    b. Wrist
    c. Elbow
    d. Shoulder

51. In which joint is the trochlea located?

    a. Hip
    b. Wrist
    c. Elbow
    d. Shoulder

52. In which joint is the trochlear notch located?

    a. Hip
    b. Knee
    c. Wrist
    d. Elbow

53. Which type of joint is the elbow?

    a. Hinge
    b. Gliding
    c. Condyloid
    d. Ball and socket

54. Where is the capitulum located?

    a. Medial side of the distal humerus
    b. Medial side of the proximal humerus
    c. Lateral side of the distal humerus
    d. Lateral side of the proximal humerus

55. With reference from the trochlea, where is the capitulum located?

    a. Distal
    b. Lateral
    c. Medial
    d. Proximal

56. What is the roughened process of the humerus superior to the intertubercular groove?

    a. Lesser tubercle
    b. Greater tubercle
    c. Lateral epicondyle
    d. Medial epicondyle

57. Which bony process is located on the anterior surface of the proximal humerus?

    a. Lesser tubercle
    b. Greater tubercle
    c. Lateral epicondyle
    d. Medial epicondyle

58. Which structure articulates with the ulna to form the humeroulnar joint?

    a. Trochlea
    b. Capitulum
    c. Radial head
    d. Humeral head

59. How many articulations does the humerus have?

    a. 2
    b. 3
    c. 4
    d. 5

60. Which structure articulates with the radius to form the humeroradial joint?

    a. Trochlea
    b. Capitulum
    c. Radial notch
    d. Humeral head

61. Which depression is located on the anterior surface of the distal humerus?

    a. Radial notch
    b. Coronoid fossa
    c. Olecranon fossa
    d. Intertubercular groove

62. Which depression is located on the posterior surface of the distal humerus?

    a. Radial notch
    b. Coronoid fossa
    c. Olecranon fossa
    d. Intertubercular groove

63. Which depression is located between the lesser and greater tubercles of the proximal humerus?

    a. Radial notch
    b. Coronoid fossa
    c. Bicipital groove
    d. Olecranon fossa

64. Which digit of the hand produces the greatest object-to-image receptor distance (OID) in the lateral projection of that digit?

    a. Thumb
    b. Index finger
    c. Ring finger
    d. Small finger

65. For lateral projections of the second through fifth digits of the hand, through which joint should the central ray be directed?

    a. Carpometacarpal
    b. Metacarpophalangeal
    c. Distal interphalangeal
    d. Proximal interphalangeal

66. From the prone position, how many degrees should a finger be rotated for the PA oblique projection of that finger?

    a. 15
    b. 30
    c. 45
    d. 90

67. Which digit of the hand produces the least OID in the lateral projection of that digit?

    a. Index finger
    b. Middle finger
    c. Ring finger

68. How should the hand be positioned for the PA medial oblique projection of the hand?

    a. From the prone position, rotate the hand ulnar side up.
    b. From the prone position, rotate the hand radial side up.
    c. From the supine position, rotate the hand ulnar side up.
    d. From the supine position, rotate the hand radial side up.

69. What is the centering point for the central ray for the PA projection of the third finger?

    a. Head of the third metacarpal
    b. Base of the third metacarpal
    c. Distal interphalangeal joint of the third digit
    d. Proximal interphalangeal joint of the third digit

70. From the prone position, how many degrees should a finger be rotated for the lateral projection of that finger?

    a. 15 degrees
    b. 30 degrees
    c. 45 degrees
    d. 90 degrees

71. For the PA projection of the hand, where should the central ray be directed?

    a. Midcarpal area
    b. Base of the third metacarpal
    c. Third metacarpophalangeal joint
    d. Proximal interphalangeal joint of the third digit

72. From the prone position, how many degrees should a hand be rotated for the PA oblique projection of that hand?

    a. 15 degrees
    b. 25 degrees
    c. 35 degrees
    d. 45 degrees

73. Which wrist-positioning maneuver opens the carpal interspaces on the lateral side of the wrist?

    a. Hyperflexion
    b. Hyperextension
    c. Ulnar deviation
    d. Radial deviation

74. Which wrist projection requires that the IR be inclined toward the elbow at an angle of 20 degrees from horizontal?

    a. PA
    b. PA oblique
    c. PA with ulnar deviation
    d. PA axial (Stecher method)

75. Which projection of the wrist corrects foreshortening of the scaphoid carpal bone?

    a. PA
    b. Lateral
    c. PA with ulnar deviation
    d. PA with radial deviation

76. In which projection of the upper limb is the fourth digit of the hand not parallel with the IR?

    a. PA projection of the hand
    b. PA projection of the wrist
    c. Lateral projection of the fourth digit
    d. PA oblique projection of the fourth digit

77. Which projection of the wrist requires that the radial styloid process be superimposed over the ulnar styloid process?

    a. PA
    b. Lateral
    c. PA oblique
    d. PA axial (Stecher method)

78. For the PA projection of the wrist, which positioning maneuver should be used to place the anterior surface of the wrist in contact with the IR?

    a. Ulnar-flex the hand.
    b. Radial-flex the hand.
    c. Slightly arch the hand.
    d. Pronate the hand in full extension.

79. How should the hand and wrist be positioned for the PA oblique projection of the wrist?

    a. With the hand pronated, rotate the wrist ulnar side up.
    b. With the hand pronated, rotate the wrist radial side up.
    c. With the hand supinated, rotate the wrist ulnar side up.
    d. With the hand supinated, rotate the wrist radial side up.

80. Which projection of the wrist best demonstrates the scaphoid carpal bone and its related articulations?

    a. Lateral projection
    b. Inferosuperior projection
    c. Ulnar deviation projection
    d. Radial deviation projection

81. How should the hand be positioned for the AP projection and for the lateral projection of the forearm?

    a. Hand supinated; hand lateral
    b. Hand supinated; hand pronated
    c. Hand pronated; hand lateral
    d. Hand pronated; hand pronated

82. Which description best explains how radial crossover occurs when the forearm is demonstrated?

    a. During the AP projection, the hand is pronated.
    b. During the AP projection, the hand is supinated.
    c. During the lateral projection, the arm is fully extended with the hand flexed.
    d. During the lateral projection, the radial and ulnar styloid processes are superimposed with each other.

83. For the AP projection of the forearm, which positioning step should be taken to prevent radial crossover?

    a. Pronate the hand.
    b. Supinate the hand.
    c. Keep the humeral epicondylar coronal plane parallel with the IR.
    d. Keep the humeral epicondylar coronal plane perpendicular with the IR.

84. In which projection of the upper limb is radial crossover a primary concern?

    a. AP projection of the elbow
    b. AP projection of the forearm
    c. Lateral projection of the elbow
    d. Lateral projection of the forearm

85. Which projection of the forearm requires that the elbow be flexed 90 degrees?

    a. AP
    b. Lateral
    c. AP lateral oblique
    d. AP medial oblique

86. When performing a radiograph of a forearm in a fiberglass cast, approximately which compensation to exposure technique should occur?

    a. Increase mAs 25% or 4 kVp
    b. Increase mAs 50% or 8 kVp
    c. Decrease mAs 25% or 4 kVp
    d. Decrease mAs 50% or 8 kVp

87. How much should the elbow be flexed for the lateral projection of the elbow?

    a. 25 degrees
    b. 45 degrees
    c. 90 degrees
    d. 180 degrees

88. Which projection of the elbow best demonstrates the radial head free of bony superimposition?

    a. AP
    b. Lateral
    c. AP lateral oblique
    d. AP medial oblique

89. With reference to the plane of the IR, how should the humeral epicondylar coronal plane be positioned for the lateral projection of the elbow?

    a. Parallel
    b. Perpendicular
    c. 45 degrees lateral rotation
    d. 45 degrees medial rotation

90. Which oblique projection of the upper limb best demonstrates the radial head free of bony superimposition?

    a. AP lateral oblique of the wrist
    b. PA medial oblique of the wrist
    c. AP lateral oblique of the elbow
    d. AP medial oblique of the elbow

91. Which oblique projection of the upper limb best demonstrates the radial head superimposed over the ulna?

    a. AP lateral oblique of the wrist
    b. PA medial oblique of the wrist
    c. AP lateral oblique of the elbow
    d. AP medial oblique of the elbow

92. With reference to the plane of the IR, how should the humeral epicondylar coronal plane be positioned for the AP projection of the elbow?

    a. Parallel
    b. Perpendicular
    c. 45 degrees lateral rotation
    d. 45 degrees medial rotation

93. Which projection of the elbow best demonstrates the olecranon process in profile?

    a. AP projection
    b. Lateral projection
    c. AP lateral oblique projection
    d. AP medial oblique projection

94. Which projection of the elbow best demonstrates the olecranon process within the olecranon fossa and the coronoid process in profile?

    a. AP projection
    b. Lateral projection
    c. AP lateral oblique projection
    d. AP medial oblique projection

95. When examining the image of the AP projection of the humerus, what determines the accuracy of the position?

    a. The centering of the central ray
    b. The placement of the epicondyles
    c. The placement of the image receptor
    d. The visualization of the lesser tubercle in profile

96. Which positioning characteristic best indicates that the humerus is properly positioned for the AP projection of the humerus?

    a. The hand is pronated on the table.
    b. The hand is true lateral on the table.
    c. The humeral epicondylar coronal plane is parallel with the IR.
    d. The humeral epicondylar coronal plane is perpendicular to the IR.

97. Which evaluation criterion indicates that the humerus was properly positioned for the AP projection?

    a. The epicondyles are superimposed.
    b. The lesser tubercle is seen in profile.
    c. The greater tubercle is superimposed over the humeral head.
    d. The humeral head and greater tubercle are both seen in profile.

98. One way that the lateral radiograph of a humerus, produced with the patient in the lateral decubitus position and the IR placed between the arm and thorax, appears different from the lateral position with the patient standing is that the former demonstrates:

    a. The humeral head in profile
    b. Less than the entire humerus
    c. The lesser tubercle in profile
    d. The greater tubercle in profile

99. With reference to the plane of the IR, how is it determined that the humerus is properly positioned in true lateral position?

    a. The hand is pronated.
    b. The hand is placed true lateral.
    c. The humeral epicondylar coronal plane is parallel.
    d. The humeral epicondylar coronal plane is perpendicular.

100. Which evaluation criterion indicates that the humerus was properly positioned for the lateral projection?

    a. The lesser tubercle is seen in profile.
    b. Beam divergence opens the elbow joint.
    c. The humeral head and greater tubercle are both seen in profile.
    d. Maximum visualization of the epicondyles without rotation is seen.

CHAPTER 5

Shoulder Girdle

SECTION 1

Osteology and Arthrology of the Shoulder Girdle

Exercise 1

Instructions: This exercise pertains to the clavicle. Identify structures, fill in missing words, choose the correct answer, or provide a short answer for each question.

1. Identify each lettered structure shown in Fig. 5-1.

   A. _____

   B. _____

   C. _____

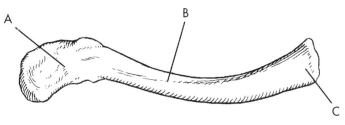

Figure 5-1 Anterior aspect of the clavicle.

2. What classification of bone is the clavicle?

   _____

3. The medial end is also known as the _____ extremity.

4. The lateral end is also known as the _____ extremity.

5. Which end—medial or lateral—articulates with part of the scapula?

   _____

6. Which end—medial or lateral—articulates with the manubrium?

   _____

7. At what level is the clavicle (with reference to the ribs)?

   _____

8. Which classification of joint are sternoclavicular joints and acromioclavicular joints?
   a. Diarthrotic
   b. Synarthrotic
   c. Amphiarthrotic

9. Which type of joint are sternoclavicular joints and acromioclavicular joints?
   a. Hinge
   b. Gliding
   c. Ball and socket

10. Which gender of adults—males or females—has the more sharply curved clavicles?

Exercise 2

Instructions: Identify each lettered structure shown in Fig. 5-2.

A. _____ (cavity)

B. _____

C. _____ (process)

D. _____ (notch)

E. _____ (border)

F. _____ (angle)

G. _____ (border)

H. _____ (angle)

I. _____ (border)

J. _____ (fossa)

Exercise 3

Instructions: Identify each lettered structure shown in Fig. 5-3.

A. _____ (angle)

B. _____

C. _____ (border)

D. _____ (angle)

E. _____ (fossa)

F. _____ (fossa)

G. _____ (border)

H. _____ (notch)

I. _____ (process)

J. _____

K. _____

L. _____ (cavity)

M. _____ (border)

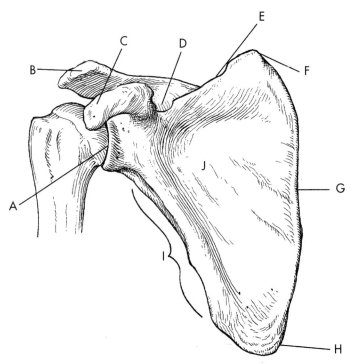

Figure 5-2 Anterior aspect of the scapula.

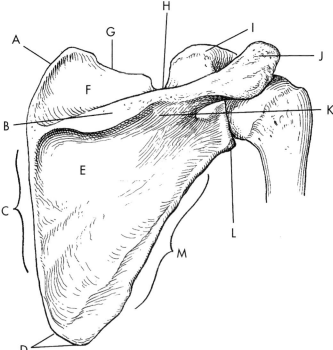

Figure 5-3 Posterior aspect of the scapula.

Exercise 4

Instructions: Identify each lettered structure shown in Fig. 5-4.

A. _____

B. _____

C. _____ (surface)

D. _____ (border)

E. _____ (angle)

F. _____ (angle)

G. _____ (process)

H. _____ (cavity)

I. _____ (surface)

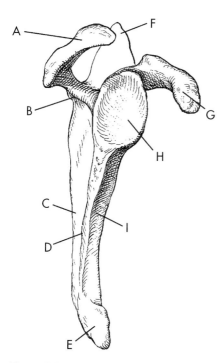

Figure 5-4 Lateral aspect of the scapula.

Exercise 5

Instructions: Match the structures located on the scapula listed in Column A with the descriptions in Column B. Not all descriptions may apply to the listed structures.

Column A

____ 1. Spine

____ 2. Acromion

____ 3. Medial border

____ 4. Glenoid cavity

____ 5. Scapular notch

____ 6. Costal surface

____ 7. Inferior angle

____ 8. Superior angle

____ 9. Lateral border

____ 10. Superior border

____ 11. Coracoid process

____ 12. Subscapular fossa

____ 13. Supraspinous fossa

____ 14. Infraspinous fossa

Column B

a. Anterior aspect of scapula

b. Also known as the sternal surface

c. Deep depression on superior border

d. Large protrusion on dorsal surface

e. Lateral extension of scapular spine

f. Large fossa at lateral angle

g. Extends from superior angle to coracoid process

h. The junction of the medial and superior borders

i. Large depression on the costal surface

j. The junction of the medial and lateral borders

k. Area above the scapular spine on dorsal surface

l. Large, broad area below the spine on dorsal surface

m. Extends from the glenoid cavity to the inferior angle

n. Extends from the superior angle to the inferior angle

o. Slender, fingerlike projection extending anteriorly and laterally from near the lateral angle

Exercise 6

Instructions: Identify each structure shown in Fig. 5-5.

A. _____

B. _____

C. _____

D. _____

E. _____

F. _____

G. _____

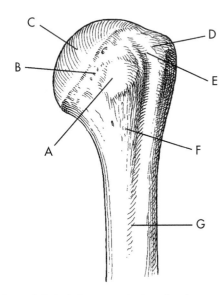

Figure 5-5 Anterior aspect of proximal humerus.

Exercise 7

Instructions: Match the structures located on the proximal portion of the humerus listed in Column A with the descriptions in Column B. Not all descriptions may apply to the listed structures.

Column A

____ 1. Head

____ 2. Surgical neck

____ 3. Anatomic neck

____ 4. Lesser tubercle

____ 5. Greater tubercle

____ 6. Intertubercular groove

Column B

a. Depression that receives the olecrano process

b. Deep depression that separates the two tubercles

c. Narrow constriction superior to the tubercles

d. Constriction of the shaft inferior to the tubercles

e. Bony process on the lateral surface of the bone

f. Rounded bony process that articulates with the radial head

g. Large, rounded eminence that articulates with the glenoid cavity

h. Bony process on the anterior surface of the shaft, inferior from the anatomic neck

Exercise 8

Instructions: Use the following clues to complete the crossword puzzle. All answers refer to the bones and joints of the shoulder girdle.

ACROSS

1. Most distal angle
3. Scapular spinal process
5. Posterior shoulder girdle bone
6. Articulates with scapula
9. Ball and socket joint
11. Scapula border
13. Scapular spine ridge
14. On superior border
16. Bone classification for humerus
17. Anterior scapular process
18. Anterior scapular fossa
19. Bone classification for scapula

DOWN

1. Posterior-inferior scapular fossa
2. Anterior part of shoulder girdle
4. Anterior scapular surface
7. Cavity for humeral head
8. Top scapular border
9. Posterior-superior scapular fossa
10. Scapular border
12. Lateral end of clavicle
15. Medial end of clavicle

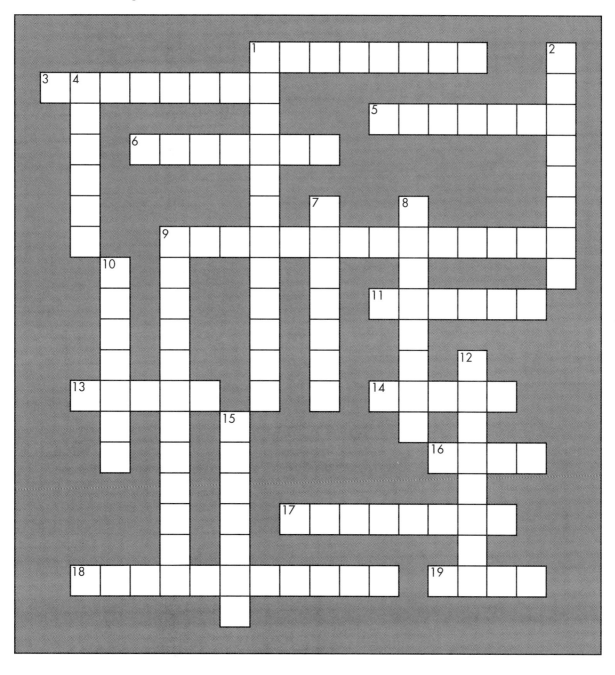

Exercise 9

Match the pathology terms in Column A with the appropriate definition in Column B. Not all choices from Column B should be selected.

Column A

_____ 1. Tumor

_____ 2. Bursitis

_____ 3. Fracture

_____ 4. Metastases

_____ 5. Dislocation

_____ 6. Osteoporosis

_____ 7. Osteoarthritis

_____ 8. Osteopetrosis

_____ 9. Chondrosarcoma

_____ 10. Rheumatoid arthritis

Column B

a. Loss of bone density

b. Inflammation of the bursa

c. Disruption in the continuity of bone

d. Benign tumor consisting of cartilage

e. Increased density of atypically soft bone

f. Displacement of a bone from the joint space

g. Malignant tumor arising from cartilage cells

h. Inflammation of bone caused by a pyogenic infection

i. Chronic, systemic, inflammatory collagen disease

j. Malignant tumor of bone arising in medullary tissue

k. Transfer of a cancerous lesion from one area to another

l. New tissue growth where cell proliferation is uncontrolled

m. Form of arthritis marked by progressive cartilage deterioration in synovial joints and vertebrae

Exercise 10

Instructions: This exercise is a comprehensive review of the osteology and arthrology of the shoulder girdle. Fill in missing words or provide a short answer for each item.

1. What bone classification is the scapula?

2. How many surfaces, borders, and angles does a scapula have?

   a. Surfaces: _____

   b. Borders: _____

   c. Angles: _____

3. Which surface (anterior; posterior) of the scapula is the costal surface?

4. Name the two fossae located on the posterior surface of the scapula.

5. What structure separates the two fossae on the posterior surface of the scapula?

6. What is the name of the lateral end of the scapular spine?

7. Where on the scapula is the scapular notch located?

8. What is the most anterior bony projection of the scapula?

9. List the names of the scapular borders.

10. List the names of the scapular angles.

11. What bone forms the anterior part of the shoulder girdle?

12. What muscle covers and attaches to the costal (anterior) surface of the scapula?

13. The portion of the humerus located between the tubercles and the head is called the _____ neck.

14. Small synovial fluid-filled sacs that relieve pressure and reduce friction in tissue are called _____.

15. How many articulations does the shoulder girdle have?

16. List the names of each shoulder girdle articulation.

17. Identify the type of movement for each articulation of the shoulder girdle.

18. What bone articulates with the glenoid cavity?

19. What bone articulates with the medial end of the clavicle?

20. What structure of the scapula articulates with the lateral end of the clavicle?

SECTION 2

Positioning of the Shoulder Girdle

Exercise 1: Positioning for the Shoulder

Instructions: This exercise pertains to radiographic images of the shoulder. Identify structures, fill in missing words, provide a short answer, choose the correct answer, or choose true or false (explaining any statement you believe to be false) for each question.

Items 1 through 5 pertain to the *AP projection*.

1. Describe how and where the central ray should be directed.

2. What positioning maneuver should be avoided if the patient possibly has a fractured humerus or dislocation of the scapulohumeral joint?

3. For AP projections, the patient's respiration should be

   _____.

4. Figs. 5-6 through 5-8 are AP projections of the shoulder. Examine the images and answer the questions that follow.

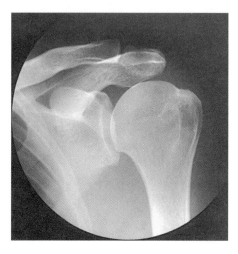

Figure 5-6 AP shoulder.

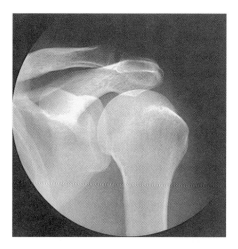

Figure 5-7 AP shoulder.

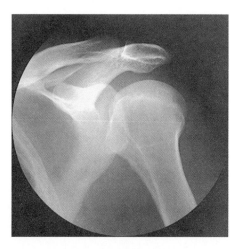

Figure 5-8 AP shoulder.

a. What positioning maneuver causes the appearance of these three images to be different?

b. Which image shows the humerus in external rotation?

c. Which image shows the humerus in internal rotation?

d. Which image shows the humerus in neutral rotation?

e. Which image was obtained by positioning the humeral epicondyles parallel to the image receptor?

f. Which image was obtained by positioning the humeral epicondyles at an angle of approximately 45 degrees with the image receptor?

g. Which image was obtained by positioning the humeral epicondyles perpendicular to the image receptor?

h. Which image shows the greater tubercle in profile on the lateral aspect of the humerus?

i. Which image shows the lesser tubercle in profile and pointing medially? Which image shows the outline of the lesser tubercle between the humeral head and the greater tubercle?

5. Identify each lettered structure shown in Fig. 5-9.

   A. _____

   B. _____

   C. _____

   D. _____

   E. _____

   F. _____

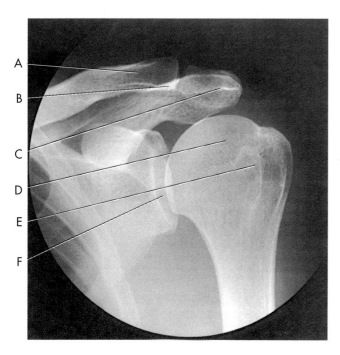

Figure 5-9 AP shoulder with external rotation of the humerus.

Items 6 through 10 pertain to the *transthoracic lateral projection (Lawrence method)*.

6. The transthoracic lateral projection may be performed with the patient positioned upright or

   a. Prone
   b. Supine
   c. Lateral recumbent

7. To what specific area of the humerus should the image receptor (IR) be centered for the transthoracic lateral projection (Lawrence method)?

   a. Epicondyles
   b. Surgical neck
   c. Distal third of the diaphysis

8. How many degrees and in which direction should the central ray be directed if it cannot be directed perpendicular to the IR because the patient is unable to elevate the unaffected shoulder?

   a. 10 to 15 degrees caudad
   b. 10 to 15 degrees cephalad
   c. 20 to 25 degrees caudad
   d. 20 to 25 degrees cephalad

9. Which change to radiographic exposure factors should be used to effectively aid the blurring of lung detail by the action of the heart when the patient is able to hold his or her breath for a sustained period?

   a. Use a low mA/long exposure time combination with the usual mAs factor.
   b. Use a high mA/short exposure time combination with the usual mAs factor.

10. Identify each lettered structure shown in Fig. 5-10.

    A. _____

    B. _____

    C. _____

    D. _____

    E. _____

    F. _____

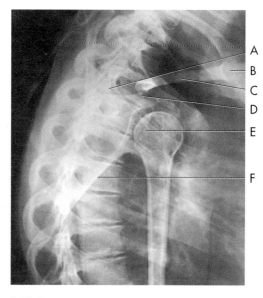

Figure 5-10 Transthoracic lateral shoulder (Lawrence method).

Items 11 through 19 pertain to the *inferosuperior axial projection (Lawrence method)*.

11. True or False. When the patient is recumbent, the IR should be placed in the Bucky tray.

12. True or False. When the patient is recumbent, the head and upper torso should be elevated 3 inches (7.6 cm).

13. True or False. When using a horizontally directed central ray, the patient should be placed in the supine body position.

14. With reference to the long axis of the body, how should the affected arm be positioned?

15. Into which rotational position should the humerus be placed?
    a. Neutral
    b. Internal
    c. External

16. Which area of the body should the central ray enter?
    a. Axilla of the affected arm
    b. Top of the affected shoulder
    c. Anterior point of the coracoid process

17. How many degrees should the central ray be directed in the medial direction?
    a. 5 to 10 degrees
    b. 15 to 30 degrees
    c. 35 to 45 degrees

18. What positioning factor determines how many degrees the central ray should be directed medially?

19. Examine Fig. 5-11, a radiograph of the inferosuperior axial projection (Lawrence method). From the following list, circle four radiographic evaluation criteria indicating that the patient was properly positioned for the inferosuperior axial projection (Lawrence method).
    a. The scapula should be seen in lateral profile.
    b. The coracoid process should be seen pointing anteriorly.
    c. The lesser tubercle should be seen in profile and pointing anteriorly.
    d. The scapulohumeral joint should be seen slightly overlapping.
    e. The scapula, clavicle, and humerus should be seen through the lung field.
    f. The greater tubercle should be seen in profile on the lateral aspect of the humerus.
    g. The AC joint, acromion, and acromial end of clavicle should be seen through the humeral head.

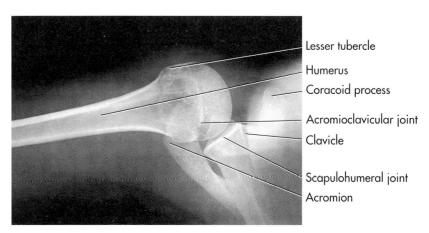

Figure 5-11 Inferosuperior axial projection (Lawrence method).

Questions 20 through 25 pertain to the *PA oblique projection (scapular Y)*.

20. True or False. The patient should be slightly rotated to place the affected shoulder in contact with the IR holder.

21. True or False. In an image of a normal shoulder, the humeral head should be directly superimposed over the junction of the scapular Y.

22. What breathing instructions should be given to the patient?

23. How much body rotation is necessary for PA oblique projections (scapular Y)?
    a. 5 to 10 degrees
    b. 15 to 20 degrees
    c. 25 to 30 degrees
    d. 45 to 60 degrees

24. With reference from the thorax, where should the scapular body be demonstrated in the image of the PA oblique projection?
    a. Superimposed with the clavicle
    b. Superimposed with ribs and lung
    c. Along the lateral aspect but not superimposed

25. Identify each lettered structure shown in Fig. 5-12.

    A. _____

    B. _____

    C. _____

    D. _____

    E. _____

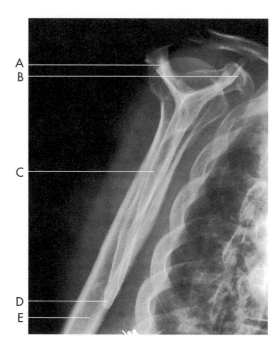

Figure 5-12 PA oblique shoulder joint.

Questions 26 through 30 pertain to the *tangential projection* for the intertubercular groove.

26. With a supine patient, describe each of the following:
    a. How the affected upper limb should be positioned
    b. The placement of the image receptor
    c. How the central ray should be directed

27. For the Fisk modification, the IR is supported on the pa-

    tient's _____.

28. For the Fisk modification, a standing patient should lean forward or backward to place the vertical humerus at an

    angle of _____ to

    _____ degrees.

29. For the Fisk modification, how should the central ray be directed?

    a. Angled 10 to 15 degrees anteriorly
    b. Angled 10 to 15 degrees posteriorly
    c. Perpendicular to the image receptor

30. Identify each lettered structure shown in Fig. 5-13.

    A. _____

    B. _____

    C. _____

    D. _____

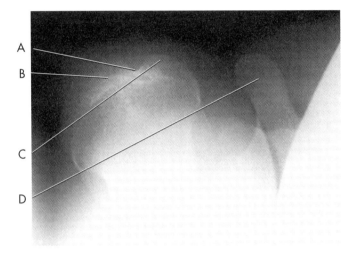

Figure 5-13 Supine tangential intertubercular groove.

Exercise 2: Positioning for the Acromioclavicular Articulations

Instructions: This exercise pertains to the bilateral AP or PA projections (Pearson method) used for demonstrating acromioclavicular (AC) joints. Provide a short answer or choose true or false (explaining any statement you believe to be false) for each question.

1. True or False. The patient may be positioned either upright or supine to demonstrate AC joints.

2. True or False. To demonstrate AC joints, both AC joints should be imaged simultaneously.

3. True or False. The central ray should be directed perpendicular to the affected acromioclavicular joint for each radiograph.

4. What procedure should be performed to demonstrate both AC joints on a patient who has wide shoulders?

5. Why should the patient hold sandbags of equal weight in each hand?

Exercise 3: Positioning for the Clavicle

Instructions: Trauma is the most frequent reason for demonstrating the clavicle. The usual projections performed to obtain a radiograph of an injured clavicle are the AP and the AP axial. The PA and PA axial projection are sometimes performed when the patient's condition permits their use (e.g., during the postreduction period to monitor the healing process). This exercise pertains to those positioning procedures that demonstrate the clavicle. Identify structures, provide a short answer, choose the correct answer, or choose true or false (explaining any statement you believe to be false) for each question.

Items 1 through 6 pertain to the AP and PA projections.

1. What size IR—and how should it be placed (lengthwise or crosswise)—should be used for the AP or PA projection?

2. What breathing instructions should be given to the patient?

3. The AP and PA projections produce similar images. Identify which projection—AP or PA—produces the best recorded detail and explain why.

4. True or False. The entire clavicle should be demonstrated with either AP or PA projection.

5. True or False. The AP and PA projections should demonstrate the entire clavicle free from superimposition with other bony structures.

6. Identify each lettered structure shown in Fig. 5-14.

A. _____

B. _____

C. _____

D. _____

E. _____

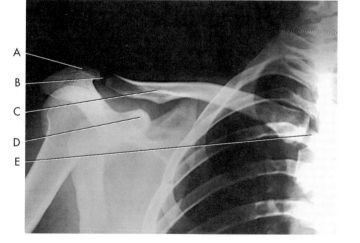

Figure 5-14 AP clavicle.

Items 7 through 12 pertain to the AP axial and *PA axial projections*.

7. How many degrees and in which direction should the central ray be directed for the following projections?

a. AP axial, with the patient supine: _____

b. PA axial, with the patient prone: _____

8. Which projection—AP or AP axial—causes the clavicle to appear horizontal in the image?

9. What positioning consideration determines how much the x-ray tube should be angled for AP axial and PA axial projections?

10. How many degrees and in which direction should the central ray be directed for the AP axial projection with the patient upright in the lordotic position?

11. True or False. For AP axial and PA axial projections, the entire clavicle should be free from superimposition with other bony structures.

12. True or False. For the AP axial projection, the exposure should occur after the patient has been instructed to suspend respiration following full expiration.

Exercise 4: Positioning for the Scapula

Instructions: This exercise pertains to AP projections and lateral projections of the scapula. Identify structures, fill in missing words, provide a short answer, choose the correct answer from a list, or choose true or false (explaining any statement you believe to be false) for each question.

1. For the AP projection, the central ray should be perpendicular to a point approximately 2 inches (5 cm) inferior to the

   _____ _____.

2. For the AP projection, which positioning maneuver of the arm will pull the scapula in a lateral direction?
   a. Abduction
   b. Adduction
   c. Internal rotation
   d. External rotation

3. Which type of respiration should the patient use to obliterate lung detail?
   a. Slow breathing
   b. Suspended full expiration
   c. Suspended full inspiration

4. Which scapular border should be demonstrated free from superimposition with the ribs for the AP projection?
   a. Lateral
   b. Medial
   c. Superior

5. True or False. AP projection images should demonstrate the area of the scapula, including the glenoid cavity and coracoid process without superimposition with the ribs.

6. True or False. AP projection images should demonstrate the acromion process and the inferior angle.

7. True or False. For the AP projection, the patient should be rotated toward the affected side to best place the scapula parallel with the IR.

8. Identify each lettered structure shown in Fig. 5-15.

   A. _____

   B. _____

   C. _____

   D. _____

   E. _____

   F. _____

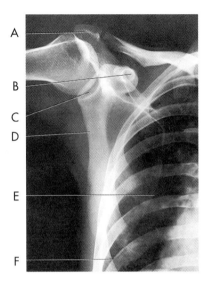

Figure 5-15 AP scapula.

9. For the lateral projection, what is the significance of arm placement?

10. Describe how and where the central ray should be directed for the lateral projection.

11. For the lateral projection, how should the affected arm be placed to best demonstrate the acromion and coracoid processes?

12. True or False. The lateral projection image should demonstrate the lateral and medial borders superimposed.

13. True or False. The lateral projection image should demonstrate the scapular body free from superimposition with the ribs.

14. True or False. The acromion process and the inferior angle should be demonstrated in the lateral projection.

15. Identify each lettered structure shown in Fig. 5-16.

A. _____

B. _____

C. _____

D. _____

E. _____

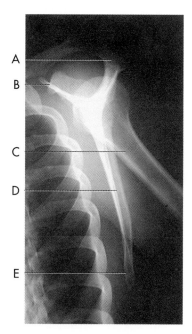

Figure 5-16 Lateral scapula.

Exercise 5: Identifying Projections of the Shoulder Girdle

Instructions: This exercise provides photographs that show patients being positioned for various projections of the shoulder girdle. Examine each photograph and identify the projection by name and the part of the shoulder girdle that is being demonstrated.

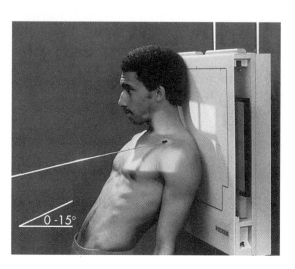

Figure 5-17

1. Fig. 5-17: _____

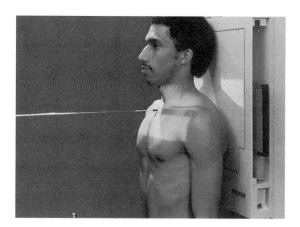

Figure 5-18

2. Fig. 5-18: _____

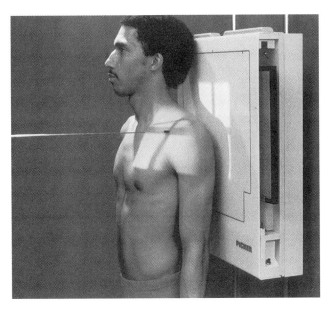

Figure 5-19

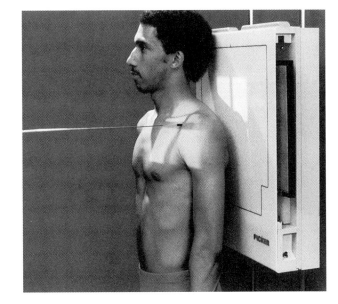

Figure 5-21

3. Fig. 5-19: _____

5. Fig. 5-21: _____

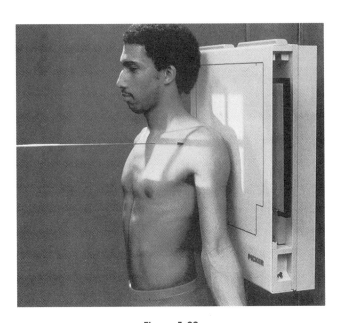

Figure 5-20

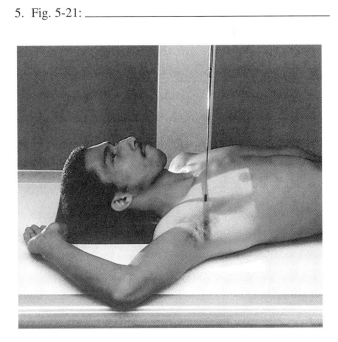

Figure 5-22

4. Fig. 5-20: _____

6. Fig. 5-22: _____

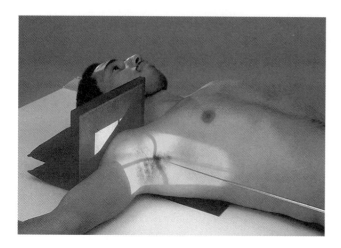

Figure 5-23

7. Fig. 5-23: _____

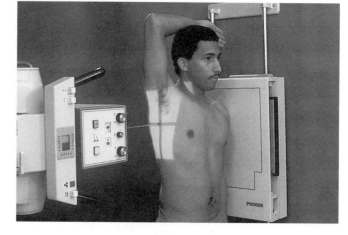

Figure 5-25

9. Fig. 5-25: _____

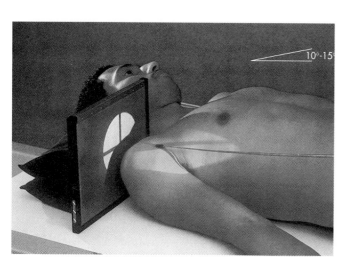

Figure 5-24

8. Fig. 5-24: _____

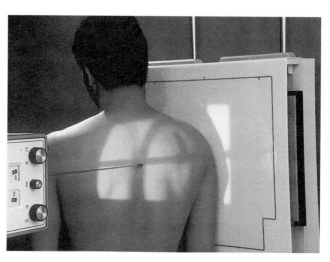

Figure 5-26

10. Fig. 5-26: _____

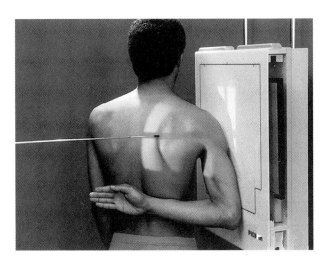

Figure 5-27

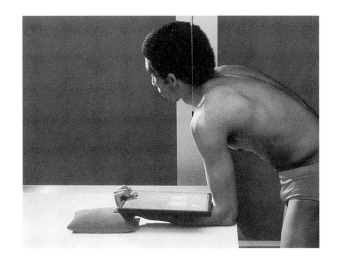

Figure 5-28

11. Fig. 5-27: _____

12. Fig. 5-28: _____

Self-Test: Osteology, Arthrology, and Positioning of the Shoulder Girdle

Instructions: Answer the following questions by selecting the best choice.

1. Which classification of bone is the scapula?

    a. Flat
    b. Long
    c. Short
    d. Irregular

2. Which classification of bone is the clavicle?

    a. Flat
    b. Long
    c. Short
    d. Irregular

3. What is the name of the fossa on the anterior surface of the scapula?

    a. Subscapular
    b. Infraspinous
    c. Supraspinous
    d. Scapular notch

4. Which border of the scapula extends from the glenoid cavity to the inferior angle?

    a. Medial
    b. Lateral
    c. Superior
    d. Vertebral

5. Which border of the scapula extends from the superior angle to the inferior angle?

    a. Lateral
    b. Medial
    c. Axillary
    d. Superior

6. Of which part of the scapula is the acromion an extension?

    a. Body
    b. Spine
    c. Glenoid cavity
    d. Coracoid process

7. With reference to the body of the scapula, where is the coracoid process located?

    a. Medial and superior
    b. Medial and inferior
    c. Lateral and superior
    d. Lateral and inferior

8. Which two borders of the scapula unite to form the medial angle?

    a. Medial and lateral
    b. Medial and superior
    c. Axillary and lateral
    d. Axillary and superior

9. Which two borders of the scapula unite to form the inferior angle?

    a. Medial and lateral
    b. Medial and superior
    c. Axillary and lateral
    d. Axillary and superior

10. Where on the scapula is the supraspinous fossa located?

    a. Anterior surface, above the scapular spine
    b. Anterior surface, below the scapular spine
    c. Posterior surface, above the scapular spine
    d. Posterior surface, below the scapular spine

11. Where on the scapula is the infraspinous fossa located?

    a. Anterior surface, above the scapular spine
    b. Anterior surface, below the scapular spine
    c. Posterior surface, above the scapular spine
    d. Posterior surface, below the scapular spine

12. On which border of the scapula is the scapular notch located?

    a. Lateral
    b. Superior
    c. Axillary
    d. Vertebral

13. Which joint is a ball and socket joint?

    a. Radiocarpal
    b. Humeroulnar
    c. Scapulohumeral
    d. Sternoclavicular

14. When performing AP projections of the shoulder, where should the central ray be directed?

    a. 1 inch medial to the coracoid process
    b. 1 inch inferior to the coracoid process
    c. 2 inches medial to the coracoid process
    d. 2 inches inferior to the coracoid process

15. With reference to the plane of the image receptor, how should the humeral epicondyles be positioned for the AP projection of the shoulder with the shoulder in external rotation?

    a. Parallel
    b. Perpendicular
    c. 45 degrees lateral oblique
    d. 45 degrees medial oblique

16. With reference to the plane of the image receptor, how should the humeral epicondyles be positioned for the AP projection of the shoulder with the shoulder in internal rotation?
    a. Parallel
    b. Perpendicular
    c. 45 degrees lateral oblique
    d. 45 degrees medial oblique

17. With reference to the plane of the image receptor, how should the humeral epicondyles be positioned for the AP projection of the shoulder with the shoulder in neutral rotation?
    a. Parallel
    b. Perpendicular
    c. 45 degrees lateral oblique
    d. 45 degrees medial oblique

18. Which projection of the shoulder best demonstrates the greater tubercle of the humerus in profile?
    a. Transthoracic lateral projection
    b. AP projection with neutral rotation
    c. AP projection with internal rotation
    d. AP projection with external rotation

19. Which projection of the shoulder best demonstrates the humeral head in profile?
    a. Transthoracic lateral projection
    b. AP projection with neutral rotation
    c. AP projection with external rotation
    d. AP projection with internal rotation

20. Which projection of the shoulder best demonstrates the lesser tubercle of the humerus in profile and pointing toward the glenoid cavity?
    a. Transthoracic lateral projection
    b. AP projection with neutral rotation
    c. AP projection with internal rotation
    d. AP projection with external rotation

21. Which projection of the shoulder is being performed when the patient is supine with the right shoulder centered on the IR, a vertical central ray is being directed perpendicular to the center of the IR, and the humeral epicondyles are parallel with the plane of the IR?
    a. Transthoracic lateral projection
    b. PA oblique (scapular Y) projection
    c. AP projection with internal rotation
    d. AP projection with external rotation

22. What should be adjusted from the regular procedure for the transthoracic lateral projection (Lawrence method) of the humerus if the patient is unable to elevate the unaffected arm?
    a. Breathing procedure
    b. Central ray angulation
    c. Placement of the film
    d. Rotation of the patient

23. Which projection of the upper limb should be performed to demonstrate a fracture of the proximal humerus when that arm cannot be abducted?
    a. Tangential projection, Fisk modification
    b. AP projection of the shoulder with internal rotation
    c. AP projection of the shoulder with external rotation
    d. Transthoracic lateral projection (Lawrence method) of the humerus

24. When performing the transthoracic lateral projection (Lawrence method) of the humerus, which breathing technique should be used to best improve the image contrast and decrease the exposure necessary to penetrate the body?
    a. Rapid breathing
    b. Shallow breathing
    c. Suspended full expiration
    d. Suspended full inspiration

25. Which projection of the shoulder requires that a horizontal central ray be directed 15 to 30 degrees medially and enter the axilla of the affected arm?
    a. AP projection
    b. PA oblique (scapular Y) projection
    c. Inferosuperior axial projection (Lawrence method)
    d. Transthoracic lateral projection (Lawrence method)

26. How should the central ray be directed for the PA oblique projection (scapular Y) of the shoulder?
    a. Cephalically 10 to 15 degrees
    b. Cephalically 15 to 25 degrees
    c. Cephalically 25 to 30 degrees
    d. Perpendicular to the image receptor

27. In which body position should the patient be placed to demonstrate the left shoulder with the PA oblique projection (scapular Y)?
    a. Left anterior oblique
    b. Left posterior oblique
    c. Right anterior oblique
    d. Right posterior oblique

28. Which projection of the shoulder joint requires the patient to be rotated until the midcoronal plane forms an angle of 45 to 60 degrees with the plane of the image receptor?

    a. Transthoracic lateral projection
    b. PA oblique projection (scapular Y)
    c. AP projection with internal rotation
    d. AP projection with external rotation

29. Which projection of the shoulder girdle is performed with the patient supine, an image receptor placed vertically against the superior surface of the shoulder, and the central ray angled 10 to 15 degrees posteriorly (downward from horizontal)?

    a. Tangential for the intertubercular groove
    b. AP axial, lordotic position, for the clavicle
    c. Transthoracic lateral, Lawrence method, for the shoulder
    d. Inferosuperior axial, Lawrence method, for the shoulder joint

30. When demonstrating the intertubercular groove with the Fisk modification of the tangential projection, how should the affected humerus be positioned?

    a. The humerus should be rotated laterally.
    b. The humerus should be rotated medially.
    c. The vertical humerus should form an angle of 10 to 15 degrees.
    d. The humerus should be abducted to a right angle with the body.

31. If the patient's condition permits, which joint should be demonstrated with the patient in an upright position?

    a. Glenohumeral
    b. Scapulohumeral
    c. Sternoclavicular
    d. Acromioclavicular

32. How many degrees and in which direction should the central ray be directed for the PA axial projection of the clavicle?

    a. 15 to 20 degrees caudad
    b. 15 to 20 degrees cephalad
    c. 25 to 30 degrees caudad
    d. 25 to 30 degrees cephalad

33. How many degrees and in which direction should the central ray be directed for the AP axial projection of the clavicle with the patient supine?

    a. 15 to 20 degrees caudad
    b. 15 to 20 degrees cephalad
    c. 25 to 30 degrees caudad
    d. 25 to 30 degrees cephalad

34. When performing the AP projection of the scapula, the central ray should be directed toward a point 2 inches (5 cm) to the coracoid process.

    a. Lateral
    b. Medial
    c. Inferior
    d. Superior

35. When performing a lateral projection of the scapula with the patient positioned right anterior oblique (RAO) or left anterior oblique (LAO), approximately how much body rotation is necessary for the average patient?

    a. 15 to 20 degrees
    b. 25 to 30 degrees
    c. 35 to 40 degrees
    d. 45 to 60 degrees

CHAPTER 6

Lower Limb

SECTION 1

Osteology and Arthrology of the Lower Limb

Exercise 1

Instructions: Identify each lettered individual bone or group of bones shown in Fig. 6-1.

A. _____

B. _____

C. _____

D. _____

E. _____

F. _____

G. _____

H. _____

I. _____

J. _____

K. _____

L. _____

M. _____

N. _____

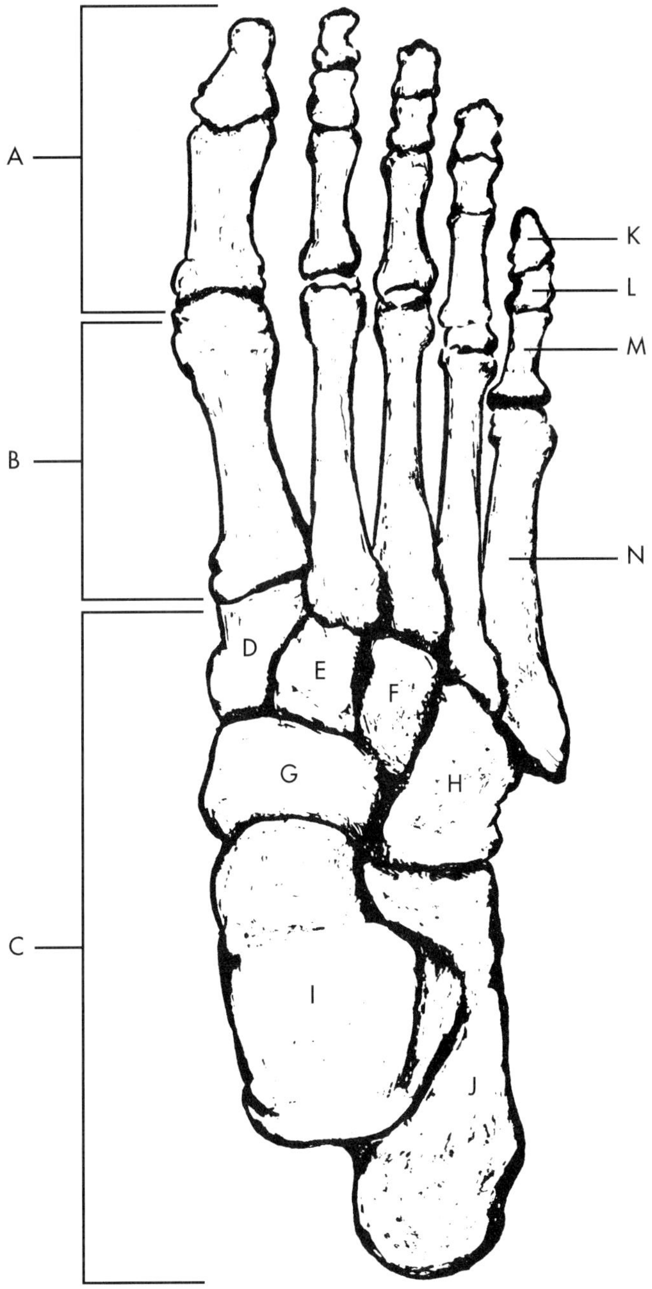

Figure 6-1 The foot.

Exercise 2

Instructions: Identify each lettered individual bone or group of bones shown in Fig. 6-2.

A. _____

B. _____

C. _____

D. _____

E. _____

F. _____

G. _____

H. _____

I. _____

J. _____

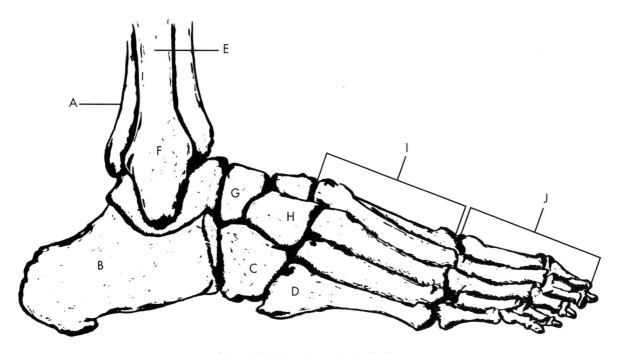

Figure 6-2 Lateral aspect of a foot.

Exercise 3

Instructions: Use the following clues to complete the crossword puzzle. All answers refer to the foot and ankle.

ACROSS

1. Lateral tarsal bone
3. Tarsal bone classification
6. Second largest tarsal
8. Toe joint
12. Number of phalanges
13. Within the forefoot
14. Number of metatarsals

DOWN

1. Largest tarsal bone
2. Comprises the toes
4. Three of these are in the tarsus
5. One toe bone
7. Between talus and cuneiforms
9. Lower limb joint
10. Number of tarsal bones
11. The ankle joint

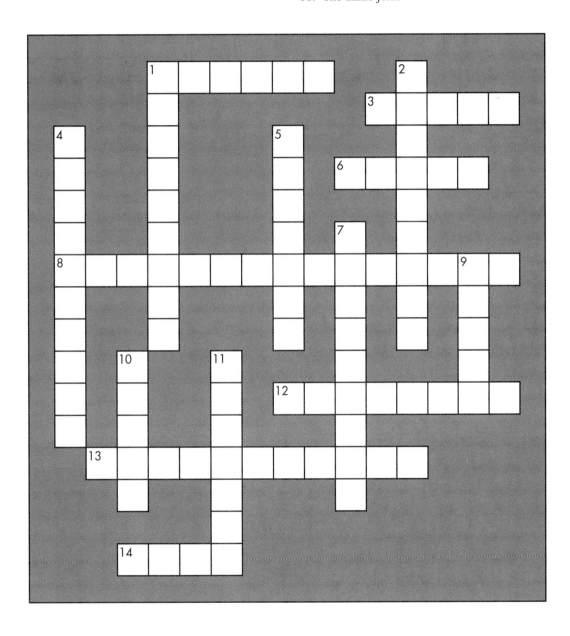

Exercise 4

Instructions: Identify each lettered structure shown in Fig. 6-3.

A. _____

B. _____

C. _____

D. _____

E. _____

F. _____

G. _____

H. _____

I. _____

J. _____

Exercise 5

Instructions: Identify each lettered structure shown in Fig. 6-4.

A. _____

B. _____

C. _____

D. _____

E. _____

F. _____

G. _____

H. _____

I. _____

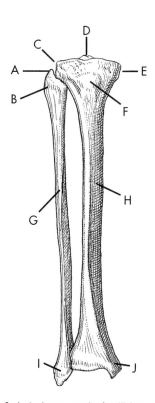

Figure 6-3 Anterior aspect of a tibia and fibula.

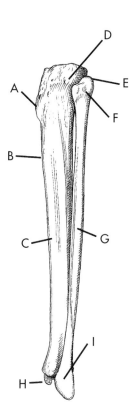

Figure 6-4 Lateral aspect of a tibia and fibula.

Exercise 6

Instructions: Match the structures found on the tibia or fibula (the bones of the leg) as listed in Column A with the descriptions in Column B. Not all descriptions may apply to the listed structures.

Column A

_____ 1. Apex

_____ 2. Crest

_____ 3. Tibia

_____ 4. Fibula

_____ 5. Condyles

_____ 6. Tubercles

_____ 7. Tuberosity

_____ 8. Lateral malleolus

_____ 9. Medial malleolus

_____ 10. Intercondylar eminence

Column B

a. Lateral bone of the leg

b. Enlarged distal end of the fibula

c. The larger of the two bones of the leg

d. Known as the anterior border of the tibia

e. Deep depression between the condyles

f. Conical projection at the head of the fibula

g. Large process at the distal end of the tibia

h. Two prominent processes on the proximal end of the tibia

i. Two peaklike processes arising from the intercondylar eminence

j. Sharp projection between the two superior articular surfaces

k. Prominent process on the anterior surface of the tibia; just below the condyles

Exercise 7

Instructions: Identify each lettered structure shown in Fig. 6-5.

A. _____

B. _____

C. _____

D. _____

E. _____

F. _____

G. _____

H. _____

I. _____

J. _____

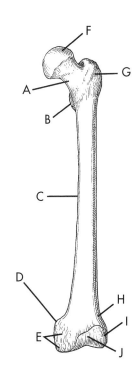

Figure 6-5 Anterior aspect of a femur.

Exercise 8

Instructions: Identify each lettered structure shown in Fig. 6-6.

A. _____

B. _____

C. _____

D. _____

E. _____

F. _____

G. _____

H. _____

I. _____

J. _____

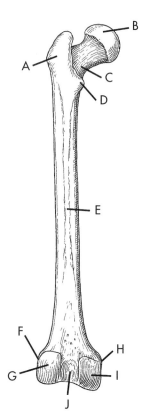

Figure 6-6 Posterior aspect of a femur.

Exercise 9

Instructions: Identify each lettered structure shown in Fig. 6-7.

A. _____

B. _____

C. _____

D. _____

E. _____

F. _____

G. _____

H. _____

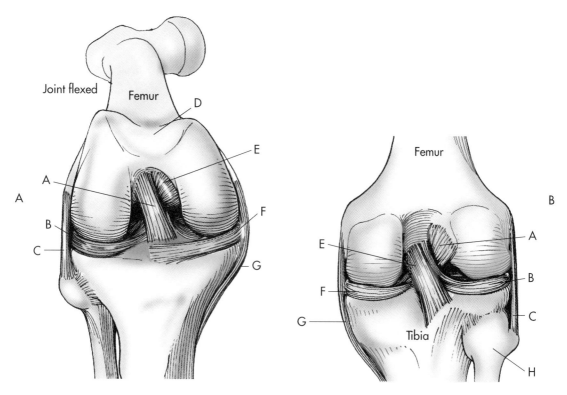

Figure 6-7 Knee joint. **A,** Anterior aspect with knee flexed. **B,** Posterior aspect.

Exercise 10

Instructions: Identify each lettered structure shown in Fig. 6-8.

A. _____

B. _____

C. _____

D. _____

E. _____

F. _____

G. _____

H. _____

I. _____

J. _____

Exercise 11

Instructions: Match the structures found on the femur as listed in Column A with the descriptions in Column B. Not all descriptions may apply to the listed structures.

Column A

____ 1. Head

____ 2. Neck

____ 3. Condyles

____ 4. Patellar surface

____ 5. Greater trochanter

____ 6. Intercondylar fossa

Column B

a. Deep depression between the condyles

b. Process located on the medial surface, distal femur

c. Constricted portion just inferior from the head

d. Large, rounded eminence on the superior end

e. Two large eminences on the distal end

f. Two large eminences on the proximal end

g. Large, prominent process superior and lateral on the shaft

h. Shallow, triangular area on the anterior surface between the condyles

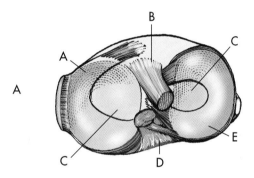

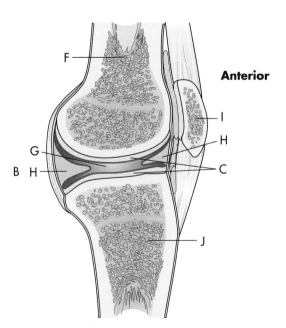

Figure 6-8 Knee joint. **A,** Superior surface of tibia. **B,** Sagittal section.

Exercise 12

Instructions: Listed following are structures found on the femur, the tibia, or the fibula. In the space provided, write *P* if that structure is closer to the proximal end or *D* if that structure is closer to the distal end of the bone on which it is located.

_____ 1. Trochanters

_____ 2. Fibular apex

_____ 3. Fibular head

_____ 4. Tibial plateau

_____ 5. Femoral neck

_____ 6. Femoral head

_____ 7. Tibial condyles

_____ 8. Patellar surface

_____ 9. Tibial tuberosity

_____ 10. Lateral malleolus

_____ 11. Medial malleolus

_____ 12. Femoral condyles

_____ 13. Intercondylar fossa

_____ 14. Femoral epicondyles

_____ 15. Intercondylar eminence

Exercise 13

Instructions: Match the structures listed in Column A with the bones on which they are found in Column B. Identify each bone if the structure is found on more than one bone.

Column A   **Column B**

_____ 1. Apex   a. Femur

_____ 2. Head   b. Tibia

_____ 3. Condyles   c. Fibula

_____ 4. Tuberosity

_____ 5. Trochanters

_____ 6. Patellar surface

_____ 7. Medial malleolus

_____ 8. Lateral malleolus

_____ 9. Intercondylar fossa

_____ 10. Intercondylar eminence

Exercise 14

Instructions: Match the articulations listed in Column A with the corresponding type of movement listed in Column B. More than one choice from Column B may be used for some articulations, but not all choices from Column B may be used.

Column A   **Column B**

_____ 1. Knee   a. Gliding

_____ 2. Ankle   b. Flexion

_____ 3. Intertarsal   c. Extension

_____ 4. Interphalangeal   d. Abduction

_____ 5. Tarsometatarsal   e. Adduction

_____ 6. Distal tibiofibular   f. Circumduction

_____ 7. Proximal tibiofibular g. Rotational (around a single axis)

_____ 8. Metatarsophalangeal   h. Syndesmosis (slight movement)

Exercise 15

Instructions: Use the following clues to complete the crossword puzzle. All answers refer to the tibia, fibula, femur, and related joints.

ACROSS

1. The ankle is this type of joint
3. Superior border of patella
5. Between femoral condyles
6. Anterior border of tibia
8. Most of tibia
11. Proximal femoral joint
12. Distal end of fibula
15. Sesamoid bone
16. Two joints in the leg
17. Interposed between tibia and femur
18. Processes on superior tibia

DOWN

1. Proximal portion of fibula
2. The femur between the head and trochanters
4. Patellar inferior tip
5. Lateral bone of the leg
7. Found superiorly on femur
9. The larger bone of the leg
10. On anterior tibial body
12. Tibia is on this side of the leg
13. Bone classification of tibia
14. Distal joint

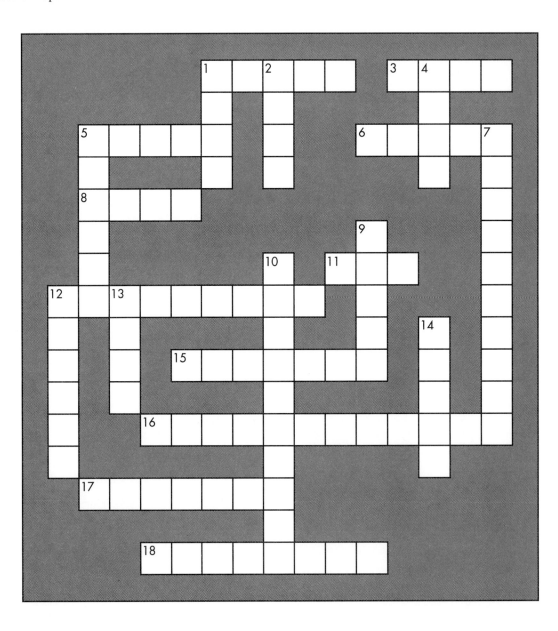

Exercise 16

Match the pathology terms in Column A with the appropriate definition in Column B. Not all choices from Column B should be selected.

Column A

____ 1. Gout

____ 2. Bone cyst

____ 3. Pott's fracture

____ 4. Paget's disease

____ 5 Osteoid osteoma

____ 6. Congenital clubfoot

____ 7. Osteomalacia (Rickets)

____ 8. Osgood-Schlatter disease

____ 9. Osteochondroma (Exostosis)

____ 10. Osteoclastoma (Giant cell tumor)

Column B

a. Loss of bone density

b. A benign lesion of cortical bone

c. Fluid-filled cyst with a wall of fibrous tissue

d. Thick, soft bone marked by bowing and fractures

e. Softening of the bones due to a vitamin D deficiency

f. Benign bone tumor projection with a cartilaginous cap

g. Incomplete separation or avulsion of the tibial tuberosity

h. Lucent lesion in the metaphysis, usually at the distal femur

i. Abnormal twisting of the foot, usually inward and downward

j. Hereditary form of arthritis where uric acid is deposited in joints

k. Avulsion fracture of the medial malleolus with the loss of the ankle mortise

Exercise 17

Instructions: This exercise is a comprehensive review of the osteology and arthrology of the lower limb. Provide a short answer for each item.

1. How many bones are found in one lower limb?

2. Identify by group name and quantity the bones found in the foot and ankle.

3. How many interphalangeal articulations does one foot have?

4. What types of movement do the interphalangeal joints permit?

5. What type of joint is an interphalangeal joint?

6. With what do the heads of metatarsals articulate?

7. How are metatarsals identified within the foot?

8. Identify by individual name or group the bones found in each section of the foot.

   a. Forefoot: _____

   b. Midfoot: _____

   c. Hindfoot: _____

9. Which metatarsal has a tuberosity that is prominent at its base?

10. List the names of the tarsal bones.

11. Which tarsal bone comprises the heel of the foot?

12. Which is the largest of the tarsal bones?

13. Which tarsal bone articulates superiorly on the calcaneus?

14. Which tarsal bone is located between the calcaneus and the fourth and fifth metatarsals?

15. Which tarsal bone is lateral from the cuneiforms?

16. Which tarsal bone is located between the talus and the cuneiforms?

17. Name the tarsal bones that articulate with metatarsals.

18. Which tarsal bone forms part of the ankle joint?

25. Name the large bony process that extends both medially and inferiorly from the distal end of the tibia.

19. Name the two bones of the leg.

26. With what bone does the undersurface of the tibia articulate?

20. Name the lateral bone of the leg.

27. List the articulations of the tibia.

21. Name the smaller of the bones of the leg.

28. Name the largest bone of the lower limb.

22. What other term refers to the tibial spine?

29. Where, exactly, is the intercondylar fossa located?

23. Which tibial condyle has a facet for articulation with the head of the fibula?

30. What are (a) the name of the "kneecap" and (b) its bone classification?

    a. _____

    b. _____

24. Specifically, where is the tibial tuberosity located?

SECTION 2

Positioning of the Lower Limb

Exercise 1: Positioning for the Toes

Instructions: When demonstrating toes, it is common to include three radiographs: an anteroposterior (AP) projection, an AP oblique projection, and a lateral projection. This exercise pertains to those projections. Identify structures, fill in missing words, provide a short answer, select the correct answer, or choose true or false (explaining any statement you believe to be false) for each item.

Items 1 through 6 pertain to the *AP and AP axial projections.*

1. Where should the central ray be directed for the AP projection?

2. How may the central ray be directed to demonstrate toes when the plantar surface of the affected foot is in contact with a horizontally placed image receptor?

   a. Perpendicularly only
   b. 15 degrees posteriorly (toward the heel) only
   c. Both a and b

3. How should the central ray be directed to demonstrate toes when the plantar surface of the affected foot is in contact with a foam wedge, which should be inclined 15 degrees so that the toes are elevated above a horizontally placed image receptor?

   a. Perpendicularly only
   b. 15 degrees posteriorly (toward the heel) only
   c. Both a and b

4. Which of the following projections for toes normally does not demonstrate open interphalangeal joints?

   a. AP projection of the toes with the central ray directed perpendicular
   b. AP axial projection of the toes with a central ray angulation of 15 degrees
   c. AP axial projection of the toes with a 15-degree foam wedge and the central ray directed perpendicular

5. Figs. 6-9 and 6-10 are AP projection radiographs. Examine the images and answer the questions that follow.

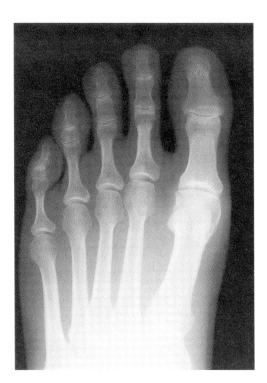

Figure 6-9 Radiograph of the toes.

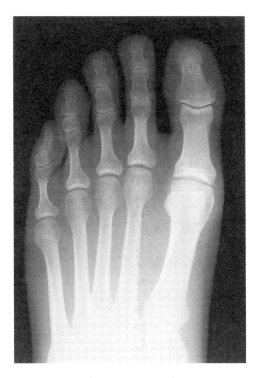

Figure 6-10 Radiograph of the toes.

a. Which image best demonstrates interphalangeal joints?

_____

b. Which image was most likely obtained with the central ray angled 15 degrees posteriorly (toward the toes)?

_____

c. Which image was most likely obtained with the foot and image receptor placed parallel with the surface of the table and the central ray directed perpendicular to the foot?

_____

d. Which image was most likely obtained with the foot inclined on a 15-degree wedge and the central ray directed perpendicular to the foot?

_____

6. Identify each lettered bone, group of bones, or joint shown in Fig. 6-11.

A. _____

B. _____

C. _____

D. _____

E. _____

F. _____

G. _____

H. _____

I. _____

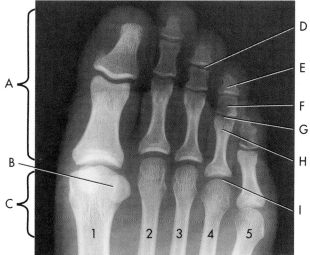

Figure 6-11 Radiograph of the toes.

Items 7 through 14 pertain to the *AP oblique projection.*

7. For the AP oblique projection demonstrating all of the toes, which way—medially or laterally—should the foot and lower leg be rotated?

_____

8. How many degrees of rotation are needed to properly rotate the foot for the AP oblique projection of toes?

_____

9. Which individual toes are best demonstrated using the AP oblique projection with the foot rotated laterally?

_____

10. Which part of the foot (proximal, middle, distal) should be centered to the image receptor?

11. For AP oblique projections, the central ray should be

_____ (perpendicular or angled).

12. For AP oblique projections, the central ray should enter the

foot at the _____

_____ joint.

13. True or False. The bases of metatarsals should be included within the image for AP oblique projections.

14. True or False. All phalanges should be seen in the image.

Items 15 through 20 pertain to the *lateral projection.*

15. For lateral projections of the toes, what can be done to prevent the superimposition of toes?

16. For lateral projections of the toes, the central ray should be

directed _____ (perpendicular or angled).

17. For the lateral projection of the great toe, the central ray

should enter at the _____ joint of the great toe.

18. For lateral projections of the lesser toes, the central ray

should enter at the _____

_____ joint.

19. True or False. For the lateral projection of the great toe, the patient should lie in the lateral recumbent position on the unaffected side.

20. True or False. Interphalangeal and metatarsophalangeal joint spaces should appear open.

Exercise 2: Positioning for the Foot

Instructions: This exercise pertains to the following radiographic procedures of the foot: the AP projection, the AP axial projection, the AP oblique projection (medial rotation), and the lateral projection. Identify structures, fill in missing words, provide a short answer, select the correct answer, or choose true or false (explaining any statement you believe to be false) for each item.

Items 1 through 7 pertain to *AP and AP axial projections.*

1. What other projection term refers to the AP projection?
   a. Axial
   b. Plantodorsal
   c. Dorsoplantar

2. Which surface of the foot should be in contact with the image receptor (IR) for AP and AP axial projections?

3. With reference to the foot, where should the IR be centered for AP and AP axial projections?

4. What two central ray angulations can be used to perform AP and AP axial projections?

5. How should the central ray be directed to best demonstrate tarsometatarsal joints with a dorsoplantar projection?

6. To what point of the foot should the central ray be directed toward for AP and AP axial projections?
   a. To the base of the third metatarsal
   b. To the head of the third metatarsal
   c. To the base of the fifth metatarsal
   d. To the head of the fifth metatarsal

7. Identify each lettered bone, joint, or group of bones shown in Fig. 6-12.

   A. _____

   B. _____

   C. _____

   D. _____

   E. _____

   F. _____

   G. _____

   H. _____

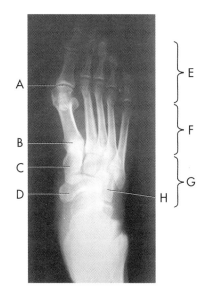

Figure 6-12 AP axial foot.

Items 8 through 14 pertain to the *AP oblique projection.*

8. In which direction—medially or laterally—should the foot be rotated for the AP oblique projection to best demonstrate the cuboid and its related articulations?

9. What projection of the foot best demonstrates the lateral tarsals with the least superimposition of structures?

   a. AP projection
   b. AP axial projection
   c. AP lateral oblique projection
   d. AP medial oblique projection

10. For the AP oblique projection, the leg should be rotated medially until the plantar surface of the foot forms an angle of _____ with the image receptor.

    a. 10 degrees
    b. 20 degrees
    c. 30 degrees
    d. 40 degrees

11. For the AP oblique projection, the central ray should be directed _____ with respect to the foot.

    a. caudally
    b. cephalically
    c. perpendicularly

12. To what point of the foot should the central ray be directed toward for the AP oblique projection?

13. What two metatarsal bases appear overlapped in the image of the AP oblique projection, medial rotation?

14. Identify each lettered bone or joint shown in Fig. 6-13.

    A. _____

    B. _____

    C. _____

    D. _____

    E. _____

    F. _____

    G. _____

    H. _____

    I. _____

    J. _____

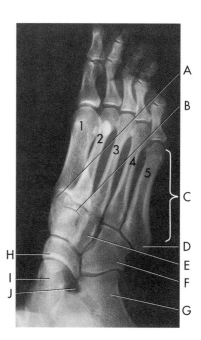

Figure 6-13 AP oblique foot, medial rotation.

Items 15 through 20 pertain to the *lateral projection.*

15. For patient comfort, which side of the foot—medial or lateral—should be placed in contact with the IR for the lateral projection?

16. With reference to the lower leg, how should the foot be positioned for the lateral projection?

17. How should the central ray be directed to the foot?

18. To what point of the foot should the central ray be directed toward for the lateral projection?

19. Where should the distal fibula be seen in images of the lateral projection of the foot?

20. Identify each lettered bone shown in Fig. 6-14.

   A. _____

   B. _____

   C. _____

   D. _____

   E. _____

   F. _____

   G. _____

   H. _____

   I. _____

   J. _____

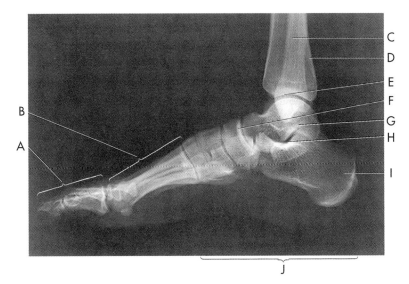

Figure 6-14 Lateral foot.

Exercise 3: Positioning for the Calcaneus

Instructions: In most cases, only two views are obtained to demonstrate the calcaneus: the axial (plantodorsal) projection and the lateral projection. This exercise pertains to those two projections. Identify structures, fill in missing words, provide a short answer, or choose true or false (explaining any statement you believe to be false) for each item.

1. The plantodorsal projection refers to the

   _____ (axial or lateral) projection.

2. With reference to the plane of the image receptor, the plantar surface of the foot should be _____.

3. How many degrees and in which direction should the central ray be directed for the axial (plantodorsal) projection?

   _____

4. At what level of the foot should the central ray enter for the axial (plantodorsal) projection?

5. What should the radiographer do to demonstrate a complete calcaneus if the anterior portion of the calcaneus is not seen in the image without it causing excessive radiographic density to the posterior portion when the calcaneus is demonstrated in the axial (plantodorsal) projection?

6. True or False. The plantar surface of the foot should be in contact with the IR for the axial (plantodorsal) projection.

7. True or False. The central ray should enter the dorsal surface of the foot for the axial (plantodorsal) projection.

8. Identify each lettered structure shown in Fig. 6-15.

   A. _____

   B. _____

   C. _____

   D. _____

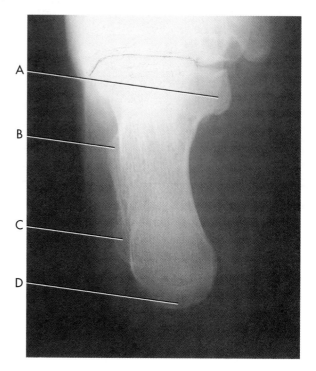

Figure 6-15 Axial (plantodorsal) calcaneus.

9. True or False. For the lateral projection, the central ray should be directed perpendicular to the midportion of the calcaneus.

10. Where on the medial surface of the foot should the central ray enter the calcaneus for the lateral projection?

11. Which projection of the calcaneus—axial or lateral—best demonstrates the sinus tarsi?

   _____

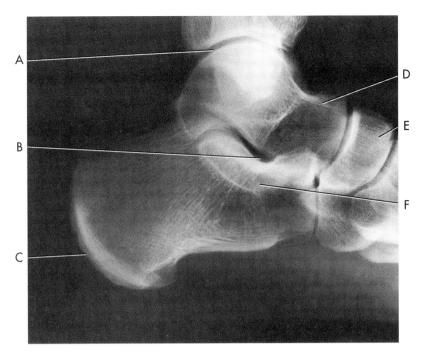

Figure 6-16 Lateral calcaneus.

12. Identify each lettered structure or joint shown in Fig. 6-16.

A. _____ D. _____

B. _____ E. _____

C. _____ F. _____

Exercise 4: Positioning for the Ankle

Instructions: This exercise pertains to the radiographic procedures that demonstrate the ankle: the AP projection, the lateral (mediolateral) projection, the AP oblique projection, and the AP stress studies. Identify structures, fill in missing words, provide a short answer, or choose true or false (explaining any statement you believe to be false) for each item.

Items 1 through 7 pertain to the *AP projection.*

1. Describe how the foot should be positioned on the IR for the AP projection.

2. Where exactly should the central ray enter the lower limb for the AP projection?

3. True or False. The central ray should be directed perpendicular to the ankle for the AP projection.

4. True or False. The AP projection should demonstrate the joint space between the medial malleolus and the talus without any overlapping of structures.

5. True or False. The AP projection should demonstrate the distal third of the fibula without superimposition with the talus or tibia.

6. True or False. The AP projection should demonstrate the lateral and medial malleoli.

7. Identify each lettered structure shown in Fig. 6-17.

A. _____

B. _____

C. _____

D. _____

E. _____

F. _____

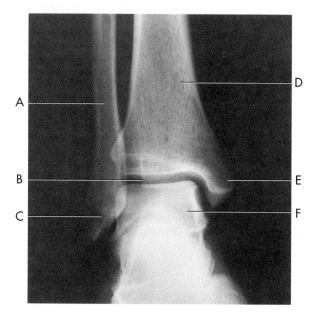

Figure 6-17 AP ankle.

Items 8 through 13 pertain to the *lateral projection.*

8. Why is dorsiflexion of the foot required for the lateral (mediolateral) projection?

9. Where should the central ray enter the patient for the lateral (mediolateral) projection?

10. For the lateral (mediolateral) projection, the central ray should be directed _____ (perpendicularly or caudally).

11. True or False. The lateral (mediolateral) projection should demonstrate the fibula over the posterior half of the tibia.

12. True or False. A radiograph of the lateral (mediolateral) projection should demonstrate the lateral malleolus free from superimposition by the talus.

13. Identify each lettered structure shown in Fig. 6-18.

    A. _____

    B. _____

    C. _____

    D. _____

    E. _____

    F. _____

    G. _____

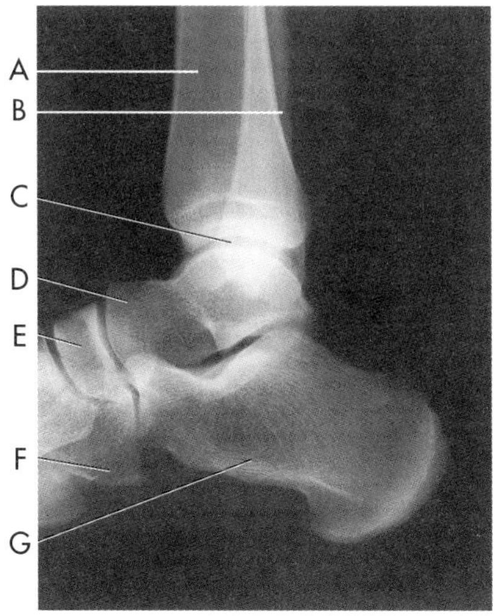

Figure 6-18 Lateral ankle.

Items 14 through 18 pertain to the *AP oblique projection (medial rotation)* of the ankle.

14. Describe the position of a patient when performing the AP oblique projection of the ankle.

15. Describe the placement of the IR relative to the patient.

16. How many degrees and in what direction should the leg and foot be rotated?

17. To where should the central ray be centered?

18. From the following list, circle the structures and articulation that should be demonstrated in the image of the AP oblique ankle.

    a. Talus
    b. Cuboid
    c. Calcaneus
    d. Distal tibia
    e. Distal fibula
    f. Tibiofibular articulation
    g. Femorotibial articulation
    h. Metatarsophalangeal articulation

Items 19 through 26 pertain to the *AP oblique projection (medial rotation)* of the ankle for demonstrating the mortise joint.

19. From the supine position, how many degrees should the leg and foot be rotated to position the ankle for this projection?

20. With reference to the position of the patient's leg and foot during the procedure, how is it determined that the leg has been rotated the correct number of degrees?

21. The image receptor should be centered midway between

    the _____.

22. How should the central ray be directed toward the ankle joint—perpendicular or angled?

23. True or False. The talofibular joint space should be demonstrated in profile without any bony superimposition.

24. True or False. The foot should be plantar-flexed to place the long axis of the foot parallel with the image receptor.

25. True or False. The affected limb should be fully extended.

26. Identify each lettered structure shown in Fig. 6-19.

    A. _____

    B. _____

    C. _____

    D. _____

    E. _____

    F. _____

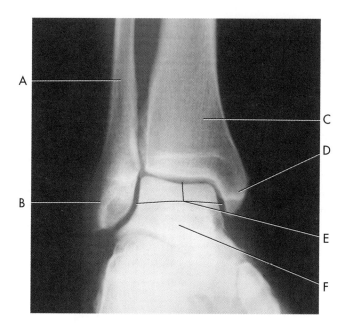

Figure 6-19 AP oblique ankle, medial rotation.

Items 27 through 30 pertain to *AP projections (stress method)*.

27. State the purpose of performing AP stress studies of the ankle.

28. Describe the stress movement that is applied to the foot in stress studies of the ankle.

29. How can the patient hold the foot in the stress position during AP stress studies?

30. How do images indicate that a patient has a torn ligament affecting the ankle?

Exercise 5: Positioning for the Leg

Instructions: This exercise pertains to radiographic procedures of the leg: the AP projection and the lateral projection. Identify structures, fill in missing words, provide a short answer, select the correct answer, or choose true or false (explaining any statement you believe to be false) for each question.

Items 1 through 5 pertain to the *AP projection.*

1. The placement of the IR should allow the top border to extend at least _____ inches above the knee joint.
   a. 1 to 1¹/₂
   b. 2 to 2¹/₂
   c. 3 to 3¹/₂

2. Which procedure should the radiographer perform if the leg is too long to demonstrate the knee and the ankle joint with the same exposure?
   a. Perform two AP projections to ensure that the entire lower limb is demonstrated.
   b. Increase the source to image receptor distance to ensure the beam covers the entire leg.
   c. Angle the central ray along the long axis of the leg to project the joint onto the image receptor.

3. To which area of the leg should the central ray be directed when only one exposure is being taken for the AP projection?
   a. Midpoint
   b. Tibial plateau
   c. Ankle mortise

4. True or False. The AP projection of the leg should demonstrate the fibula without any overlapping with the tibia.

5. Identify each lettered structure shown in Fig. 6-20.

   A. _____

   B. _____

   C. _____

   D. _____

   E. _____

   F. _____

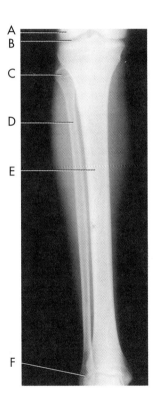

Figure 6-20 AP tibia and fibula.

Items 6 through 10 pertain to the *lateral projection.*

6. For the lateral projection of the leg, how should the patella be positioned with reference to the plane of the image receptor—perpendicular or parallel?

7. What procedure should the radiographer perform if the patient is unable to turn from the supine position toward the affected side to position a fractured leg on the image receptor for the lateral projection?

8. If a radiographer positions the lower limb very carefully to ensure that femoral condyles are physically superimposed, but they do not appear to be well superimposed on the radiograph, what could have caused the image to appear that way?

9. True or False. The lateral projection should demonstrate some interosseous space between the shafts of the fibula and tibia.

10. Identify each lettered structure shown in Fig. 6-21.

A. _____

B. _____

C. _____

D. _____

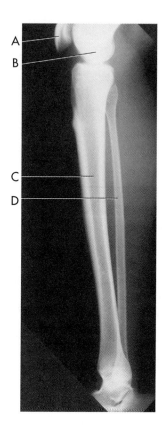

Figure 6-21 Lateral tibia and fibula.

Exercise 6: Positioning for the Knee

Instructions: A variety of radiographs are obtained to demonstrate the knee, the largest joint in the body. This exercise pertains to those radiographic images. Identify structures, fill in missing words, provide a short answer, select the correct answer, or choose true or false (explaining any statement you believe is false) for each question.

Items 1 through 10 pertain to the *AP projection.*

1. List three factors that should be considered when deciding whether or not to use a grid for AP projections.

2. With reference to the knee, where is the centering point used for positioning the image receptor to the knee?

   a. To the apex of the patella
   b. To the most superior point of the patella
   c. $^1/_2$ inch (1.2 cm) below the apex of the patella
   d. 2 inches (5 cm) below the apex of the patella

3. Where should the patella be positioned on the knee for the AP projection?

   a. Slightly off center to the lateral side of the tibia
   b. Slightly off center to the medial side of the tibia
   c. Slightly off center to the lateral side of the femur
   d. Slightly off center to the medial side of the femur

4. For the following three situations, choose the central ray angulation that best demonstrates the joint space based on the anterior superior iliac spine (ASIS)-to-tabletop measurement by writing in the space provided the corresponding letter from the following choices:

   ____ 1. Less than 19 cm   a. Perpendicular

   ____ 2. Between 19 and 24 cm   b. 3 to 5 degrees
                                       caudad

   ____ 3. More than 24 cm   c. 3 to 5 degrees
                                       cephalad

                                    d. 10 degrees
                                       caudad

                                    e. 10 degrees
                                       cephalad

5. How should the central ray be directed when the distal femur or proximal ends of the tibia and fibula, rather than the joint space, are of primary interest?

   a. Perpendicular
   b. 3 to 5 degrees caudad
   c. 3 to 5 degrees cephalad
   d. 10 degrees caudad
   e. 10 degrees cephalad

6. The patella should be demonstrated completely superimposed on the _____.

   a. tibia
   b. fibula
   c. femur

7. True or False. The central ray should be directed to a point $^1/_2$ inch (1.2 cm) below the apex of the patella.

8. True or False. The AP projection image of a normal knee should demonstrate a femorotibial joint space with equal distances on both sides.

9. Identify each lettered structure shown in Fig. 6-22.

   A. _____

   B. _____

   C. _____

   D. _____

   E. _____

   F. _____

   G. _____

   H. _____

   I. _____

   J. _____

   K. _____

   L. _____

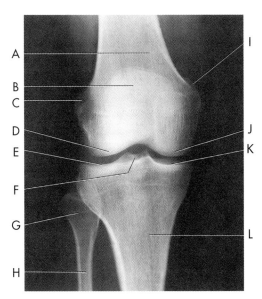

Figure 6-22 AP knee.

10. Fig. 6-23 is another AP projection radiograph of the knee. Compare this image with Fig. 6-22 and answer the questions that follow.

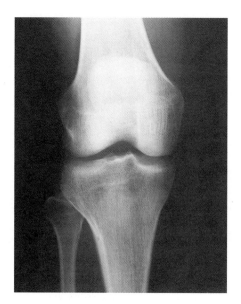

Figure 6-23 AP knee.

  i. How does Fig. 6-23 appear different?

    a. The patella does not superimpose the femur.
    b. The femorotibial joint space is not fully open.
    c. The fibular head does not slightly superimpose the tibia.

  ii. How did the positioning procedures most likely differ to produce these images?

  iii. Assuming that the ASIS-to-tabletop measurement for the patient in Fig. 6-22 is greater than 24 cm, describe how you believe the central ray was directed to produce the image. Explain why.

  iv. Assuming that the patient in Fig. 6-23 is the same patient seen in Fig. 6-22, describe how you believe the central ray was directed to produce the image in Fig. 6-23. Explain why.

  v. Which image best demonstrates the femorotibial joint space?

Items 11 through 21 pertain to the *lateral projection.*

11. With reference to the plane of the IR, the patella should be

    _____ (parallel or perpendicular).

12. The knee should be flexed _____ degrees.

13. When a new or healing fracture is present, the knee should

    be flexed no more than _____ degrees.

14. What could occur if a patient with a healing fracture flexes the knee more than the recommended number of degrees?

15. How many degrees and in what direction should the central ray be directed?

16. Why is the central ray angled cephalad for the lateral projection?

17. The central ray should enter the patient 1 inch (2.5 cm) distal to the _____ _____.

18. Which positioning maneuver relaxes the muscles and shows the maximum volume of the joint cavity?
    a. Fully extending the lower limb
    b. Flexing the knee 20 to 30 degrees
    c. Placing support pads under the ankle to elevate the lower leg

19. True or False. The femoral condyles should appear superimposed.

20. True or False. The lateral projection demonstrates the patella with slight overlapping with the femoral condyles.

21. Identify each lettered structure shown in Fig. 6-24.

    A. _____

    B. _____

    C. _____

    D. _____

    E. _____

    F. _____

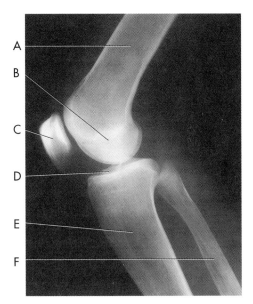

Figure 6-24 Lateral knee.

Items 22 through 27 pertain to the *weight-bearing AP projection* of the knees.

22. Which physical condition affecting knees is often the reason that weight-bearing AP projections are performed?
    a. Arthritis
    b. Fracture
    c. Torn ligament

23. What size IR should be used and how should it be placed (lengthwise or crosswise) when demonstrating both knees with one exposure?

24. To what level of the patient should the IR be centered?

25. Describe how and where the central ray should be directed.

26. True or False. The patient should slightly flex both knees to maximize the knee joint space.

27. True or False. Both knees should be demonstrated without rotation.

Items 28 through 35 pertain to the *AP oblique projections.*

28. How many degrees should the leg be rotated?

    a. 15 degrees
    b. 30 degrees
    c. 45 degrees
    d. 60 degrees

29. How many degrees and in what direction should the central ray be directed if the patient measures less than 19 cm from the ASIS to the tabletop?

    a. 0 degrees (perpendicular)
    b. 3 to 5 degrees caudal
    c. 3 to 5 degrees cephalic

30. How many degrees and in what direction should the central ray be directed if the patient measures between 19 to 24 cm from the ASIS to the tabletop?

    a. 0 degrees (perpendicular)
    b. 3 to 5 degrees caudal
    c. 3 to 5 degrees cephalic

31. How many degrees and in what direction should the central ray be directed if the patient measures more than 24 cm from the ASIS to the tabletop?

    a. 0 degrees (perpendicular)
    b. 3 to 5 degrees caudal
    c. 3 to 5 degrees cephalic

32. Where on the knee should the central ray enter?

    a. $1/2$ inch inferior to the patellar apex
    b. $1/2$ inch superior to the patellar apex
    c. $1\,1/2$ inches inferior to the patellar apex
    d. $1\,1/2$ inches superior to the patellar apex

33. Listed following are evaluation criteria for AP oblique projections. In the space provided, write *M* if the statement refers to the medial oblique projection, *L* if the statement refers to the lateral oblique projection, or *B* if the statement refers to both oblique projections.

    ____ a. Tibial plateaus should be visualized.

    ____ b. Knee joint should be seen and open.

    ____ c. Soft tissue around the knee should be seen.

    ____ d. Medial femoral and tibial condyles should be demonstrated.

    ____ e. Lateral femoral and tibial condyles should be demonstrated.

    ____ f. Fibula should be superimposed over the lateral half of the tibia.

    ____ g. Tibia and fibula should be separated at their proximal articulation.

    ____ h. Bony detail of the distal femur and proximal tibia should be demonstrated.

    ____ i. Margin of the patella should project slightly beyond the edge of the femoral lateral condyle.

    ____ j. Margin of the patella should project slightly beyond the edge of the femoral medial condyle.

34. Identify each lettered structure shown in Fig. 6-25.

A. _____

B. _____

C. _____

D. _____

E. _____

F. _____

G. _____

H. _____

I. _____

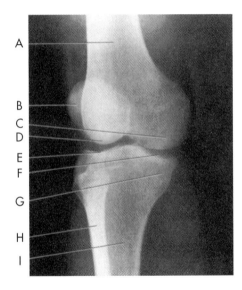

Figure 6-25 AP oblique knee, lateral rotation.

35. Identify each lettered structure shown in Fig. 6-26.

A. _____

B. _____

C. _____

D. _____

E. _____

F. _____

G. _____

H. _____

I. _____

J. _____

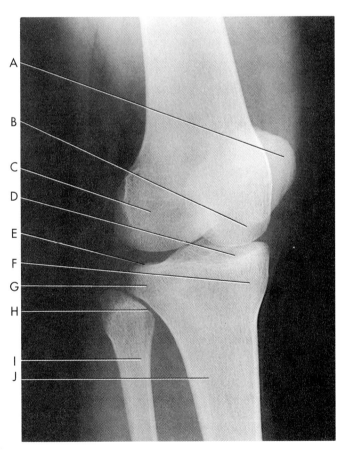

Figure 6-26 AP oblique knee, medial rotation.

Exercise 7: Positioning for the Intercondylar Fossa

Instructions: Two PA axial projections, the Holmblad method and the Camp-Coventry method, are performed to demonstrate specific structures within the knee. This exercise pertains to those two projections. Identify structures, fill in missing words, provide a short answer, choose the correct answer from a list, or choose true or false (explaining any statement you believe to be false) for each item.

Items 1 through 7 pertain to the *PA axial projection (the Holmblad method).*

1. The PA axial projection, first described by Holmblad in 1937, requires the patient to assume a

   _____ position.

2. Describe the three ways patients can be positioned.

3. Describe how the image receptor should be placed.

4. Describe how and where the central ray should be directed.

5. What angle should be formed between the femur and the plane of the IR when the patient is correctly positioned?

6. What structures of the knee are demonstrated with this type of projection?

7. Identify each lettered structure in Fig. 6-27.

   A. _____

   B. _____

   C. _____

   D. _____

   E. _____

   F. _____

   G. _____

   H. _____

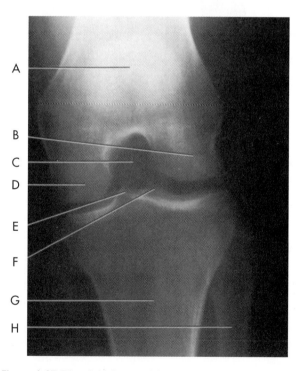

Figure 6-27 PA axial intercondylar fossa, Holmblad method.

Examine Fig. 6-28 as you answer items 8 through 15, which pertain to the *PA axial projection (Camp-Coventry method).*

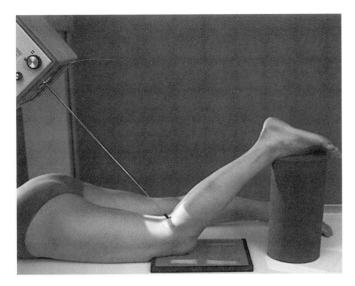

Figure 6-28 PA axial intercondylar fossa, Camp-Coventry method.

8. Which patient body position should be used when performing this projection?

   a. Prone
   b. Supine
   c. Upright

9. Approximately how many degrees should the knee be flexed?

   a. 20 or 30
   b. 40 or 50
   c. 60 or 70

10. What should the radiographer do to make maintaining the proper flexion of the knee more comfortable for the patient?

11. The central ray should be directed perpendicular to the

    long axis of the _____.

12. How many degrees and in what direction should the central ray be directed?

13. What factor determines the number of degrees the central ray should be angled?

14. What structure of the knee is demonstrated with this projection?

15. Both PA axial projections—the Holmblad method and the Camp-Coventry method—produce similar results and have identical evaluation criteria. From the following list, circle the seven evaluation criteria that refer to both projections.

    a. Patella should be seen in lateral profile.
    b. Femoral condyles should be superimposed.
    c. Fossa should be open and visualized.
    d. Apex of the patella should not superimpose the fossa.
    e. Soft tissue in the fossa and interspaces should be seen.
    f. Intercondylar eminences and knee joint space should be seen.
    g. No rotation is evident by slight tibiofibular overlap being seen.
    h. Posteroinferior surface of the femoral condyles should be demonstrated.
    i. Bony detail on the tibial eminences, distal femur, and proximal tibia should be demonstrated.

Exercise 8: Positioning for the Patella

Instructions: Three projections—the PA projection, the lateral projection, and a tangential projection—are often used in some combination to comprise a series of radiographs demonstrating the patella. This exercise pertains to those projections. Identify structures, fill in missing words, provide a short answer, or choose true or false (explaining any statement you believe to be false) for each item.

Examine Fig. 6-29 as you answer items 1 through 6, which pertain to the *PA projection.*

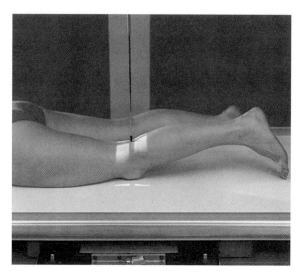

Figure 6-29 PA patella.

1. The patient should be placed in the

   _____ (supine or prone) position.

2. With reference to the plane of the image receptor, the plane

   of the patella should be _____ (parallel or perpendicular).

3. Why is the PA projection preferred over the AP projection?

4. What can be done to alleviate the pressure on the patella caused by the patient's weight?

5. How should the lower limb be adjusted to place the patella parallel with the image receptor?

6. Describe how and where the central ray should be directed.

Items 7 through 10 pertain to the *lateral projection.*

7. True or False. The lateral side of the affected knee should be in contact with the table or image receptor.

8. The knee should be flexed no more than _____ degrees.

9. What might occur if the patient flexes the knee more than the recommended number of degrees?

10. Describe the projection of the central ray.

Items 11 through 20 pertain to the *tangential projection (Settegast method).*

11. Describe three ways the patient can be positioned on a radiographic table for the tangential projection (Settegast method).

12. Why is it preferable to place the patient in the prone position for the tangential projection?

13. What projection of the patella should be performed before a tangential projection is attempted? Explain why.

14. When the patient is placed in the prone position and is unable to maintain a steady lower leg after flexing the knee, what can be done to help the patient hold the position?

15. Describe how and where the central ray should be directed.

16. What determines the number of degrees the central ray is angled?

17. True or False. The patellofemoral articulation is seen in slight overlap with the anterior surfaces of the femoral condyles.

18. True or False. The patella should be seen in profile.

19. True or False. The bony detail of the femoral condyles should be demonstrated.

20. Identify each lettered structure shown in Fig. 6-30.

    A. _____

    B. _____

    C. _____

    D. _____

    E. _____

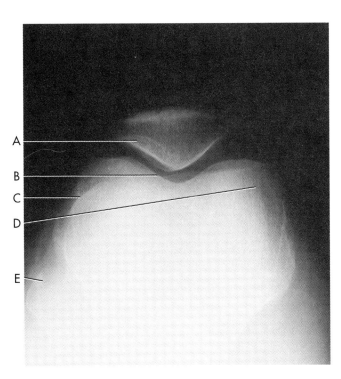

Figure 6-30 Tangential patella, Settegast method.

Exercise 9: Positioning for the Femur

Instructions: AP and lateral projections are usually obtained to adequately demonstrate the femur. This exercise pertains to those two types of projection. Identify structures, fill in missing words, provide a short answer, choose the correct answer from a list, or choose true or false (explaining any statement you believe to be false) for each item.

Items 1 through 11 pertain to the *AP projection.*

1. How many degrees should the lower limb be rotated?

    a. 3 to 5 degrees
    b. 10 to 15 degrees
    c. 20 to 30 degrees

2. In which direction should the lower limb be rotated?

    a. Externally (laterally)
    b. Internally (medially)

3. Why should the lower limb be rotated?

4. Describe how and where the central ray should be directed.

5. What factor determines which femoral joint should be demonstrated if only one joint needs to be seen?

6. What should the radiographer do if both femoral joints need to be demonstrated on a typical adult?

7. How should the femoral neck appear in the AP projection of the proximal femur?

8. Describe how the lesser trochanter should appear in the AP projection of the proximal femur.

9. What portion of an orthopedic appliance should be demonstrated on the radiograph?

10. True or False. Gonadal shielding should not be used because it may superimpose the femoral head.

11. Identify each lettered structure shown in Fig. 6-31.

A. _____

B. _____

C. _____

D. _____

E. _____

F. _____

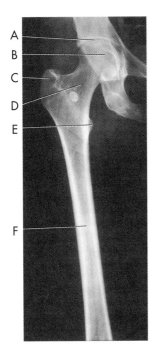

Figure 6-31 AP proximal femur.

Items 12 through 20 pertain to the *lateral projection.*

12. How should the pelvis be positioned to demonstrate the proximal femur?

   a. True lateral
   b. From true lateral, the pelvis should be rolled anteriorly about 10 to 15 degrees
   c. From true lateral, the pelvis should be rolled posteriorly about 10 to 15 degrees

13. How should the pelvis be positioned to demonstrate the distal femur?

   a. True lateral
   b. From true lateral, the pelvis should be rolled anteriorly about 10 to 15 degrees
   c. From true lateral, the pelvis should be rolled posteriorly about 10 to 15 degrees

14. Concerning image receptor placement, (a) to what level on the patient should the upper border of an IR be placed when demonstrating the proximal femur, and (b) to what level of the patient should the lower border of the IR be placed when demonstrating the distal femur?

15. Concerning the placement of the unaffected (uppermost) limb, (a) where should it be placed when demonstrating the proximal femur, and (b) where should it be placed when demonstrating the distal femur?

16. When demonstrating the distal femur and including the knee, how many degrees should the knee be flexed?

17. Describe how and where the central ray should be directed.

18. Describe placement of the image receptor if it is suspected that a patient has a fracture of the distal femur.

19. From the following list, circle the four evaluation criteria that indicate the femur was correctly positioned when including the knee in a lateral projection of the distal femur.

   a. The patella should be seen in profile.
   b. The patella should superimpose the femur.
   c. The patellofemoral joint space should be open.
   d. The greater trochanter should be seen in profile.
   e. The anterior surface of the femoral condyles should be superimposed.
   f. The inferior surface of the femoral condyles will not be superimposed.

20. Identify each lettered structure shown in Fig. 6-32.

   A. _____

   B. _____

   C. _____

   D. _____

   E. _____

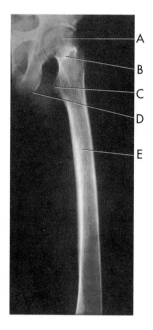

Figure 6-32 Lateral proximal femur.

Exercise 10: Evaluating Radiographs of the Lower Limb

Instructions: This exercise consists of radiographs of the lower extremity to give you practice in evaluating extremity positioning. These images are not from *Merrill's Atlas of Radiographic Positions and Radiologic Procedures*. Each radiograph shows at least one positioning error. Examine each image and answer the questions that follow by providing a short answer or choosing the correct answer from a list.

1. Fig. 6-33 shows an AP oblique projection radiograph of the toes. Examine the image and state why it does not meet the evaluation criteria for this projection.

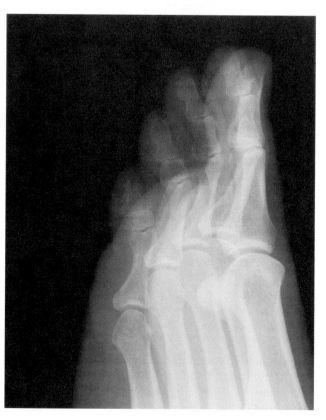

Figure 6-33 AP oblique toes with improper positioning.

2. Fig. 6-34 is an inferior-quality AP projection radiograph of the ankle. Examine the image and state (a) why the image does not meet the evaluation criteria for this type of projection and (b) what positioning error most likely produced this image.

3. Fig. 6-35 is an AP oblique projection radiograph of inferior quality demonstrating the mortise joint. Examine the image and state why it does not meet the evaluation criteria for this projection.

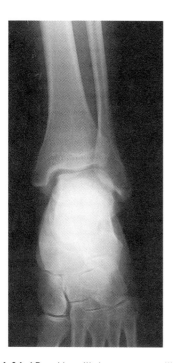

Figure 6-34 AP ankle with improper positioning.

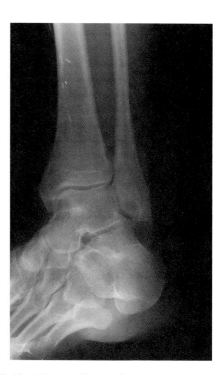

Figure 6-35 AP oblique ankle, medial rotation, with improper positioning.

4. Fig. 6-36 is a lateral projection radiograph of the knee that does not meet all the evaluation criteria for this type of projection. Examine the image and answer the questions that follow.

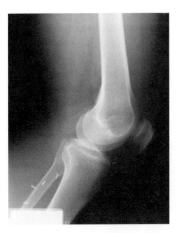

Figure 6-36 Lateral knee with improper positioning.

i. From the following list, circle the three evaluation criteria for lateral projections that this image does not meet.

a. The femoropatellar space should be open.

b. The femoral condyles should be superimposed.

c. The knee should be flexed approximately 20 to 30 degrees.

d. The fibular head and tibia should be slightly superimposed.

e. The joint space between femoral condyles and tibia should be open.

ii. What central ray angulation was most likely used to make this image? Explain your answer.

Self-Test: Osteology, Arthrology, and Positioning of the Lower Limb

Instructions: Answer the following questions by selecting the best choice.

1. How many and what kind of bones comprise the foot and ankle?
    a. 14 phalanges, 5 metatarsals, and 7 tarsals
    b. 14 phalanges, 7 metatarsals, and 5 tarsals
    c. 7 phalanges, 5 metatarsals, and 14 tarsals
    d. 7 phalanges, 14 metatarsals, and 5 tarsals

2. Which bone classification are tarsals?
    a. Flat
    b. Long
    c. Short
    d. Irregular

3. What is the most distal part of a metatarsal?
    a. Base
    b. Head
    c. Tuberosity
    d. Styloid process

4. Where in the foot is the tuberosity that is easily palpable?
    a. Distal portion of the first metatarsal
    b. Distal portion of the fifth metatarsal
    c. Proximal portion of the first metatarsal
    d. Proximal portion of the fifth metatarsal

5. Which tarsal bone is the most superior tarsal bone?
    a. Talus
    b. Cuboid
    c. Navicular
    d. Calcaneus

6. Which tarsal bone is the largest of the tarsal bones?
    a. Talus
    b. Cuboid
    c. Navicular
    d. Calcaneus

7. Which tarsal bone is located on the lateral side of the foot between the calcaneus and the fourth and fifth metatarsals?
    a. Talus
    b. Cuboid
    c. Navicular
    d. Lateral cuneiform

8. Which tarsal bone is located on the medial side of the foot between the talus and the three cuneiforms?
    a. Talus
    b. Cuboid
    c. Navicular
    d. Calcaneus

9. Which bone articulates medially with the cuboid?
    a. First metatarsal
    b. Medial cuneiform
    c. Intermediate cuneiform
    d. Lateral cuneiform

10. Which bones comprise the midfoot?
    a. Talus and cuboid
    b. Talus and calcaneus
    c. Metatarsals and toes
    d. Navicular, cuboid, and cuneiforms

11. Which bone articulates superiorly with the calcaneus?
    a. Tibia
    b. Talus
    c. Fibula
    d. Navicular

12. Which bones articulate distally with the tarsal navicular?
    a. Phalanges
    b. Cuneiforms
    c. Metatarsals
    d. Talus and calcaneus

13. Which bones articulate distally with the three cuneiforms?
    a. Navicular
    b. Phalanges
    c. Metatarsals
    d. Talus and calcaneus

14. Which bones articulate with the metatarsals?
    a. Calcaneus and cuboid
    b. Calcaneus and navicular
    c. Cuneiforms and cuboid
    d. Cuneiforms and navicular

15. Which cuneiform is the largest cuneiform?
    a. Medial
    b. Intermediate
    c. Third
    d. Lateral

16. Where in the foot are the cuneiforms located?

    a. Between the cuboid and the calcaneus
    b. Between the cuboid and the metatarsals
    c. Between the navicular and the calcaneus
    d. Between the navicular and the metatarsals

17. Which articulation is a condyloid-type joint?

    a. Intertarsal
    b. Interphalangeal
    c. Tarsometatarsal
    d. Metatarsophalangeal

18. Which articulation of the foot is a gliding-type joint?

    a. Mortise
    b. Intertarsal
    c. Interphalangeal
    d. Tarsometatarsal

19. Which two tarsal bones articulate with each other by way of three facets?

    a. Talus and cuboid
    b. Talus and calcaneus
    c. Navicular and cuboid
    d. Navicular and calcaneus

20. Which part of the talus articulates with the distal tibia?

    a. Styloid
    b. Tubercle
    c. Trochlea
    d. Epicondyle

21. Which type of joint is the ankle joint?

    a. Hinge
    b. Gliding
    c. Condyloid
    d. Ball-and-socket

22. Where is the medial malleolus located in the leg?

    a. Distal tibia
    b. Distal fibula
    c. Proximal tibia
    d. Proximal fibula

23. Where is the lateral malleolus located in the leg?

    a. Distal tibia
    b. Distal fibula
    c. Proximal tibia
    d. Proximal fibula

24. What structure is located on the proximal end of the fibula?

    a. Base
    b. Apex
    c. Tuberosity
    d. Trochanter

25. Where is the intercondylar eminence located?

    a. Distal tibia
    b. Distal femur
    c. Proximal tibia
    d. Proximal femur

26. Where are the tibial plateaus located?

    a. Distal tibia
    b. Distal femur
    c. Proximal tibia
    d. Proximal femur

27. On which border of the tibia is the crest located?

    a. Lateral
    b. Medial
    c. Anterior
    d. Posterior

28. Which term refers to the sharp ridge on the anterior border of the tibia?

    a. Apex
    b. Crest
    c. Tubercle
    d. Eminence

29. Which term refers to the prominent process on the anterior surface of the proximal tibia that is just inferior to the condyles?

    a. Apex
    b. Styloid
    c. Eminence
    d. Tuberosity

30. Which joint is formed by the articulation of the head of the fibula with the lateral condyle of the tibia?

    a. Knee
    b. Ankle
    c. Distal tibiofibular
    d. Proximal tibiofibular

31. Which type of joint is the proximal tibiofibular joint?

    a. Hinge
    b. Gliding
    c. Condyloid
    d. Ball-and-socket

32. Which structure is located on the head of the fibula?

    a. Apex
    b. Condyle
    c. Lateral malleolus
    d. Medial malleolus

33. With which structure does the head of the fibula articulate?

    a. Lateral malleolus
    b. Medial malleolus
    c. Lateral tibial condyle
    d. Medial tibial condyle

34. Which term refers to the inferior tip of the patella?

    a. Base
    b. Apex
    c. Styloid
    d. Tubercle

35. Which part of the patella is the base?

    a. Apex
    b. Lateral border
    c. Medial border
    d. Superior border

36. Where on the femur is the greater trochanter located?

    a. Lateral and inferior
    b. Lateral and superior
    c. Medial and inferior
    d. Medial and superior

37. Where on the femur is the lesser trochanter located?

    a. Lateral and anterior
    b. Lateral and posterior
    c. Medial and anterior
    d. Medial and posterior

38. Where is the fovea capitis located?

    a. Distal tibia
    b. Distal femur
    c. Proximal tibia
    d. Proximal femur

39. Where is the intercondylar fossa located?

    a. Distal tibia
    b. Distal femur
    c. Proximal tibia
    d. Proximal femur

40. Which femoral structures articulate with the tibia?

    a. Condyles
    b. Tubercles
    c. Trochanters
    d. Epicondyles

41. With which structure does the head of the femur articulate?

    a. Condyle
    b. Trochanter
    c. Epicondyle
    d. Acetabulum

42. When an angled central ray is used to perform the AP projection of the toes, how many degrees and in what direction should the central ray be directed?

    a. 10 degrees caudad (toward the toes)
    b. 10 degrees cephalad (toward the heel)
    c. 15 degrees caudad (toward the toes)
    d. 15 degrees cephalad (toward the heel)

43. How many degrees and in what direction should the foot be rotated for the AP oblique projection to demonstrate the second toe?

    a. 15 to 25 degrees medially
    b. 15 to 25 degrees laterally
    c. 30 to 45 degrees medially
    d. 30 to 45 degrees laterally

44. How and toward what centering point should the central ray be directed for the AP oblique projection to demonstrate all five toes?

    a. Perpendicular to the proximal interphalangeal (PIP) joint of the third digit
    b. Perpendicular to the third metatarsophalangeal joint
    c. 15 degrees posterior (toward the heel) to the PIP of the third digit
    d. 15 degrees posterior (toward the heel) to the third metatarsophalangeal joint

45. How many degrees and in what direction should the foot be rotated for the AP oblique projection to best demonstrate the great toe?

    a. 10 to 15 degrees medially
    b. 10 to 15 degrees laterally
    c. 30 to 45 degrees medially
    d. 30 to 45 degrees laterally

46. What other projection term refers to the AP projection of the foot?

    a. Plantodorsal
    b. Dorsoplantar
    c. Inferosuperior
    d. Superoinferior

47. How many degrees and in what direction should the central ray be directed for the AP axial projection of the foot?

    a. 10 degrees caudad (toward the toes)
    b. 10 degrees cephalad (toward the heel)
    c. 15 degrees caudad (toward the toes)
    d. 15 degrees cephalad (toward the heel)

48. Which projection of the foot best demonstrates the cuboid and its articulations?

    a. Lateral
    b. Dorsoplantar
    c. AP lateral oblique
    d. AP medial oblique

49. How many degrees and in what direction should the foot be rotated for the AP oblique projection of the foot?

    a. 15 degrees laterally
    b. 30 degrees medially
    c. 45 degrees laterally
    d. 45 degrees medially

50. How many degrees and in what direction should the foot be rotated for the AP oblique projection to best demonstrate the cuboid and its articulations?

    a. 30 degrees laterally
    b. 30 degrees medially
    c. 45 degrees laterally
    d. 45 degrees medially

51. How and toward what centering point should the central ray be directed for the AP oblique projection of the foot?

    a. Perpendicular to the head of the third metatarsal
    b. Perpendicular to the base of the third metatarsal
    c. 10 degrees posterior (toward the heel) to the head of the third metatarsal
    d. 10 degrees posterior (toward the heel) to the base of the third metatarsal

52. Where should the central ray be directed for the AP oblique projection of the foot?

    a. To the base of the third metatarsal
    b. To the head of the third metatarsal
    c. To the metatarsophalangeal joint of the third digit
    d. To the proximal interphalangeal joint of the third digit

53. Regardless of the condition of the patient, which positioning maneuver should be performed to position the foot for the lateral projection?

    a. Plantar-flex the foot.
    b. Rotate the leg laterally until the knee is against the table.
    c. Ensure that the plantar surface is in contact with the image receptor.
    d. Ensure that the plantar surface is perpendicular to the image receptor.

54. How should the central ray be directed to best demonstrate the tarsometatarsal joint spaces of the midfoot for the AP projection of the foot?

    a. Perpendicularly
    b. 10 degrees posteriorly (toward the heel)
    c. 15 degrees posteriorly (toward the heel)
    d. 20 degrees posteriorly (toward the heel)

55. Which projection of the foot best demonstrates the sinus tarsi?

    a. AP projection
    b. Lateral projection
    c. AP oblique projection (lateral rotation)
    d. AP oblique projection (medial rotation)

56. Which projection of the foot best demonstrates most of the tarsals with the least amount of superimposition?

    a. AP projection
    b. Lateral projection
    c. AP oblique projection (lateral rotation)
    d. AP oblique projection (medial rotation)

57. Which projection of the foot best demonstrates the bases of the fourth and fifth metatarsals free from superimposition?

    a. AP projection
    b. Lateral projection
    c. AP oblique projection (lateral rotation)
    d. AP oblique projection (medial rotation)

58. Which projection of the foot should demonstrate metatarsals nearly superimposed on each other?

    a. AP projection
    b. Lateral projection
    c. AP oblique projection (lateral rotation)
    d. AP oblique projection (medial rotation)

59. Which two projections comprise the typical series that best demonstrates the calcaneus?

    a. AP (dorsoplantar) and lateral projections
    b. AP (dorsoplantar) and medial oblique projections
    c. Axial (plantodorsal) and lateral projections
    d. Axial (plantodorsal) and medial oblique projections

60. How many degrees and in what direction should the central ray be directed for the axial (plantodorsal) projection of the calcaneus?

    a. 10 degrees caudad
    b. 10 degrees cephalad
    c. 40 degrees caudad
    d. 40 degrees cephalad

61. At which level on the plantar surface should the central ray enter the foot for the axial (plantodorsal) projection of the calcaneus?

   a. Midpoint of the calcaneus
   b. Tuberosity of the calcaneus
   c. Base of the third metatarsal
   d. Head of the third metatarsal

62. Where should the central ray be directed for the lateral projection of the calcaneus?

   a. Toward the midpoint of the foot
   b. Toward the midpoint of the calcaneus
   c. Toward the base of the third metatarsal
   d. Toward the head of the third metatarsal

63. Where should the central ray enter for the lateral projection of the ankle?

   a. At the lateral malleolus
   b. At the medial malleolus
   c. At the midpoint of the calcaneus
   d. At the base of the third metatarsal

64. How many degrees and in which direction should the foot and leg be rotated to best demonstrate the mortise joint for the AP oblique projection of the ankle?

   a. 15 to 20 degrees laterally
   b. 15 to 20 degrees medially
   c. 40 to 45 degrees laterally
   d. 40 to 45 degrees medially

65. Which projection of the ankle best demonstrates the talofibular joint space free from bony superimposition?

   a. AP projection
   b. Lateral projection
   c. AP oblique projection (lateral rotation)
   d. AP oblique projection (medial rotation)

66. Which articulation should be seen in profile with the AP oblique projection (medial rotation) of the ankle?

   a. Subtalar
   b. Talofibular
   c. Talocalcaneal
   d. Distal tibiofibular

67. With reference to the plane of the image receptor, how should the malleoli be positioned for the AP oblique projection of the ankle to best demonstrate the mortise joint spaces open?

   a. Parallel
   b. Perpendicular
   c. 45 degrees lateral rotation
   d. 45 degrees medial rotation

68. Which projection of the ankle should be performed to best demonstrate a ligamentous tear?

   a. AP projection with inversion
   b. AP projection with dorsiflexion
   c. AP oblique projection (lateral rotation)
   d. AP oblique projection (medial rotation)

69. Which projection of the knee best demonstrates the femorotibial joint space open if the patient measures more than 24 cm between the ASIS and the tabletop?

   a. AP oblique projection (medial rotation)
   b. AP projection with perpendicular central ray
   c. AP projection with the central ray angled 3 to 5 degrees caudad
   d. AP projection with the central ray angled 3 to 5 degrees cephalad

70. For the lateral projection of the knee, how many degrees should the knee be flexed?

   a. 10 to 20 degrees
   b. 20 to 30 degrees
   c. 30 to 40 degrees
   d. 40 to 50 degrees

71. With reference to the knee, where should the image receptor be centered for the PA axial projection (Holmblad method) of the knee?

   a. To the apex of the patella
   b. To the most superior point of the patella
   c. 2 inches (5 cm) below the apex of the patella
   d. 2 inches (5 cm) above the femorotibial joint space

72. How many degrees of angulation should be formed between the femur and the radiographic table for the PA axial projection (Holmblad method) of the knee?

   a. 20 degrees
   b. 45 degrees
   c. 70 degrees
   d. 90 degrees

73. Which of the following projections of the knee best demonstrates the intercondylar fossa?

   a. AP projection
   b. Lateral projection
   c. AP oblique projection (medial rotation)
   d. PA axial projection (Holmblad method)

74. How many degrees and in what direction should the central ray be directed for the lateral projection of the knee?

   a. Perpendicular
   b. 5 to 7 degrees caudad
   c. 5 to 7 degrees cephalad
   d. 10 degrees cephalad

75. Which structure of the knee is best demonstrated with the tangential projection?

    a. Patella
    b. Intercondylar fossa
    c. Joint space of the knee
    d. Intercondylar eminence

76. Which structure of the knee is best demonstrated with the PA axial projection (the Holmblad method)?

    a. Patella
    b. Tibial crest
    c. Tibiofibular articulation
    d. Femoral intercondylar fossa

77. Which projection of the knee best demonstrates the proximal tibiofibular articulation without bony superimposition?

    a. AP projection
    b. Lateral projection
    c. AP oblique projection (lateral rotation)
    d. AP oblique projection (medial rotation)

78. Which projection of the knee best demonstrates the femoropatellar space open?

    a. Lateral projection
    b. AP oblique projection (lateral rotation)
    c. AP oblique projection (medial rotation)
    d. PA axial projection (the Holmblad method)

79. Which of the following evaluation criteria indicates that the knee is properly positioned for a lateral projection?

    a. The femoral condyles are superimposed.
    b. The proximal tibiofibular articulation is open.
    c. The patella is parallel with the image receptor.
    d. The femoral condyles are parallel with the image receptor.

80. What should be done to prevent the knee joint space from being obscured by the magnified shadow of the medial femoral condyle when the lateral projection of the knee is performed?

    a. Use foam wedges to support the leg.
    b. Direct the central ray perpendicularly.
    c. Direct the central ray 5 to 7 degrees cephalad.
    d. Decrease the source-to-image receptor distance.

81. Which of the following evaluation criteria indicates that the knee is properly positioned for the AP projection?

    a. The femorotibial joint space is open.
    b. The femoral condyles are perpendicular.
    c. The proximal tibiofibular articulation is open.
    d. The patella is perpendicular to the image receptor.

82. Where should the patella be demonstrated on the radiograph of the AP oblique projection of the knee with medial rotation?

    a. Over the lateral condyle of the femur
    b. Over the medial condyle of the femur
    c. Centered between the femoral condyles
    d. Superimposed with the tibiofibular articulation

83. Where should the patella be demonstrated on the radiograph of the AP oblique projection of the knee with lateral rotation?

    a. Over the lateral femoral condyle
    b. Over the medial femoral condyle
    c. Centered between the femoral condyles
    d. Superimposed with the femorotibial joint

84. For the lateral projection of the patella, which positioning maneuver reduces the femoropatellar joint space?

    a. Straightening the leg
    b. Superimposing the tibial condyles
    c. Superimposing the femoral condyles
    d. Flexing the knee more than 10 degrees

85. Which area of the knee should the central ray enter for the PA axial projection (Holmblad method)?

    a. Anterior
    b. Posterior
    c. Lateral condyle
    d. Medial condyle

86. Which of the following projections of the knee best demonstrates the femoral intercondylar fossa?

    a. AP projection
    b. Lateral projection
    c. AP oblique projection (medial rotation)
    d. PA axial projection (Camp-Coventry method)

87. Which projection of the knee should be used to demonstrate the patella completely superimposed on the femur?

    a. AP projection
    b. Lateral projection
    c. AP oblique projection (lateral rotation)
    d. AP oblique projection (medial rotation)

88. Which projection of the knee should be used to demonstrate the patella in profile?

    a. AP projection
    b. Lateral projection
    c. AP oblique projection (lateral rotation)
    d. AP oblique projection (medial rotation)

89. For a patient prone on the radiographic table with the knee centered to the midline and the knee flexed until the lower leg forms a 40-degree angle with the table, how should the central ray be directed to demonstrate the femoral inter-condylar fossa?

    a. Caudally 3 to 5 degrees
    b. Cephalically 3 to 5 degrees
    c. Caudally 40 degrees
    d. Cephalically 40 degrees

90. For which projection of the knee should the patient be prone on the table, with the knee flexed until the leg forms an angle of 40 degrees with the table, and the central ray directed perpendicular to the long axis of the leg, entering the back side of the knee?

    a. Tangential projection (Settegast method)
    b. PA oblique projection (medial rotation)
    c. PA axial projection (Holmblad method)
    d. PA axial projection (Camp-Coventry method)

91. How should the central ray be directed for the bilateral weight-bearing AP projection of the knees?

    a. Perpendicularly
    b. Caudally 3 to 5 degrees
    c. Cephalically 3 to 5 degrees
    d. Cephalically 10 degrees

92. Which projection of the knee can be accomplished with the patient upright, the affected knee flexed and its anterior surface in contact with a vertically placed image receptor, and the horizontally directed central ray entering the posterior aspect of the knee?

    a. Tangential projection (Settegast method)
    b. AP projection, weight-bearing
    c. PA axial projection (Holmblad method)
    d. PA axial projection (Camp-Coventry method)

93. Which positioning factor determines the number of degrees the central ray should be angled for the tangential projection (Settegast method) to demonstrate the patella?

    a. Part thickness
    b. Degree of knee flexion
    c. Object-to-image distance
    d. Source-to-image receptor distance

94. How should the central ray be directed for the AP projection of the femur?

    a. Perpendicularly
    b. Caudally 3 to 5 degrees
    c. Cephalically 3 to 5 degrees
    d. Cephalically 15 degrees

95. Which positioning maneuver should be performed to place the femoral neck in profile for the AP projection of the femur?

    a. Flex the lower limb.
    b. Rotate the lower limb laterally 10 to 15 degrees.
    c. Rotate the lower limb medially 10 to 15 degrees.
    d. Elevate the unaffected side of the pelvis 10 to 15 degrees.

96. Which positioning maneuver should be performed to prevent the femoral neck from appearing foreshortened in the AP projection of the femur?

    a. Angle the central ray 10 to 15 degrees caudad.
    b. Angle the central ray 10 to 15 degrees cephalad.
    c. Rotate the lower limb laterally 10 to 15 degrees.
    d. Rotate the lower limb medially 10 to 15 degrees.

97. For the AP projection of the femur on typical adults, what should be done to ensure that both joints of the femur are demonstrated?

    a. Rotate the lower limb laterally 15 degrees.
    b. Increase the source-to-image receptor distance.
    c. Use lead masking to divide the image receptor in half.
    d. Perform a second exposure with another image receptor.

98. For which lower limb projection should the lower limb be rotated medially 10 to 15 degrees?

    a. AP projection of the femur
    b. Lateral projection of the femur
    c. AP medial oblique projection of the foot
    d. AP medial oblique projection of the knee

99. For which lower limb projection should the pelvis be rotated 10 to 15 degrees from true lateral?

    a. AP projection of the leg
    b. AP projection of the femur
    c. Lateral projection of the leg
    d. Lateral projection of the femur

100. For the lateral projection of the femur, how should the pelvis be positioned to demonstrate only the knee joint with the distal femoral shaft?

    a. True lateral
    b. From supine, unaffected side elevated 15 degrees
    c. From true lateral, rotated anteriorly 10 to 15 degrees
    d. From true lateral, rotated posteriorly 10 to 15 degrees

CHAPTER 7

Pelvis and Upper Femora

SECTION 1

Osteology and Arthrology of the Pelvis and Upper Femora

Exercise 1

Instructions: Identify each lettered structure shown in Fig. 7-1.

A. _____

B. _____

C. _____

D. _____

E. _____

F. _____

G. _____

H. _____

I. _____

J. _____

K. _____

L. _____

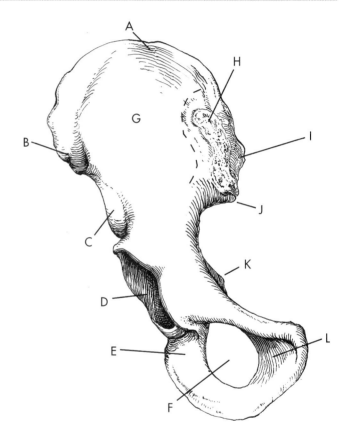

Figure 7-1 Anterior aspect of the right os coxae (hip bone).

Exercise 2

Instructions: Identify each lettered structure shown in Fig. 7-2.

A. _____

B. _____

C. _____

D. _____

E. _____

F. _____

G. _____

H. _____

I. _____

J. _____

K. _____

L. _____

M. _____

N. _____

O. _____

P. _____

Q. _____

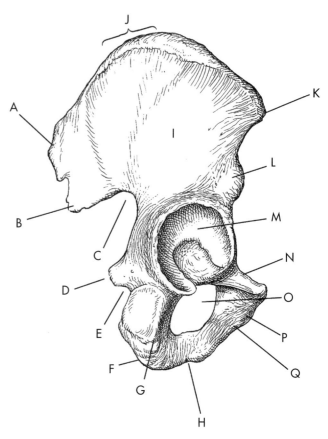

Figure 7-2 Lateral aspect of the right os coxae (hip bone).

Exercise 3

Instructions: Identify each lettered structure shown in Fig. 7-3.

A. _____

B. _____

C. _____

D. _____

E. _____

F. _____

G. _____

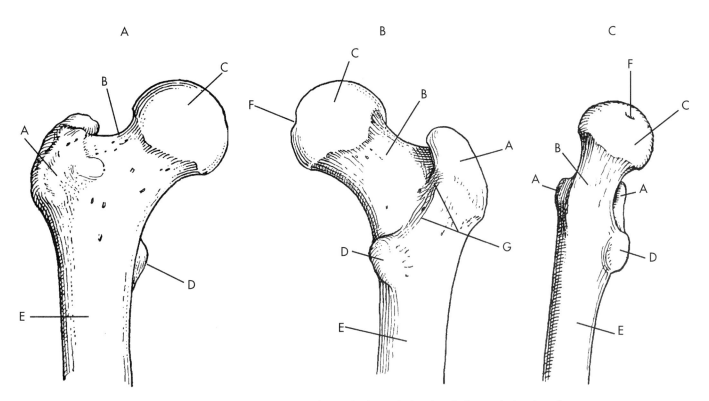

Figure 7-3 Three views of the proximal femur. **A,** the anterior view. **B,** the posterior view. **C,** a view of the medial aspect.

Exercise 4

Instructions: Identify each lettered structure shown in Fig. 7-4.

A. _____   H. _____

B. _____   I. _____

C. _____   J. _____

D. _____   K. _____

E. _____   L. _____

F. _____   M. _____

G. _____   N. _____

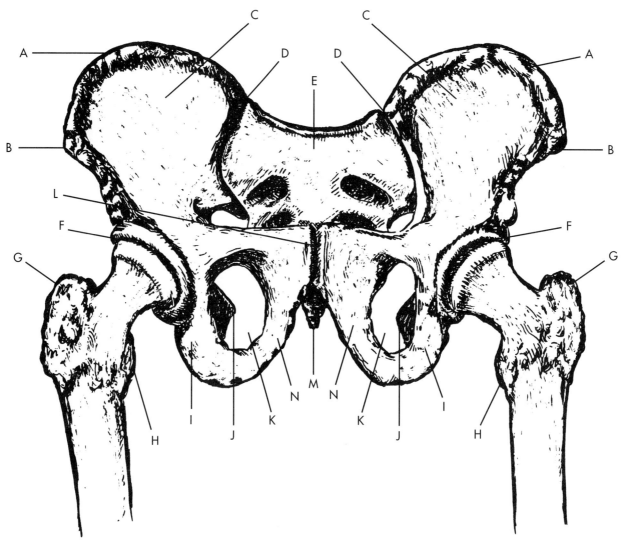

Figure 7-4 Anterior view of the pelvis and upper femora.

Exercise 5

Instructions: Use the following clues to complete the crossword puzzle. All answers refer to the bones and joints of the pelvis.

ACROSS

2. Femoral process
4. Serves as a base for the trunk
8. Inferior process
9. Posterior pelvic articulations
13. Large opening
14. Ridgelike process
16. Hip bone
18. Projects from the pubic bone

DOWN

1. Superior process
3. Hip socket
5. Articulation
6. Forms posterior aspect of pelvis
7. Found above the acetabulum
10. Opening in bone
11. Articulates with the sacrum
12. Has a body and two rami
15. Sharp bony process
17. Winglike portion of ilium

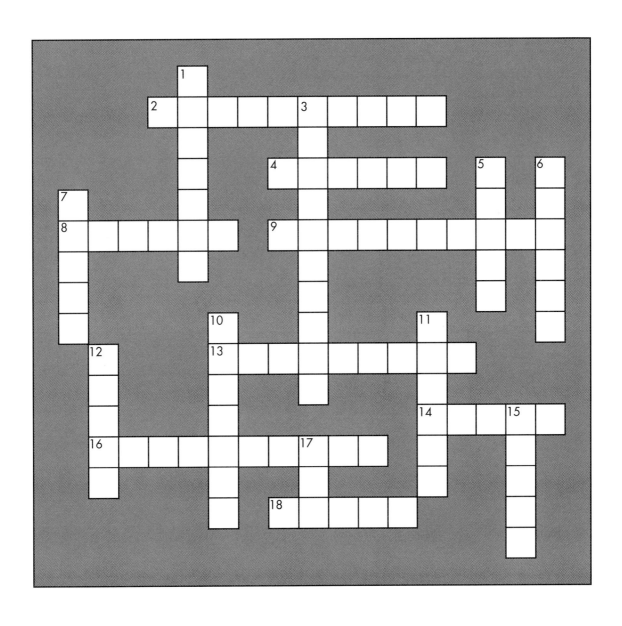

Exercise 6

Match the pathology terms in Column A with the appropriate definition in Column B. Not all choices from Column B should be selected.

Column A

_____ 1. Osteoporosis

_____ 2. Osteopetrosis

_____ 3. Osteoarthritis

_____ 4. Paget's disease

_____ 5. Chondrosarcoma

_____ 6. Slipped epiphysis

_____ 7. Multiple myeloma

_____ 8. Ankylosing spondylitis

_____ 9. Congenital hip dysplasia

_____ 10. Legg-Calve-Perthes disease

Column B

a. Loss of bone density

b. Benign tumor consisting of cartilage

c. Increased density of atypically soft bone

d. Malignant tumor arising from cartilage cells

e. Thick, soft bone marked by bowing and fractures

f. Flattening of the femoral head due to vascular interruption

g. Rheumatoid arthritis variant involving the sacroiliac (SI) joints and spine

h. Malformation of the acetabulum causing displacement of the femoral head

i. Proximal portion of femur dislocated from distal portion at the proximal epiphysis

j. Form of arthritis marked by progressive cartilage deterioration in synovial joints and vertebrae

k. Malignant neoplasm of plasma cells involving the bone marrow and causing destruction of bone

Exercise 7

Instructions: This exercise is a comprehensive review of the osteology and arthrology of the pelvis and the proximal femur. Fill in missing words, provide a short answer, select the answer from a list, or choose true or false (explaining any statement you believe to be false) for each item.

1. The structure of the body that serves as a base for the trunk and as a girdle for the attachment of the lower limbs is

   known as the _____.

2. Which bones form the pelvis?
   a. Two hip bones only
   b. Two hip bones and sacrum only
   c. Two hip bones, sacrum, and coccyx only
   d. Two hip bones, sacrum, coccyx, and femurs

3. Which three names refer to the major bone that makes up the right or left half of the pelvis?
   a. Ilium, hip bone, and ischium
   b. Ilium, pubis, and innominate
   c. Os coxae, pubis, and ischium
   d. Os coxae, hip bone, and innominate

4. Which two prominent structures found on the ilium are frequently used as radiographic positioning reference points?
   a. Iliac crest and inferior superior iliac spine
   b. Iliac crest and anterior superior iliac spine
   c. Symphysis pubis and inferior superior iliac spine
   d. Symphysis pubis and anterior superior iliac spine

5. Which bone/portion of the hip bone consists of a body and two rami?
   a. Ala
   b. Ilium
   c. Pubis
   d. Ischium

6. Which bone/portion of the hip bone extends inferiorly from the acetabulum and joins with the inferior ramus of the pubic bone?
   a. Ilium
   b. Pubis
   c. Ischium
   d. Acetabulum

7. What part of the hip bone forms the broad, curved portion called the ala?

8. What bones of the hip bone form the obturator foramen?

9. What structure of the hip bone is formed by the fusion of three bones?

10. What structures form the posterior part of the pelvis?

11. Name the two parts a pelvis is divided into by the brim of the pelvis.

12. With reference to the brim of the pelvis, identify the location of the greater (false) pelvis and the lesser (true) pelvis as either "above" or "below."

    a. Greater pelvis: _____

    b. Lesser pelvis: _____

13. The region between the inlet and the outlet of the true

    pelvis is called the _____

    _____.

14. Which gender—male or female—has a pelvis with larger and more rounded outlet?

15. Which gender—male or female—has a broader and shallower pelvis?

16. Which two large processes are located at the proximal end of the femur?

    a. Greater tubercle and lesser tubercle
    b. Greater tubercle and lesser trochanter
    c. Greater trochanter and lesser tubercle
    d. Greater trochanter and lesser trochanter

17. Which process is located at the superolateral aspect of the proximal femoral shaft?

    a. Lesser tubercle
    b. Lesser trochanter
    c. Greater tubercle
    d. Greater trochanter

18. Name the two areas of the proximal femur that are common sites for fractures in elderly patients.

19. In a typical adult, in which direction—anterior or posterior—does the femoral neck project away from the long axis of the femur?

20. Identify the major articulations of the pelvis and give the quantity for each.

21. What are the two palpable bony points of localization for the hip joint?

22. Describe how to use the two points identified in question 21 to locate the femoral neck.

23. True or False. The greater sciatic notch is located on the anterior border of the ilium.

24. True or False. In the seated position, the weight of the body rests on two ischial tuberosities.

25. True or False. The highest point of the greater trochanter is in the same transverse plane as the midpoint of the hip joint.

SECTION 2

Positioning of the Pelvis and Upper Femora

Exercise 1: Positioning for the Pelvis

Instructions: The anteroposterior (AP) projection of the pelvis demonstrates the pelvic girdle and the head, neck, trochanters, and upper third or fourth of the shaft of the femora. This exercise pertains to the AP projection of the pelvis. Provide a short answer, select the answer from a list, or identify structures for each item.

1. Describe how the patient's lower limbs should be positioned.

2. Why should the patient's lower limbs be rotated medially?

3. How can it be determined that a pelvis has not been rotated when the patient is positioned for the AP projection?

   a. Ask the patient to ensure he or she is comfortable.
   b. Ensure that the lower limbs are fully extended and rotated medially 15 degrees.
   c. Ensure that the distance from the ASIS to the tabletop on each side of the pelvis is the same.

4. Which plane of the body should be positioned on the midline of the table and grid?

   a. Horizontal
   b. Midsagittal
   c. Midcoronal

5. With reference to the patient, where should the image receptor be centered?

6. With reference to the patient, where should the upper border of the image receptor be placed when the patient has a deep pelvis?

7. State how and where the central ray should be directed.

8. Examine the AP images in Figs. 7-5 and 7-6 and answer the questions that follow.

a. Which structures in these two images appear different?

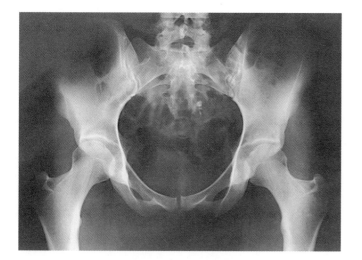

Figure 7-5 AP pelvis.

b. Which image demonstrates correct positioning of the upper femora? State the image characteristics that lead you to believe the patient was properly positioned for that image.

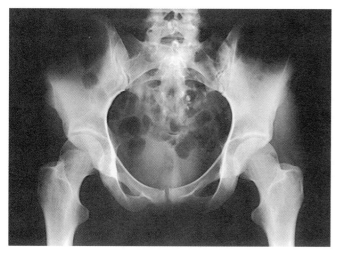

Figure 7-6 AP pelvis.

c. Describe how the lower limbs were positioned in Fig. 7-5.

d. Describe how the lower limbs were positioned in Fig. 7-6.

9. From the following list, circle the 11 evaluation criteria that indicate the pelvis was properly positioned for an AP projection.

 a. The iliac alae should be symmetric.

 b. The obturator foramina should be symmetric.

 c. The ischial spines should be equally demonstrated.

 d. The greater trochanters should be fully demonstrated.

 e. Both ilia should be equidistant to the edge of the radiograph.

 f. The entire pelvis should be included along with the proximal femurs.

 g. The sacrum and coccyx should be aligned with the symphysis pubis.

 h. The lower vertebral column should be centered to the middle of the radiograph.

 i. Both greater trochanters should be equidistant to the edge of the radiograph.

 j. Each greater trochanter should be seen superimposed with the femoral neck.

 k. The femoral necks should be demonstrated in their full extent without superimposition.

 l. The femoral necks should not be well demonstrated to their full extent because of superimposition.

 m. If seen, the lesser trochanters should be demonstrated on the lateral borders of the femurs.

 n. If seen, the lesser trochanters should be demonstrated on the medial borders of the femurs.

10. Identify each lettered structure shown in Fig. 7-7.

 A. _____

 B. _____

 C. _____

 D. _____

 E. _____

 F. _____

 G. _____

 H. _____

 I. _____

 J. _____

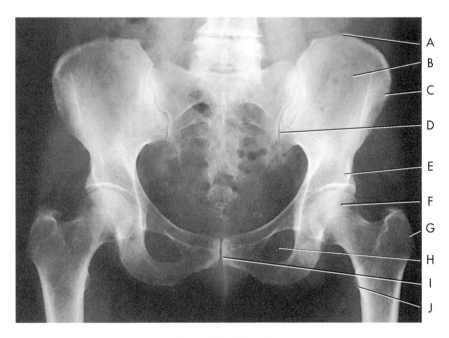

Figure 7-7 AP pelvis

Exercise 2: AP Oblique Projection (Modified Cleaves Method)

Instructions: The AP oblique projection is often performed to compare both upper femora with one projection. This exercise pertains to the AP oblique projection. Provide a short answer, select the answer from a list, or choose true or false (explaining any statement you believe to be false) for each item.

Examine Fig. 7-8 as you answer the following questions.

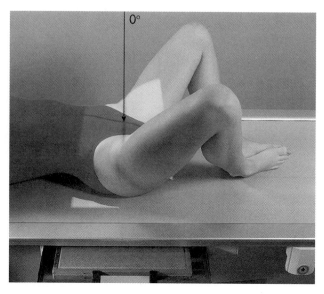

Figure 7-8 AP oblique femoral necks, modified Cleaves method.

1. What other name commonly refers to the AP oblique projection, modified Cleaves method?

2. How much should the hips and knees be flexed?

3. After the patient's knees and hips are flexed, how many degrees from vertical should the thighs be abducted?

4. What is the purpose of abducting the thighs as required?

5. What breathing instructions should be given to the patient?

6. Describe how and where the central ray should be directed.

7. Where should each lesser trochanter appear in the image?
   a. Superimposed on the femur
   b. On the lateral side of the femur
   c. On the medial side of the femur

8. True or False. The patient may be positioned either supine or upright.

9. True or False. The gonads should not be shielded for the AP oblique projection.

10. True or False. The image receptor size should be 35 cm × 43 cm.

11. True or False. The IR should be placed on the tabletop.

12. True or False. The IR should be positioned crosswise.

13. True or False. The AP oblique projection should not be performed on a patient who is suspected of having a fractured femoral neck.

14. True or False. The greater trochanter should be seen in profile on the lateral side of the proximal femur.

15. True or False. This projection can be modified to demonstrate only one hip area.

Exercise 3: Projections for Demonstrating the Hip

Instructions: A typical radiographic series demonstrating the hip structures usually includes the AP projection and either the lateral projection or an axiolateral projection. This exercise pertains to those projections. Identify structures, provide a short answer, select from a list, or choose true or false (explaining any statement you believe to be false) for each item.

Examine Fig. 7-9 as you answer the following items. Items 1 through 10 pertain to the *AP projection.*

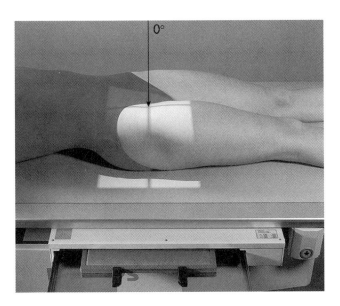

Figure 7-9 AP hip.

1. Why should a radiographer ensure that the distance from the ASIS to the tabletop on each side of the pelvis is the same?
   a. To ensure that the pelvis is not rotated
   b. To align the midsagittal plane to the midline of the table
   c. To demonstrate the lesser trochanter beyond the medial border of the femur

2. Which positioning maneuver should be performed to place the femoral neck parallel with the plane of the image receptor?
   a. Abduct the femur laterally 15 to 20 degrees.
   b. Abduct the femur medially 15 to 20 degrees.
   c. Rotate the foot and lower limb laterally 15 to 20 degrees.
   d. Rotate the foot and lower limb medially 15 to 20 degrees.

3. What procedure should help the patient keep the affected lower leg in the required position?
   a. Place a compression band across the pelvis.
   b. Place a foam cushion or folded blanket under the pelvis.
   c. Place a support under the knee and a sandbag across the ankle.

4. Describe how to find the centering point where the central ray should enter the patient.

5. With reference to the patient, where should the image receptor be centered?

6. Which trochanter—greater or lesser—is not usually demonstrated beyond the border of the femur?

7. True or False. The entire pubis of the affected side should be demonstrated.

8. True or False. The exposure should be performed with the patient breathing shallowly.

9. True or False. An initial radiographic study of a fractured hip may include an AP projection of the pelvic girdle and proximal femora to demonstrate bilateral hip joints.

10. Identify each lettered structure shown in Fig. 7-10.

A. _____

B. _____

C. _____

D. _____

E. _____

F. _____

G. _____

H. _____

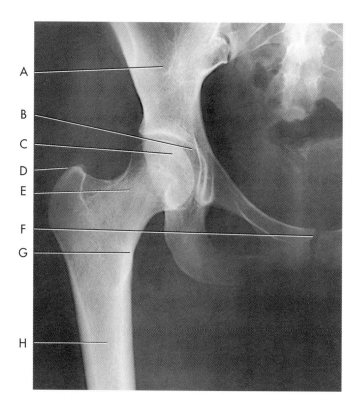

Figure 7-10 AP hip.

Examine Fig. 7-11 as you answer the following questions. Items 11 through 17 pertain to the *Lauenstein method and Hickey method for lateral projections.*

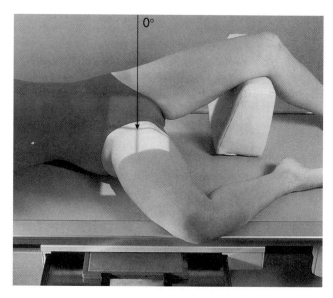

Figure 7-11 Mediolateral hip, Lauenstein method.

11. A lateral projection radiograph obtained by the Lauenstein method or the Hickey method is used to demonstrate the hip joint and the relationship of the head of the femur with the _____.

    a. Acetabulum
    b. Femoral shaft
    c. Greater trochanter

12. Describe how the affected thigh and leg should be positioned for lateral projections of the hip.

13. Describe how the unaffected lower limb should be positioned.

14. With reference to the patient, where should the IR be centered?

15. How should the central ray be directed for the Lauenstein method of a lateral hip projection?

    a. Perpendicularly
    b. Caudally 20 to 25 degrees
    c. Medially 20 to 25 degrees
    d. Cephalically 20 to 25 degrees

16. How should the central ray be directed for the Hickey method of a lateral hip projection?

    a. Perpendicularly
    b. Caudally 20 to 25 degrees
    c. Medially 20 to 25 degrees
    d. Cephalically 20 to 25 degrees

17. Identify each lettered structure shown in Fig. 7-12.

    A. _____

    B. _____

    C. _____

    D. _____

    E. _____

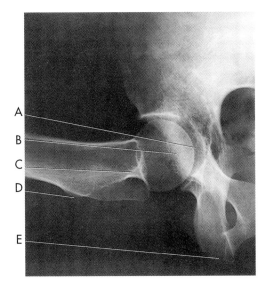

Figure 7-12 Mediolateral hip, Lauenstein method.

Examine Fig. 7-13 as you answer the following questions. Items 18 through 30 pertain to the *axiolateral projection, Danelius-Miller modification of the Lorenz method.*

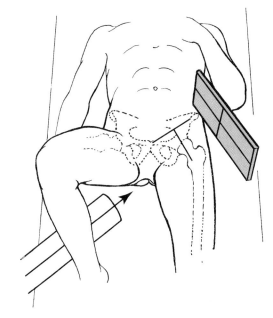

Figure 7-13 Axiolateral hip, Danelius-Miller modification.

18. Describe an acceptable method for locating the femoral neck.

19. Why should a firm pillow or folded blanket be placed under the pelvis?

20. Describe how the unaffected lower limb should be positioned.

21. Describe the placement of the image receptor.

22. Describe how and where the central ray should be directed.

23. With reference to the femoral neck, how should the lead strips of the grid be placed?

   a. Horizontally, parallel with the long axis of the femoral neck
   b. Vertically, perpendicular with the long axis of the femoral neck

24. What breathing instructions should be given to the patient?

   a. Breathe slowly and deeply.
   b. Stop breathing for the exposure.

25. What is the general rule concerning demonstration of any orthopedic appliance with this projection?

   a. Any orthopedic appliance should be completely demonstrated.
   b. Ensure that the orthopedic appliance does not overly the acetabulum.

26. True or False. The pelvis should be rotated approximately 15 to 20 degrees.

27. True or False. The foot and lower limb should be rotated laterally 15 to 20 degrees.

28. True or False. The entire lesser trochanter should be demonstrated on the lateral surface of the femur.

29. True or False. A small area of soft-tissue overlap from the thigh of the unaffected lower limb is permitted.

30. Identify each lettered structure shown in Fig. 7-14.

   A. _____

   B. _____

   C. _____

   D. _____

   E. _____

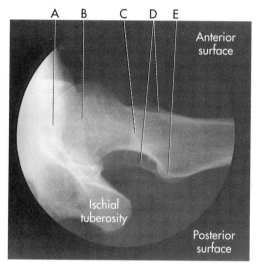

Figure 7-14 Axiolateral hip, Danelius-Miller modification.

Self-Test: Osteology, Arthrology, and Positioning of the Pelvis and Upper Femora

Instructions: Answer the following questions by selecting the best choice.

1. Which structure of the pelvis articulates with the femur?
   a. Acetabulum
   b. Inferior aperture
   c. Auricular surface
   d. Obturator foramen

2. Which bones of the pelvis compose the acetabulum?
   a. Ilium and pubis only
   b. Ilium and ischium only
   c. Pubis and ischium only
   d. Pubis, ischium, and ilium

3. On which bone is the ala located?
   a. Ilium
   b. Pubis
   c. Femur
   d. Ischium

4. Which of the following pelvic structures is not used as a positioning palpation point?
   a. Iliac crest
   b. Ischial spine
   c. Pubic symphysis
   d. Anterior superior iliac spine

5. Which portions of the hip bone join to form the obturator foramen?
   a. Ilium and pubis only
   b. Ilium and ischium only
   c. Pubis and ischium only
   d. Pubis, ischium, and ilium

6. What is the name of the border that extends on the hip bone from the posterior superior iliac spine to the anterior superior iliac spine?
   a. Iliac crest
   b. Greater sciatic notch
   c. Iliac auricular surface
   d. Brim of the lesser pelvis

7. What is the name of the process that separates the greater sciatic notch from the lesser sciatic notch on the hip bone?
   a. Ischial spine
   b. Ischial ramus
   c. Inferior ramus of the pubis
   d. Superior ramus of the pubis

8. Which parts of the hip bones support the weight of the body when a person is in the sitting position?
   a. Ischial spines
   b. Ischial tuberosities
   c. Inferior rami of the pubes
   d. Posterior inferior iliac spines

9. Where in the pelvis is the body of the pubis located?
   a. It forms part of the acetabulum.
   b. It forms part of the symphysis pubis.
   c. It is between the inferior and superior rami of the pubis.
   d. It is between the ischial ramus and the inferior ramus of the pubis.

10. Where should the image receptor be centered for the AP projection of the pelvis?
    a. To the level of the iliac crest
    b. To the level of the pubic symphysis
    c. 2 inches (5 cm) below the greater trochanter
    d. Midway between the ASIS and the pubic symphysis

11. Where on the midline of the patient should the central ray enter for the AP projection of the pelvis?
    a. 2 inches (5 cm) above the iliac crest
    b. 2 inches (5 cm) above the pubic symphysis
    c. At the level of the anterior superior iliac spines
    d. 2 inches (5 cm) above the level of the anterior superior iliac spines

12. Which positioning maneuver should be performed to place the femoral necks parallel with the IR for an AP projection of the pelvis?
    a. Rotate the lower limbs laterally 15 to 20 degrees.
    b. Rotate the lower limbs medially 15 to 20 degrees.
    c. Flex the hips 15 to 20 degrees and extend the lower limbs.
    d. Flex the hips and abduct the femurs laterally 15 to 20 degrees.

13. How should the central ray be directed for the AP oblique projection (modified Cleaves method) to demonstrate bilateral hips?
    a. Perpendicularly
    b. Cephalically 20 degrees
    c. Cephalically 40 degrees
    d. Parallel with the long axis of the femurs

14. For which projection of the lower limbs or pelvis should the hips be flexed and the femurs be abducted from the midline of the patient?

    a. AP projection of the hip
    b. AP projection of the pelvis
    c. AP oblique projection (modified Cleaves method) for femoral necks
    d. Axiolateral projection (Danelius-Miller modification of the Lorenz method) of the hip

15. Where on the midline of the patient should the central ray be directed for the AP oblique projection (modified Cleaves method)?

    a. To the level of the iliac crests
    b. 1 inch (2.5 cm) above the symphysis pubis
    c. To the level of the anterior superior iliac spines
    d. 2 inches (5 cm) above the anterior superior iliac spines

16. Which projection of the hip or pelvis should not be performed if the patient is suspected to have an intertrochanteric fracture?

    a. AP projection of the hip
    b. AP projection of the pelvis
    c. Lateral projection (Lauenstein method) of the hip
    d. Axiolateral projection (Danelius-Miller modification of the Lorenz method) of the hip

17. For the AP oblique projection (modified Cleaves method), what is the purpose of abducting the femurs the required number of degrees?

    a. To position the pelvis in the true lateral position
    b. To prevent superimposing the acetabulum with the pelvis
    c. To position the femoral necks parallel with the image receptor
    d. To prevent superimposing the femoral head with the acetabulum

18. Which structure should be centered to the midline of the table when the AP oblique projection (modified Cleaves method) is adapted to demonstrate only one hip?

    a. Femoral body
    b. Symphysis pubis
    c. Greater trochanter
    d. Anterior superior iliac spine

19. For which projection of an individual hip should the unaffected hip be flexed and the thigh be raised out of the way of the central ray?

    a. AP projection
    b. Lateral projection (Lauenstein method)
    c. AP oblique projection (modified Cleaves method)
    d. Axiolateral projection (Danelius-Miller modification of the Lorenz method)

20. For which projection of the hip should the central ray be directed horizontally into the medial aspect of the affected thigh?

    a. AP projection
    b. Lateral projection (Lauenstein method)
    c. AP oblique projection (modified Cleaves method)
    d. Axiolateral projection (Danelius-Miller modification, of the Lorenz method)

CHAPTER 8

Vertebral Column

SECTION 1

Osteology and Arthrology of the Vertebral Column

Exercise 1

Instructions: Refer to Fig. 8-1 and match the vertebral curvatures listed in Column A with the characteristic or classification terms in Column B. Each curvature will have three terms associated with it. Terms will be used more than once.

Column A

_____ ____ ____ 1. Cervical

_____ ____ ____ 2. Thoracic

_____ ____ ____ 3. Lumbar

_____ ____ ____ 4. Pelvic

Column B

a. Primary curve

b. Secondary curve

c. Lordotic curve

d. Kyphotic curve

e. Convex anteriorly

f. Concave anteriorly

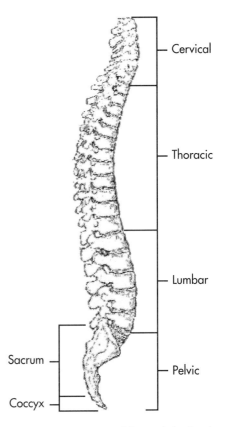

Figure 8-1 Lateral aspect of the vertebral column.

Exercise 2

Instructions: Examine Fig. 8-2 and identify the abnormal curvatures of the vertebral column.

1. Identify each abnormal curvature shown in Fig. 8-2.

   A. _____

   B. _____

   C. _____

Exercise 3

Instructions: This exercise pertains to the cervical vertebrae. Identify structures for each question.

1. Identify each lettered structure shown in Fig. 8-3.

   A. _____

   B. _____

   C. _____

   D. _____

   E. _____

   F. _____

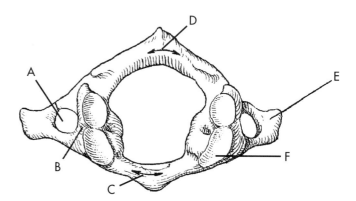

Figure 8-3 Superior aspect of atlas (C1).

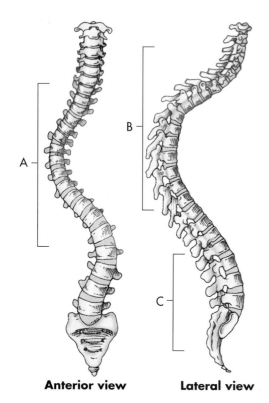

Figure 8-2 Two views of the vertebral column showing abnormal curvatures.

2. Identify each lettered structure shown in Fig. 8-4.

A. _____

B. _____

C. _____

D. _____

E. _____

3. Identify each lettered structure shown in Fig. 8-5.

A. _____

B. _____

C. _____

D. _____

E. _____

F. _____

G. _____

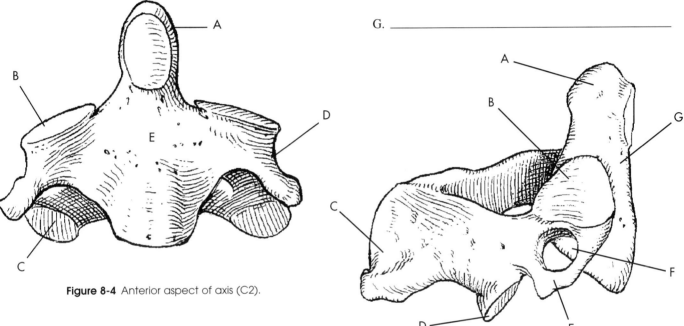

Figure 8-4 Anterior aspect of axis (C2).

Figure 8-5 Lateral aspect of axis (C2).

4. Identify each lettered structure shown in Fig. 8-6.

A. _____   E. _____

B. _____   F. _____

C. _____   G. _____

D. _____   H. _____

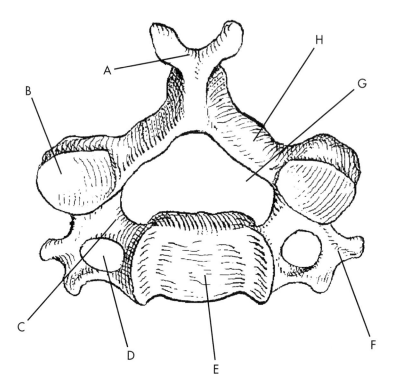

Figure 8-6 Superior aspect of a typical cervical vertebra.

5. Identify each lettered structure shown in Fig. 8-7.

A. _____

B. _____

C. _____

D. _____

E. _____

F. _____

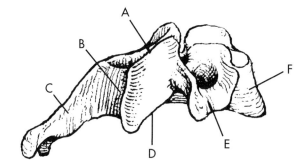

Figure 8-7 Lateral aspect of a typical cervical vertebra.

Exercise 4

Instructions: This exercise pertains to the thoracic vertebrae. Identify structures for each question.

1. Identify each lettered structure shown in Fig. 8-8.

   A. _____

   B. _____

   C. _____

   D. _____

   E. _____

   F. _____

   G. _____

   H. _____

   I. _____

2. Identify each lettered structure shown in Fig. 8-9.

   A. _____

   B. _____

   C. _____

   D. _____

   E. _____

   F. _____

   G. _____

   H. _____

   I. _____

   J. _____

   K. _____

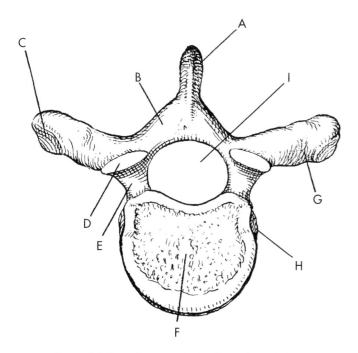

Figure 8-8 Superior aspect of a thoracic vertebra.

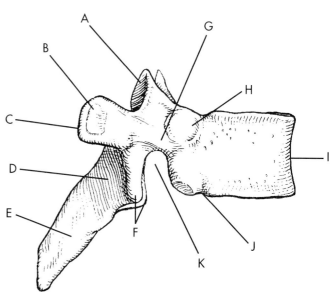

Figure 8-9 Lateral aspect of a thoracic vertebra.

Exercise 5

Instructions: This exercise pertains to the lumbar vertebrae. Identify structures for each question.

1. Identify each lettered structure shown in Fig. 8-10.

A. _____

B. _____

C. _____

D. _____

E. _____

F. _____

G. _____

H. _____

I. _____

2. Identify each lettered structure shown in Fig. 8-11.

A. _____

B. _____

C. _____

D. _____

E. _____

F. _____

G. _____

H. _____

I. _____

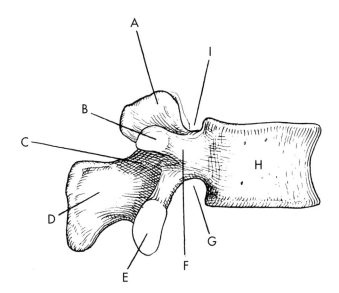

Figure 8-11 Lateral aspect of a lumbar vertebra.

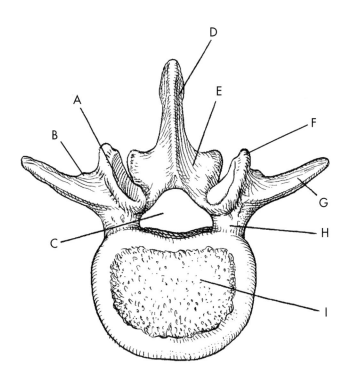

Figure 8-10 Superior aspect of a lumbar vertebra.

Exercise 6

Instructions: This exercise pertains to the sacrum and coccyx. Identify structures for each question.

1. Identify each lettered structure shown in Fig. 8-12.

   A. _____

   B. _____

   C. _____

   D. _____

   E. _____

   F. _____

2. Identify each lettered structure shown in Fig. 8-13.

   A. _____

   B. _____

   C. _____

   D. _____

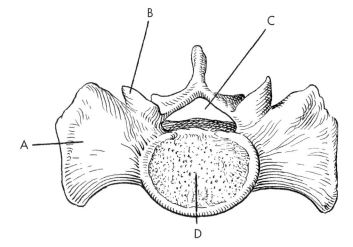

Figure 8-13 Base of the sacrum.

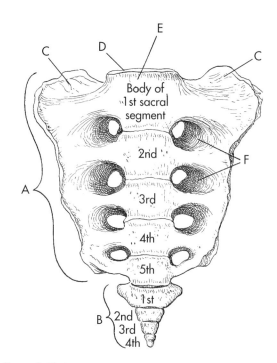

Figure 8-12 Anterior aspect of the sacrum and coccyx.

Exercise 7

Instructions: Use the following clues to complete the crossword puzzle. All answers refer to the vertebral column.

ACROSS

3. Thoracic depressions
6. C2 name
8. Number of cervical vertebrae
10. Articular processes
12. Holds up the skull
13. Articulates with thoracic vertebrae
15. Lumbar curvature
17. Forms posterior vertebral arch
20. Two tips
21. Inferior to the sacrum
22. Between thoracic and sacrum

DOWN

1. Number of lumbar vertebrae
2. Extends posteriorly from a vertebral body
4. Lateral vertebral curvature
5. Cylindrical vertebral portion
6. Occipitocervical joint
7. Most superior vertebrae
9. Thoracic curvature
11. Just below cervical
14. Odontoid process
16. Number of thoracic vertebrae
18. Vertebral cartilage pad
19. Articulates with both ilia

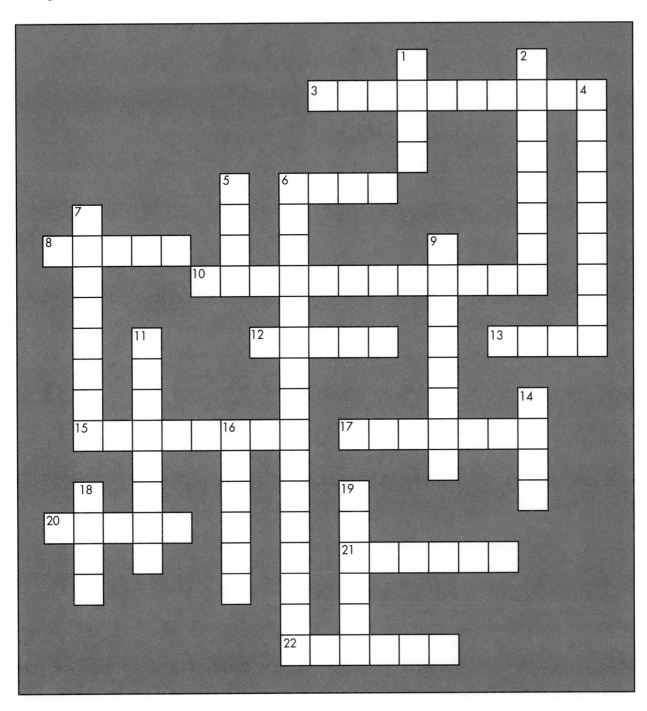

Exercise 8

Instructions: Match the parts of the vertebra listed in Column A with the descriptions in Column B.

Column A

____ 1. Body

____ 2. Laminae

____ 3. Pedicles

____ 4. Zygapophyses

____ 5. Spinous process

____ 6. Transverse process

Column B

a. Process extending laterally and posteriorly from the body

b. Process extending posteriorly from the junction of both laminae

c. Process extending laterally from the pedicle-lamina junction

d. Articular processes

e. Solid anterior part of a vertebra

f. Connects the transverse process with the spinous process

Exercise 9

Match the pathology terms in Column A with the appropriate definition in Column B. Not all choices from Column B should be selected.

Column A

_____ 1. Tumor

_____ 2. Fracture

_____ 3. Lordosis

_____ 4. Scoliosis

_____ 5. Kyphosis

_____ 6. Metastases

_____ 7. Subluxation

_____ 8. Spina bifida

_____ 9. Osteoporosis

_____ 10. Spondylolysis

_____ 11. Paget's disease

_____ 12. Jefferson fracture

_____ 13. Spondylolisthesis

_____ 14. Multiple myeloman.

_____ 15. Hangman's fracture

_____ 16. Compression fracture

_____ 17. Ankylosing spondylitis

_____ 18. Scheuermann's disease

_____ 19. Clay shoveler's fracture

_____ 20. Herniated nucleus pulposus

Column B

a. Loss of bone density

b. Breaking down of a vertebra

c. Incomplete or partial dislocation

d. Kyphosis with onset in adolescence

e. Disruption in the continuity of bone

f. Comminuted fracture of the ring of C2

g. Increased density of atypically soft bone

h. Abnormal forward curvature of the spine

i. Malignant tumor arising from cartilage cells

j. Thick, soft bone marked by bowing and fractures

k. Transfer of a cancerous lesion from one area to another

l. Fracture of the anterior arch of C2 due to hyperextension

m. Abnormally increased convexity in the thoracic curvature

n. New tissue growth where cell proliferation is uncontrolled

o. Rheumatoid arthritis variant involving the SI joints and spine

p. Lateral deviation of the spine with possible vertebral rotation

q. Failure of the posterior encasement of the spinal cord to close

r. Rupture or prolapse of the nucleus pulposus into the spinal canal

s. Forward displacement of a vertebra over a lower vertebra, usually L5-S1

t. Fracture that causes compaction of bone and a decrease in the length or width

u. Avulsion fracture of the spinous process in the lower cervical and upper thoracic region

v. Malignant neoplasm of plasma cells involving the bone marrow and causing destruction of bone

Exercise 10

Instructions: This exercise is a comprehensive review of the osteology and arthrology of the vertebral column. Provide a short answer for each question.

1. List four functions of the vertebral column.

2. As viewed from the lateral aspect, name (from superior to inferior) the four vertebral curvatures.

3. State how vertebral curvatures are classified as either primary or secondary curvatures.

4. Name the two vertebral curvatures that are classified as primary curvatures.

5. Name the two vertebral curvatures that are classified as secondary curvatures.

6. What is the name of the opening formed by the vertebral arch and the body of a vertebra?

7. What other name refers to C1?

8. What other name refers to C2?

9. What other name refers to C7?

10. What two typical vertebral parts are missing from the first cervical vertebra?

11. How are the transverse processes of cervical vertebrae significantly different from those of other typical vertebrae?

12. Which cervical vertebra has the dens?

13. What other term refers to the dens?

14. How many cervical vertebrae are in the vertebral column?

15. With reference to the midsagittal plane, how do zygapophyseal articulations of the cervical vertebrae open?

16. With reference to the midsagittal plane, how do cervical intervertebral foramina open?

17. Which section of the vertebral column has costovertebral joints?

18. Which section of the vertebral column has facets and demifacets?

19. Which bones articulate with thoracic facets and demifacets?

20. With reference to the midsagittal plane, how do zygapophyseal articulations of the thoracic vertebrae open?

21. With reference to the midsagittal plane, how do thoracic intervertebral foramina open?

22. With reference to the midsagittal plane, how do zygapophyseal articulations of the lumbar vertebrae open?

23. With reference to the midsagittal plane, how do lumbar intervertebral foramina open?

24. What structure of the vertebral column articulates with both ilia?

25. With reference to the midsagittal plane, how many degrees and in which direction do sacroiliac joints open?

SECTION 2

Positioning of the Vertebral Column

Exercise 1: Positioning for the Cervical Spine

Instructions: Many projections are used to demonstrate the cervical vertebrae, including anteroposterior (AP) projections (open mouth), AP axial projections, AP and posteroanterior (PA) axial oblique projections, lateral projections, and hyper-extension and hyperflexion lateral projections. This exercise pertains to those projections. Identify structures, fill in missing words, provide a short answer, select the correct answer from a list, or choose true or false (explaining any statement you believe to be false) for each item.

Items 1 through 6 pertain to the *AP projection (Fuchs method).* Examine Fig. 8-14 as you answer the following items.

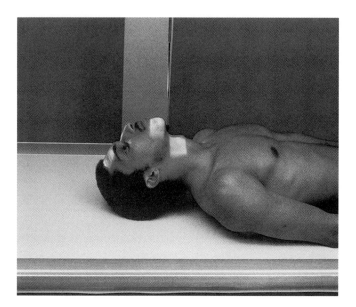

Figure 8-14 AP dens: Fuchs method.

1. To what level of the patient should the image receptor be centered?

2. Describe how the patient should be positioned and how the head should be adjusted.

3. How and where should the central ray be directed?

4. True or False. The AP projection (Fuchs method) should be used to demonstrate an upper cervical fracture in trauma patients.

5. True or False. In the image of the AP projection (Fuchs method), the entire dens should be seen within the foramen magnum.

6. Identify each lettered structure shown in Fig. 8-15.

A. _____

B. _____

C. _____

D. _____

E. _____

F. _____

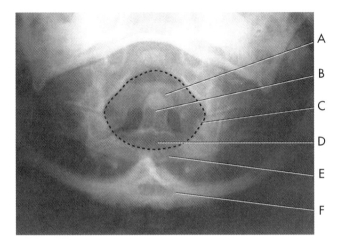

Figure 8-15 AP dens: Fuchs method.

Items 7 through 14 pertain to the *AP projection (open mouth)*. Examine Fig. 8-16 as you answer the following items.

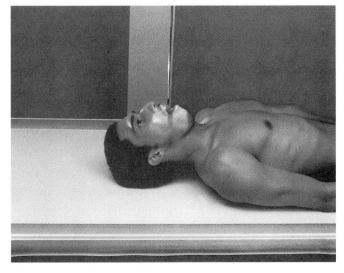

Figure 8-16 AP atlas and axis.

7. Which body position placement should be used for the patient?

   a. Prone
   b. Supine
   c. Upright

8. Describe how the patient's mouth should be adjusted.

9. How and where should the central ray be directed?

10. Why should the patient be asked to softly phonate *ah* during the exposure?

11. To which level of the patient should the image receptor be centered?

    a. C2 vertebra
    b. C4 vertebra
    c. C7 vertebra

12. In the image produced by the AP projection (open mouth), which cranial structure should be superimposed with the occlusal surface of the upper central incisors?

    a. Mastoid process
    b. Base of the skull
    c. External occipital protuberance

13. Which areas of cervical vertebrae should be clearly demonstrated with the AP projection (open mouth)?

    a. Intervertebral foramina
    b. Zygapophyseal articulations
    c. Articulations between C1 and C2

14. Identify each lettered structure shown in Fig. 8-17.

   A. _____

   B. _____

   C. _____

   D. _____

   E. _____

15. What should the patient be instructed to do to prevent superimposition of the mandible and the midcervical vertebrae?

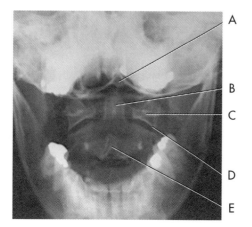

Figure 8-17 Open-mouth atlas and axis.

16. How is it determined that the chin has been correctly extended?

Items 15 through 22 pertain to the *AP axial projection.* Examine Fig. 8-18 as you answer the following items.

17. How many degrees and in what direction should the central ray be directed?

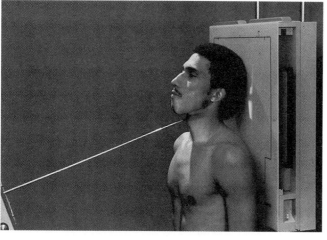

Figure 8-18 AP axial cervical vertebrae.

18. Which cervical vertebra should be the centering point for the central ray?

19. Where on the surface of the patient's neck should the central ray enter?

20. Which cervical vertebrae are usually not shown in the image produced by the AP axial projection?

21. The AP axial projection for cervical vertebrae should demonstrate the vertebrae from _____ to _____ .
    a. C1; C7
    b. C1; T2
    c. C3; C7
    d. C3; T2

22. From the following list, circle the two evaluation criteria indicating that the patient was properly positioned without rotation for the AP axial projection.
    a. The spinous processes should be equidistant to the pedicles.
    b. The mandibular angles should be equidistant to the vertebrae.
    c. The intervertebral foramina farthest from the IR should be "open."
    d. The superimposed rami of the mandible should be anterior to vertebral bodies.

Items 23 through 30 pertain to the *lateral projection, Grandy method*. Examine Fig. 8-19 as you answer the following items.

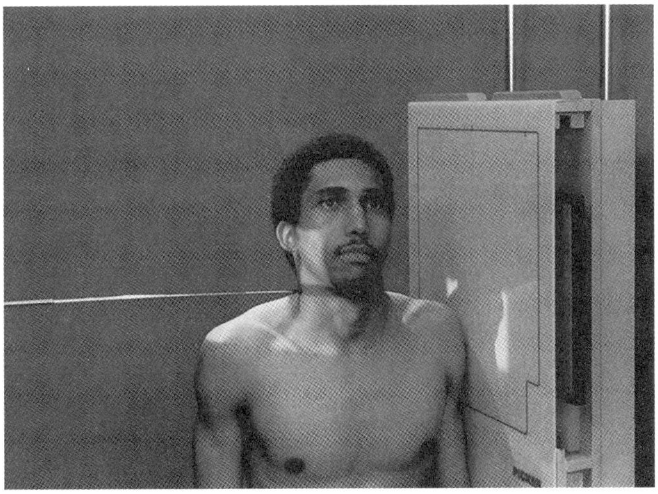

Figure 8-19 Lateral cervical vertebrae, Grandy method.

23. Which of the cervical vertebrae should be demonstrated with lateral projections?

24. To what level of the patient should the image receptor be centered?

25. To what level of the patient should the top border of the image receptor be located?

26. How should the patient be positioned to prevent the mandible from superimposing the vertebrae?

27. What breathing instructions should be given to the patient?

28. What should the radiographer do to help overcome the effects of a large object-to-image receptor distance created with the lateral projection?

29. What should the radiographer do if the C7 vertebra is not well visualized on a lateral projection radiograph?

30. Identify each lettered structure shown in Fig. 8-20.

A. _____

B. _____

C. _____

D. _____

E. _____

F. _____

G. _____

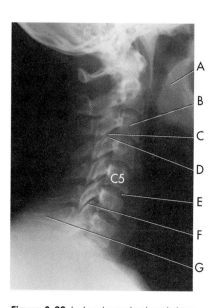

Figure 8-20 Lateral cervical vertebrae.

Items 31 through 37 pertain to *hyperextension and hyperflexion lateral projections.* Examine Figs. 8-21 and 8-22 as you answer the following items.

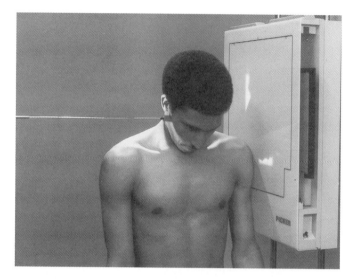

Figure 8-21 Lateral cervical vertebrae, hyperflexion.

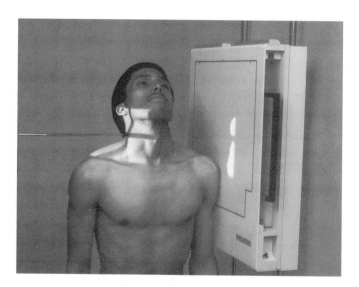

Figure 8-22 Lateral cervical vertebrae, hyperextension.

31. To what level of the patient should the top border of the image receptor be located?

32. Describe how the patient's head and neck should be adjusted from the neutral lateral position for the hyperflexion position.

33. Describe how the patient's head and neck should be adjusted from the neutral lateral position for the hyperextension position.

34. In an image with the patient in the hyperflexion position, how is it determined that the patient's neck has been flexed far enough?

35. In an image with the patient in the hyperextension position, how is it determined that the patient's neck has been extended far enough?

36. What cervical vertebrae should be clearly demonstrated in images produced with the patient in the hyperflexion and hyperextension positions?

37. Indicate how the cervical spinous processes should appear in radiographs with the patient in the (a) hyperflexion lateral position and (b) hyperextension lateral position.

a. _____

_____

b. _____

_____

Items 38 through 51 pertain to the *AP axial oblique projection.* Examine Fig. 8-23 as you answer the following items.

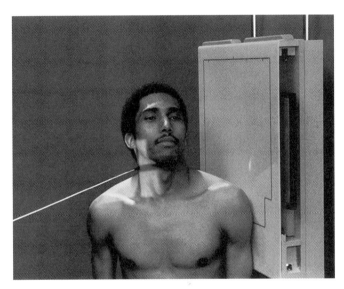

Figure 8-23 AP axial oblique intervertebral foramina.

38. AP axial oblique projections are used to best demonstrate

the pedicles and _____.
a. zygapophyseal joints
b. intervertebral foramina
c. superior articular facets

39. How many degrees should the patient be rotated?

40. With reference to the patient, where should the image receptor be centered?

41. Why should the patient be instructed to lift and extend the chin?

42. Explain how the positioning of the cervical vertebrae is affected if the patient turns the head until the midsagittal plane of the skull is parallel with the plane of the image receptor.

43. Through which cervical vertebra should the central ray be directed?

44. How many degrees and in what direction should the central ray be directed?

45. Why is the central ray directed in the manner indicated in the answer to question 44?

46. If an AP axial oblique projection is performed with the patient in a semisupine position, should the direction and angulation of the central ray be different from that recommended for an upright patient?

47. Why should a support be placed under the patient's head for the AP axial oblique projection with the patient in a semisupine body position?

48. What breathing instructions should be given to the patient?

49. Which of the following procedures should be avoided when positioning a patient for an AP axial oblique projection?
    a. Slightly protruding the chin
    b. Turning the chin to the side
    c. Rotating the body 45 degrees

50. From the following list, circle the five evaluation criteria indicating that the patient was properly positioned for an AP axial oblique projection.

   a. The occipital bone should not overlap C1.
   b. The zygapophyseal joints should be well demonstrated.
   c. The chin should be elevated and not overlap C1 and C2.
   d. All seven cervical vertebrae and T1 should be included.
   e. The intervertebral disk spaces should be open and well demonstrated.
   f. The intervertebral foramina should be open, with those nearest the IR well demonstrated.
   g. The intervertebral foramina should be open, with those farthest from the IR well demonstrated.

51. Fig. 8-24 shows an AP axial oblique projection radiograph. Examine the image and answer the questions that follow.

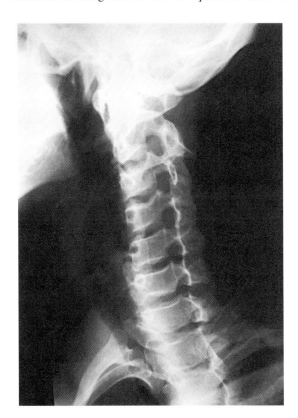

Figure 8-24 AP axial oblique intervertebral foramina.

   a. In what body position is the patient?

   b. The intervertebral foramina of which side-left or right-are best demonstrated?

   c. Are they the ones closer to or the ones farther from the image receptor?

Items 52 through 60 pertain to *PA axial oblique projections.* Examine Fig. 8-25 as you answer the following items.

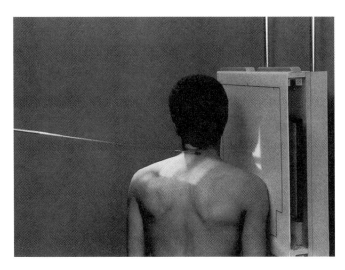

Figure 8-25 PA axial oblique intervertebral foramina.

52. With the patient positioned in the right anterior oblique (RAO) position, the intervertebral foramina best demonstrated are those on the patient's _____ (right or left) side.

53. When the patient is in the standing position, to what level of the patient should the IR be centered?

   a. C3
   b. C5
   c. C7

54. How many degrees should the entire body of the patient be rotated?

   a. 25
   b. 35
   c. 45

55. In which direction should the central ray be directed?

   a. Caudad
   b. Cephalad
   c. Perpendicular

56. How many degrees should the central ray be angled?

   a. 5 to 10 degrees
   b. 15 to 20 degrees
   c. 25 to 30 degrees
   d. 35 to 40 degrees

57. Through which cervical vertebra should the central ray be directed?

    a. C3
    b. C4
    c. C5

58. True or False. Radiographs of the cervical vertebrae with the patient in the anterior oblique body position should be displayed on an illuminator as if the patient were standing facing the person viewing the radiograph.

59. True or False. PA axial oblique projections should demonstrate the intervertebral foramina closer to the image receptor.

60. Fig. 8-26 shows a PA axial oblique projection radiograph. Examine the image and answer the questions that follow.

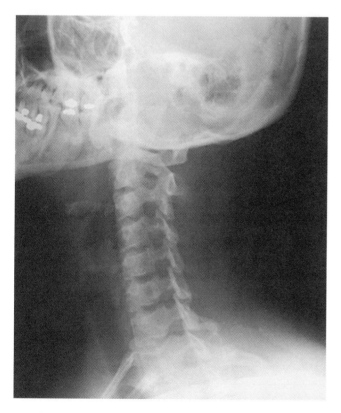

Figure 8-26 PA axial oblique intervertebral foramina.

    a. What position is shown in the image?

    b. The intervertebral foramina of which side-left or right-are best demonstrated?

    c. Are they closer to or farther from the image receptor compared with the intervertebral foramina that are not opened in this image?

Exercise 2: Positioning for the Cervicothoracic Region

Instructions: A lateral projection using either of two methods, the Twining method or the Pawlow method, can be performed to demonstrate the cervicothoracic region. This exercise pertains to those two projections. Identify structures, fill in missing words, provide a short answer, select an answer from a list, or choose true or false (explain any statement you believe to be false) for each item.

Items 1 through 7 pertain to the Twining method for demonstrating the cervicothoracic region. Examine Fig. 8-27 as you answer the following items.

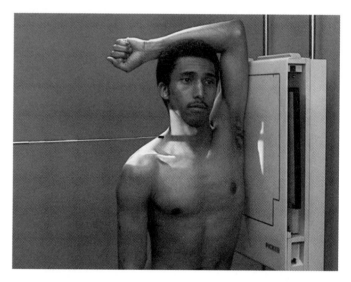

Figure 8-27 Lateral cervicothoracic projection, Twining method.

1. The Twining method is also known as the

   _____ lateral.

2. Which body plane should be centered to the midline of the grid?

3. With reference to the patient, where should the IR be centered?

4. Describe how the patient's arms should be positioned.

5. Describe how the patient's shoulders should be positioned.

6. List the two ways that the patient's respiration can be controlled.

7. Which two ways can the central ray be directed for the Twining method?
   a. Perpendicular or 5 degrees caudad
   b. Perpendicular or 5 degrees cephalad
   c. 5 degrees caudad or 5 degrees cephalad

Questions 8 through 15 pertain to the Pawlow method for demonstrating the cervicothoracic region. Examine Fig. 8-28 as you answer the following questions.

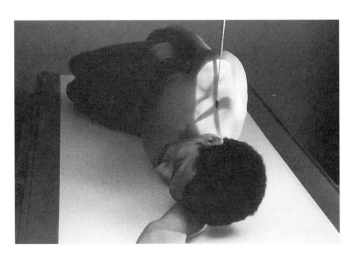

Figure 8-28 Lateral cervicothoracic region, Pawlow method.

8. For the Pawlow method, the patient should be positioned in the _____ body position.

9. Which body plane should be centered to the midline of the grid?

10. Under what two areas of the body should supports be placed to maintain the long axis of the cervicothoracic vertebrae horizontal?

11. With reference to the patient, to what specific location should the central ray be directed?
    a. Disk space of C1 and C2
    b. Disk space of C4 and C5
    c. Disk space of C7 and T1
    d. Disk space of T1 and T2

12. How many degrees and in which direction should the central ray be directed?
    a. 3 to 5 degrees caudad
    b. 3 to 5 degrees cephalad
    c. 7 to 10 degrees caudad
    d. 7 to 10 degrees cephalad

13. True or False. For the Pawlow method with the patient in the left lateral recumbent position, the right humeral head should superimpose the left humeral head.

14. From the following list, circle the four evaluation criteria indicating that the patient was properly positioned for a lateral projection of the cervicothoracic region.

   a. The exposure must have penetrated the shoulder area.

   b. The shoulders should be seen separated from each other.

   c. The area from approximately C5 to T4 should be included.

   d. The vertebrae should be lateral and not appreciably rotated.

   e. The spinous processes should be seen centered on vertebral bodies.

   f. The intervertebral foramina should be open, with those nearest the image receptor (IR) well demonstrated.

   g. The intervertebral foramina should be open, with those farthest from the IR well demonstrated.

15. Identify each lettered structure shown in Fig. 8-29.

A. _____

B. _____

C. _____

D. _____

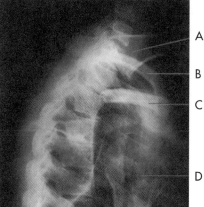

Figure 8-29 Lateral cervicothoracic region.

Exercise 3: Positioning for the Thoracic Vertebrae

Instructions: A typical series demonstrating the thoracic vertebrae usually includes the AP projection and the lateral projection. This exercise pertains to those two projections. Identify structures, fill in missing words, provide a short answer, select an answer from a list, or choose true or false (explaining any statement you believe to be false) for each question.

Items 1 through 14 pertain to the AP projection. Examine Fig. 8-30 as you answer the following questions.

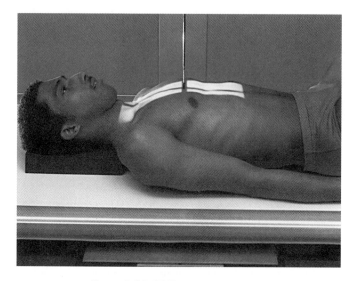

Figure 8-30 AP thoracic vertebrae.

1. Which body plane should be centered on the midline of the table or vertical grid device?

   a. Oblique
   b. Horizontal
   c. Midsagittal
   d. Midcoronal

2. If the supine position is used, what should be done to reduce the normal thoracic kyphosis of the patient?

   a. Flex the patient's hips and knees.
   b. Extend the patient's lower extremities.
   c. Place cushions under the patient's lower back.

3. To which vertebra should a 35 cm × 43 cm IR be centered?

   a. T3
   b. T5
   c. T7
   d. T12

4. Where exactly on the anterior side of the patient's chest should the central ray enter?

5. With reference to the patient, where should the upper edge of the IR be placed?

6. If the patient is unable to sustain shallow breathing, what other breathing instructions should be given? Explain why.

7. Which part of the x-ray tube—the anode or cathode—should be positioned over the patient's head? Explain why.

8. For the supine patient, why should the patient's head rest directly on the table or on a thin pillow instead of a thick foam cushion or thick pillow?

9. What should the radiographer do if the AP projection does not adequately demonstrate all 12 thoracic vertebrae because of a poor exposure latitude that results in an image of uneven densities?

10. True or False. The central ray should be directed perpendicular to T7.

11. True or False. If the patient's condition permits, he or she may be requested to take shallow breaths to blur lung markings.

12. Figs. 8-31 and 8-32 both show AP projection radiographs; however, they are not identical in appearance. Compare the images and answer the questions that follow.

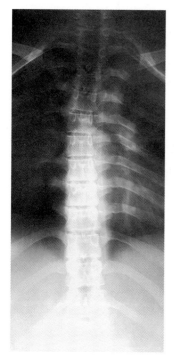

Figure 8-31 AP thoracic vertebrae.

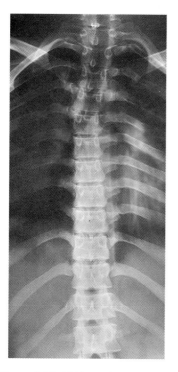

Figure 8-32 AP thoracic vertebrae.

a. Which image best demonstrates all 12 thoracic vertebrae?

_____

b. Which image used the anode heel effect of the x-ray tube to its maximum advantage?

_____

c. In which image was the anode of the x-ray tube positioned above the patient's head?

_____

d. In which image was the cathode of the x-ray tube positioned above the patient's head?

_____

13. From the following list, circle the five evaluation criteria indicating that the patient was correctly positioned and the exposure was properly performed for the AP projection.
   a. The ribs should appear posteriorly superimposed.
   b. All 12 thoracic vertebrae should be included.
   c. The zygapophyseal joints should be best demonstrated.
   d. The x-ray beam should be collimated to the thoracic spine.
   e. The spinous processes should appear at the midline of the patient.
   f. The vertebral column should be aligned to the middle of the radiograph.
   g. The spinous processes should appear without superimposition of vertebral bodies.
   h. A wide latitude of exposure should exist, or two radiographs can be taken for the upper and lower vertebrae.

14. Identify each lettered structure shown in Fig. 8-33.

A. _____

B. _____

C. _____

D. _____

E. _____

F. _____

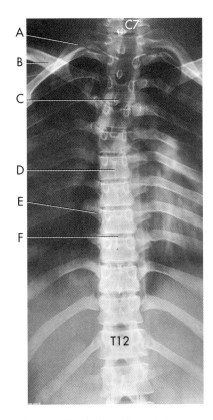

Figure 8-33 AP thoracic vertebrae.

Items 15 through 35 pertain to the *lateral projection.* Examine Fig. 8-34 as you answer the following items.

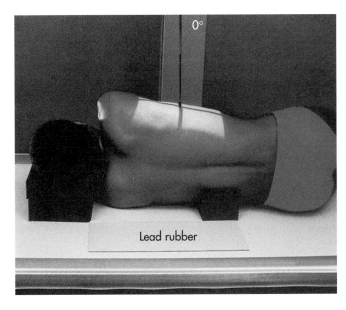

Figure 8-34 Lateral thoracic vertebrae.

15. Why is it preferable to place the patient in the left lateral position instead of the right lateral position?

16. For the lateral recumbent position, what is the purpose of placing a firm pillow under the patient's head?

17. To what level of the patient should the superior border of the IR be placed?

18. Which posterior body landmark coincides with T7 for centering the IR?

19. Describe how the patient's arms should be positioned.

20. Why should the patient's arms be placed in the manner described for question 19?

21. What is the purpose of placing a radiolucent support under the lower thoracic region when the patient is in the lateral recumbent position?

22. How many degrees and in which direction should the central ray be directed if the thoracic vertebrae are not parallel with the table when a female patient is in the lateral recumbent position? For male patients?

23. If an angled central ray is used, why should it be angled more for men than for women?

24. With reference to the patient's breathing, when should the exposure be made?

25. Why should a sheet of leaded rubber be placed on the table posterior to the patient when the IR is exposed and the patient is in a lateral recumbent position?

26. How can it be determined by looking at ribs in the image that the patient was rotated?

27. What additional projection may be performed if the upper thoracic vertebrae are not well demonstrated with a routine lateral projection?

28. When the thoracic vertebrae are parallel with the plane of the IR, the central ray should be directed

    _____ (perpendicularly; cephalad; caudad).

29. True or False. A lead apron should be placed over the patient's pelvis.

30. True or False. The central ray should be directed to enter the posterior half of the thorax at the level of T7.

31. True or False. Normal breathing by the patient reduces the amount of scattered radiation that reaches the image receptor.

32. True or False. Scattered radiation may cause the automatic exposure control system to terminate the exposure prematurely.

33. True or False. If the exposure is terminated prematurely, the vertebral bodies will appear too light in the image.

34. True or False. The upper thoracic vertebrae, specifically T1 and T2, are not usually demonstrated in the full lateral view.

35. From the following list, circle the six evaluation criteria indicating that the patient was correctly positioned and the exposure was properly performed for the lateral projection.
    a. The zygapophyseal joints should be open.
    b. A wide latitude of exposure should be seen.
    c. The intervertebral disk spaces should be open.
    d. The ribs should appear posteriorly superimposed.
    e. The spinous processes should appear at the midline of the patient.
    f. The vertebrae should be clearly seen through rib and lung shadows.
    g. Twelve thoracic vertebrae should be centered on the image receptor.
    h. The x-ray beam should be tightly collimated to reduce scatter radiation.

Exercise 4: Positioning for the Lumbar Vertebrae

Instructions: Projections used to demonstrate lumbar vertebrae include the AP projection, the AP axial projection, the AP oblique projection, and the lateral projection. This exercise pertains to those projections. Identify structures, fill in missing words, provide a short answer, select an answer from a list, or choose true or false (explaining any statement you believe to be false) for each question.

Items 1 through 12 pertain to the *AP projection* with the patient in the supine position. Examine Fig. 8-35 as you answer the following items.

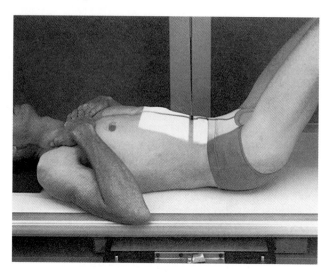

Figure 8-35 AP lumbar vertebrae.

1. Why should the patient empty the urinary bladder before the AP projection is performed?

2. What source-to-image receptor distance (SID) is recommended? Why?

3. What body plane should be centered to the midline of the table?

4. How should the patient's arms be positioned to prevent the forearms from inadvertently superimposing the lower abdomen?

5. Why should the patient be instructed to flex the hips and knees?

6. To what level of the patient should a 35 cm × 43 cm IR be centered?

7. Describe how and where the central ray should be directed and centered.

8. List the parts of the lumbar vertebrae that should be demonstrated in the image of the AP projection.

9. How much of the vertebral column should be clearly demonstrated in the image?

10. To what area of the body should the edge of collimation be adjusted?

11. Explain why a patient wearing a pair of undershorts with an elastic waistband should be asked to remove or lower the garment.

12. Identify each lettered structure of the lumbar vertebrae in Fig. 8-36.

A. _____

B. _____

C. _____

D. _____

E. _____

F. _____

G. _____

H. _____

I. _____

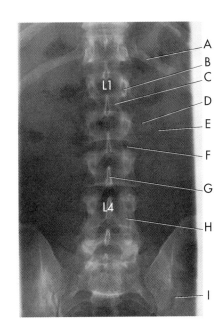

Figure 8-36 AP lumbar vertebrae.

Items 13 through 26 pertain to the *lateral projection* with the patient in the left lateral recumbent body position. Examine Fig. 8-37 as you answer the following items.

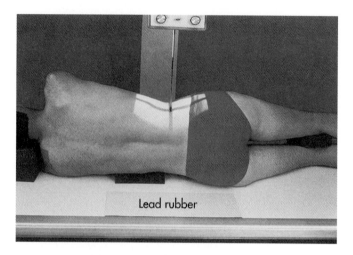

Figure 8-37 Lateral lumbar vertebrae.

13. What body plane should be centered to the midline of the table?

14. Describe how the patient's lower limbs (extremities) should be situated on the table.

15. For a patient with a thin body build and a narrow waist, what can a radiographer do to make the lumbar vertebral column closer to parallel with the table?

16. When using a 35 cm × 43 cm IR, to what level of the patient should it be centered?
    a. Iliac crests
    b. L1 vertebra
    c. L3 vertebra

17. Which breathing instruction should be given to the patient?
    a. Breathe slowly.
    b. Stop breathing after expiration.
    c. Stop breathing after inspiration.

18. How should the central ray be directed when the long axis of the lumbar vertebral column is parallel with the table?
    a. Caudad
    b. Cephalad
    c. Perpendicular

19. For males, how many degrees and in what direction should the central ray be directed when the long axis of the lumbar vertebral column is not parallel with the table? For females?

20. How much of the vertebral column should be included in the image?

21. Should lumbar intervertebral foramina be demonstrated with the lateral projection?

22. How should lumbar intervertebral disk spaces appear in the image of the lateral projection?

23. True or False. The patient's knees should be exactly superimposed to prevent rotation.

24. True or False. A sheet of leaded rubber should be placed on the table just posterior to the patient's lumbar column.

25. True or False. Collimation should extend to the borders of a 35 cm × 43 cm IR.

26. Identify each lettered structure of the vertebral column shown in Fig. 8-38.

    A. _____

    B. _____

    C. _____

    D. _____

    E. _____

    F. _____

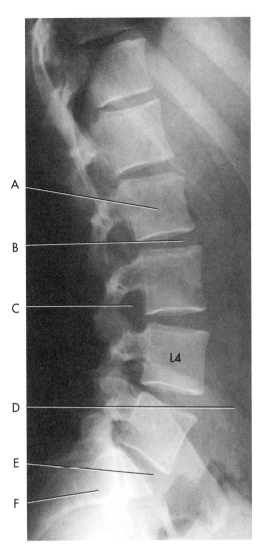

Figure 8-38 Lateral lumbar vertebrae.

Items 27 through 34 pertain to the *localized lateral projection* that demonstrates the lumbosacral junction. Refer to Fig. 8-39, which shows a patient in the lateral recumbent position for a lateral projection of L5-S1, as you answer the following items.

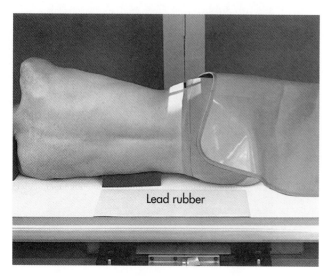

Figure 8-39 Lateral L5-S1.

27. Which position should the patient be placed in for the lateral projection of L5-S1 junction?

   a. Supine
   b. Upright
   c. Lateral recumbent

28. When positioning the typical patient, where is the lumbosacral junction located?

29. To what level of the patient should the IR be centered?

30. What positioning factor determines whether the central ray needs to be angled or directed perpendicularly?

   a. Whether the legs are extended or hips flexed
   b. Whether or not the vertebral column is horizontal with the table
   c. Whether or not the arms are perpendicular to the long axis of the torso

31. Where should the perpendicular central ray enter the patient?

   a. At the level of the iliac crests
   b. 2 inches (5 cm) superior to the iliac crest
   c. 2 inches (5 cm) posterior to the anterior superior iliac spine (ASIS) and $1^3/_4$ inches (4.4 cm) inferior to the iliac crest

32. When the central ray needs to be angled, how many degrees and in what direction should it be directed for males? For females?

33. How much of the vertebral column should be included in the image?

34. Identify each lettered structure of the vertebral column shown in Fig. 8-40.

   A. _____

   B. _____

   C. _____

   D. _____

   E. _____

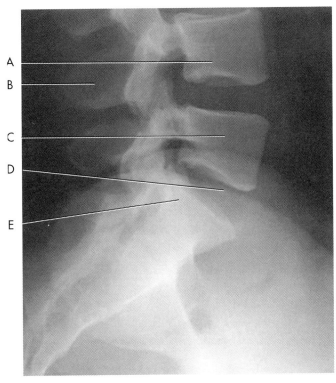

Figure 8-40 Lateral L5-S1.

Items 35 through 54 pertain to *AP oblique projections* with the patient recumbent. Examine Figs. 8-41 and 8-42 as you answer the following items.

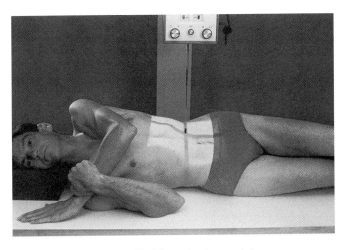

Figure 8-41 AP oblique lumbar vertebrae.

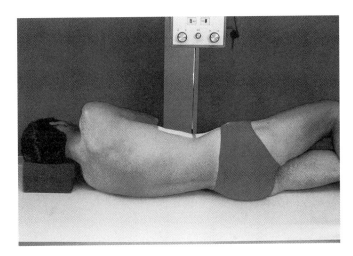

Figure 8-42 AP oblique lumbar vertebrae.

35. Lumbar articular facets for vertebrae L1 through L4 form

   an angle of _____ to

   _____ degrees.

36. The last lumbar vertebra's articular facets form an angle of

   _____ degrees.

37. To which side—right or left—are the lumbar zygapophyseal articulations being demonstrated when the patient is rotated with the left side elevated away from the table?

38. On what vertebra should the IR be centered for demonstrating the lumbar region?

39. How many degrees from the supine position should the patient be rotated to demonstrate the zygapophyseal articulations of the lumbar region?
    a. 10 to 20 degrees
    b. 25 to 30 degrees
    c. 45 degrees
    d. 60 degrees

40. How should the central ray be directed?
    a. Perpendicular
    b. 5 to 8 degrees caudad
    c. 5 to 8 degrees cephalad

41. Where exactly should the central ray enter the patient?

42. What is the significance of seeing the "Scottie dog" in the image?

43. Identify each lettered structure of the "Scottie dog" in Fig. 8-43.

    A. _____

    B. _____

    C. _____

    D. _____

    E. _____

    F. _____

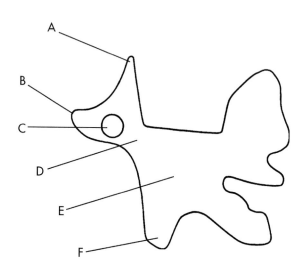

Figure 8-43 Parts of the "Scottie dog."

44. On which side—right or left—are the lumbar zygapophyseal joints best demonstrated when the patient is positioned left posterior oblique (LPO)?

45. How much of the vertebral column should be included in the image?

46. What positioning error most likely occurred if the zygapophyseal joint is not well demonstrated and the pedicle is quite anterior on the vertebral body?
    a. The patient was rotated too much.
    b. The patient was not rotated enough.
    c. The vertebral column was not parallel with the table.

47. What positioning error most likely occurred if the zygapophyseal joint is not well demonstrated and the pedicle is quite posterior on the vertebral body?
    a. The patient was rotated too much.
    b. The patient was not rotated enough.
    c. The vertebral column was not parallel with the table.

48. True or False. The vertebral column should remain parallel with the tabletop to keep T12-L1 and L1-L2 joint spaces open.

49. True or False. The patient should be instructed to breathe slowly and deeply to blur overlying soft tissue shadows.

50. True or False. Demonstrating the "Scottie dog" means that the lumbar intervertebral foramina are open and well demonstrated.

51. True or False. The "eye" in the "Scottie dog" is the pedicle on the side closer to the image receptor.

52. True or False. The central ray should be directed caudally when the vertebral column is not parallel with the plane of the image receptor.

53. True or False. The pelvis should be rotated approximately 30 degrees from the supine position to demonstrate the lumbosacral articular facets.

54. Identify each lettered structure of the vertebral column shown in Fig. 8-44.

    A. _____

    B. _____

    C. _____

    D. _____

    E. _____

    F. _____

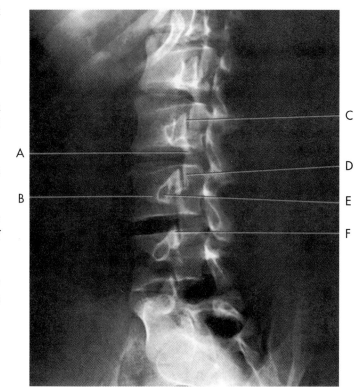

Figure 8-44 AP oblique lumbar vertebrae.

Questions 55 through 60 pertain to the *AP axial projection.* Examine Fig. 8-45 as you answer the following questions.

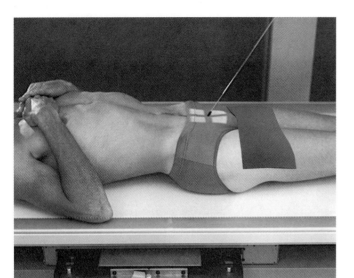

Figure 8-45 AP axial projection of the lumbosacral junction and sacroiliac joints.

55. How should the patient's lower limbs be positioned?

56. What vertebral joints are demonstrated with the AP axial projection?

57. Through what joint should the central ray be directed?

58. Where on the midsagittal plane of the patient's anterior surface should the central ray enter?

59. How many degrees and in what direction should the central ray be directed for adult males? For adult females?

60. What breathing instructions should be given to the patient?

Exercise 5: Positioning for the Sacroiliac Joints, the Sacrum, and the Coccyx

Instructions: Usually only two radiographs are needed to image the sacroiliac joints, the sacrum, or the coccyx. This exercise pertains to those structures. Identify structures, fill in missing words, provide a short answer, select an answer from a list, or choose true or false (explaining any statement you believe to be false) for each item.

Items 1 through 8 pertain to the *AP oblique projection* for the sacroiliac joints. Examine Fig. 8-46 as you answer the following items.

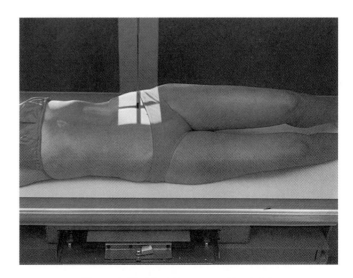

Figure 8-46 AP oblique sacroiliac joint.

1. True or False. Positioning for AP oblique projections should begin with the patient supine.

2. True or False. The affected side of the patient should be elevated.

3. One side of the pelvis should be elevated

_____ to _____ degrees.

4. Where is the sagittal plane located that should be used to position the patient to the midline of the table?

5. To what level of the patient should the IR be centered?

6. What breathing instructions should be given to the patient?

7. How should the central ray be directed for the AP oblique projection?

8. Where on the patient's body should the central ray enter?

Items 9 through 19 pertain to *projections for the sacrum.* Examine Figs. 8-47 and 8-48 as you answer the following items.

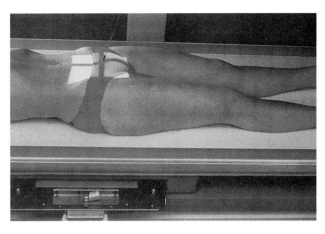

Figure 8-47 AP axial sacrum.

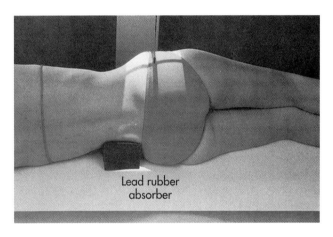

Figure 8-48 Lateral sacrum.

9. Why is the AP axial projection preferred to the PA axial projection?

10. How many degrees and in which direction should the central ray be directed for the AP axial projection?

11. Why should the central ray be directed at a certain angle for the AP axial projection instead of being perpendicular to the IR?

12. Where on the midline of the patient should the central ray enter for the AP axial projection?

13. When the patient is in the lateral recumbent position for the lateral projection, where should the coronal plane that needs to be centered to the IR pass through the patient?

14. Where on the patient's body should the central ray enter for the lateral projection?

15. For the lateral projection, where should the IR be centered on the patient?

16. What breathing instructions should be given to the patient?

17. What scale of contrast—long-scale (low) contrast or short-scale (high) contrast—is desired for any radiograph of the sacrum?

18. The central ray should be directed _____ to the IR for the lateral projection.

19. Identify each lettered structure of the sacrum shown in Fig. 8-49.

A. _____

B. _____

C. _____

D. _____

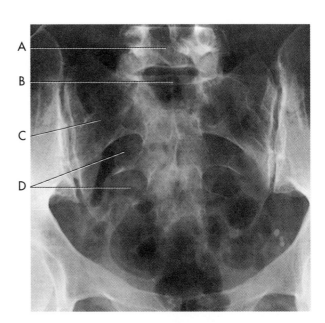

Figure 8-49 The sacrum.

Items 20 through 30 pertain to *projections for the coccyx.* Examine Figs. 8-50 and 8-51 as you answer the following items.

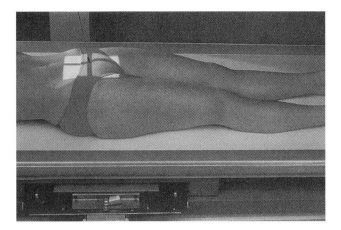

Figure 8-50 AP coccyx.

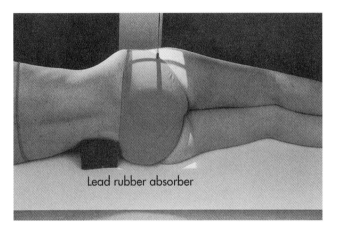

Lead rubber absorber

Figure 8-51 Lateral coccyx.

20. To center the coccyx on the IR for the AP projection, which body plane should overlie the midline of the table?

 a. Horizontal
 b. Midsagittal
 c. Midcoronal

21. Why is the AP projection preferred to the PA projection?

22. How many degrees and in what direction should the central ray be directed for the AP projection?

23. Where on the patient's body should the central ray enter?

24. Should gonadal shielding be used for female patients? Explain your answer.

25. How should coccygeal segments appear in the AP image?

 a. They should overlie the sacral segments.
 b. They should be superimposed with the symphysis pubis.
 c. They should be centered on the IR without rotation or superimposition.

26. For the lateral projection, which object should be placed behind the patient on the tabletop to improve image quality?

 a. Foam cushion
 b. Folded blanket
 c. Sheet of leaded rubber

27. When the patient is in the lateral recumbent position for the lateral projection, approximately how far posterior from the ASIS should the patient be centered on the image receptor?

28. To what level of the patient should the IR be centered for the lateral projection?

29. What breathing instructions should be given to the patient?

30. True or False. The central ray should be perpendicularly directed to the IR for the lateral projection of the coccyx.

Exercise 6: Scoliosis Series (Ferguson Method)

Instructions: This exercise pertains to the Ferguson method of radiographing patients with scoliosis. Provide a short answer, select an answer from a list, or choose true or false (explaining any statement you believe to be false) for each item. Examine Fig. 8-52 as you answer the following items.

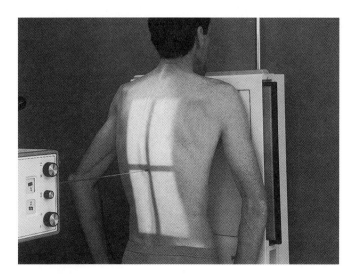

Figure 8-52 PA thoracic and lumbar vertebrae for scoliosis.

1. How many radiographs are necessary to complete the Ferguson series?
   a. 2
   b. 3
   c. 4

2. True or False. The patient should be in the supine position for the Ferguson series.

3. True or False. The projection may be either AP or PA.

4. True or False. In the first radiograph the patient should be standing with a support block under the convex side of the vertebral curve.

5. True or False. Lead-impregnated gonadal shielding is not required when the patient is standing in the PA body position.

6. True or False. A compression band may be used to firmly hold the patient against the grid.

7. How much of the vertebral column should be demonstrated on the radiographs?

8. Why is a PA projection preferred to an AP projection?

9. To expose the length of the 36-inch (90-cm) IR, what recommended SID should be used?

10. Fig. 8-53 shows a frontal view of a patient who has scoliosis. If this is the first radiograph obtained with the Ferguson method for performing a scoliosis series, under which side of the patient should a support block be placed for the patient to stand on for the second radiograph?

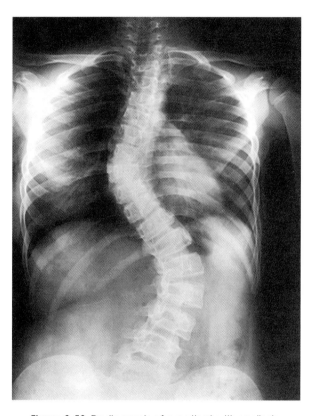

Figure 8-53 Radiograph of a patient with scoliosis.

Exercise 7: Identifying Projections of the Vertebral Column

Instructions: This exercise has photographs that show patients being positioned for various projections of the vertebral column. Examine each photograph and identify the projection by name and the part of the vertebral column that is being demonstrated.

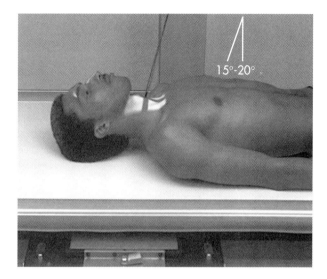

Figure 8-54

1. Fig. 8-54: _____

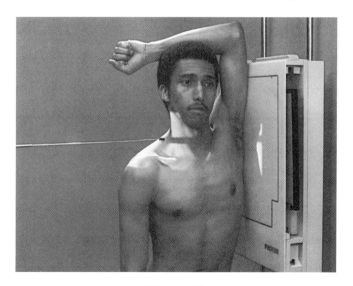

Figure 8-55

2. Fig. 8-55: _____

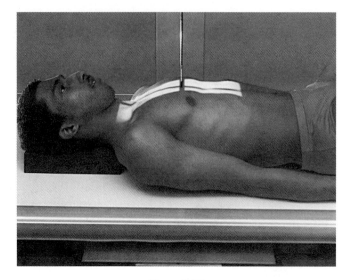

Figure 8-56

3. Fig. 8-56:

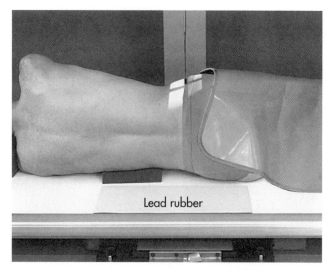

Figure 8-58

5. Fig. 8-58:

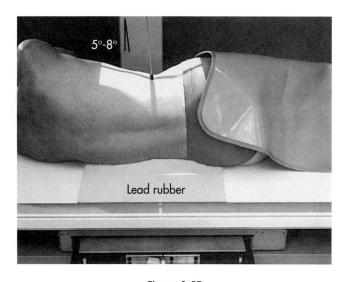

Figure 8-57

4. Fig. 8-57:

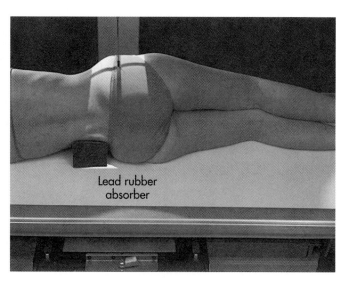

Figure 8-59

6. Fig. 8-59:

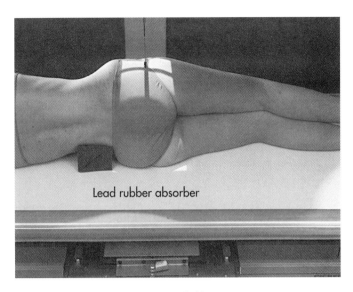

Figure 8-60

7. Fig. 8-60:

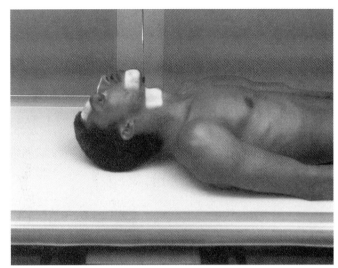

Figure 8-62

9. Fig. 8-62:

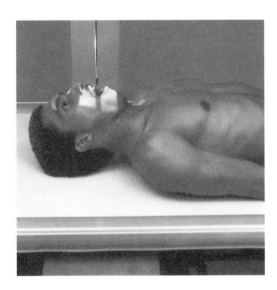

Figure 8-61

8. Fig. 8-61:

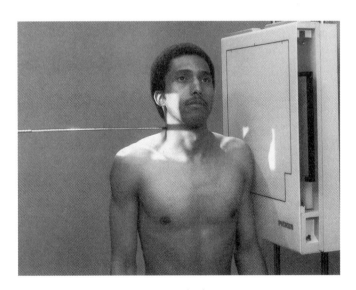

Figure 8-63

10. Fig. 8-63:

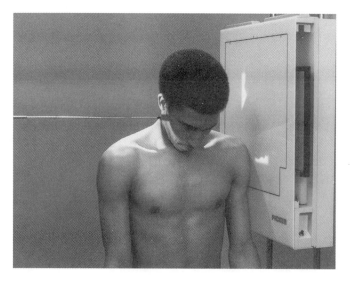

Figure 8-64

11. Fig. 8-64:

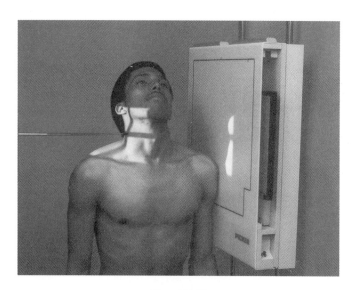

Figure 8-65

12. Fig. 8-65:

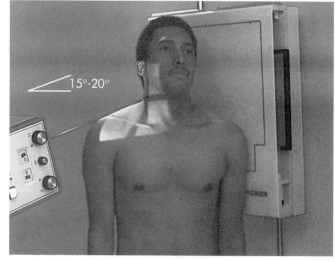

Figure 8-66

13. Fig. 8-66:

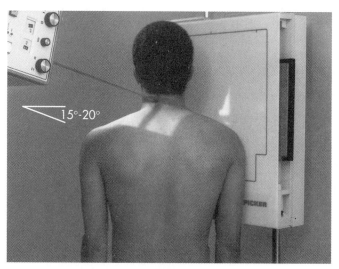

Figure 8-67

14. Fig. 8-67:

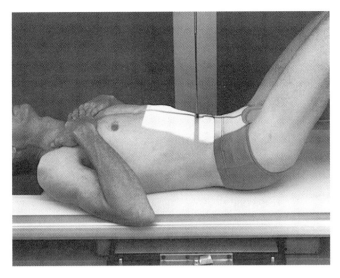

Figure 8-68

15. Fig. 8-68:

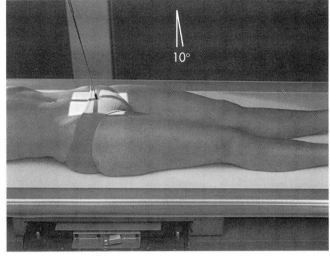

Figure 8-70

17. Fig. 8-70:

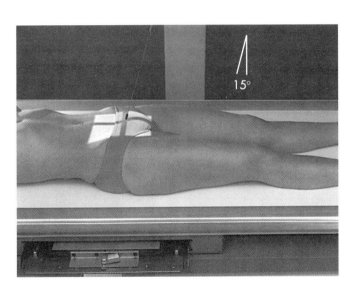

Figure 8-69

16. Fig. 8-69:

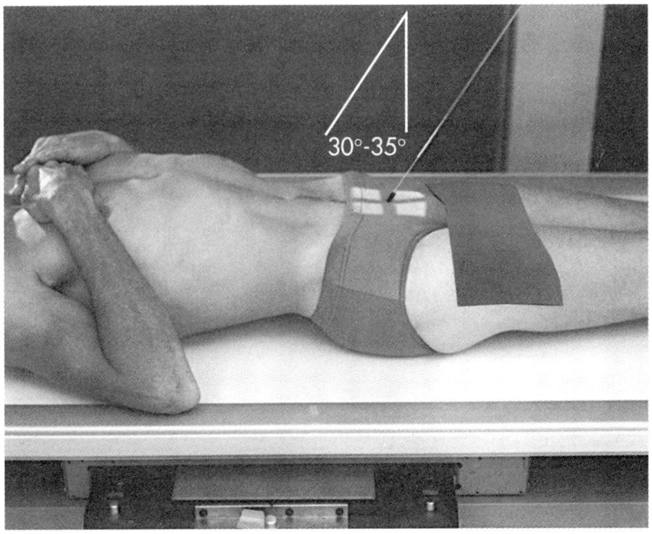

Figure 8-71

18. Fig. 8-71:

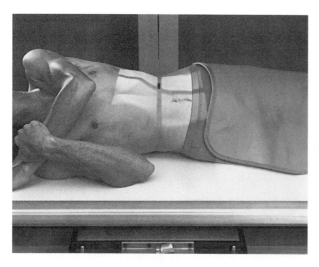

Figure 8-72

19. Fig. 8-72:

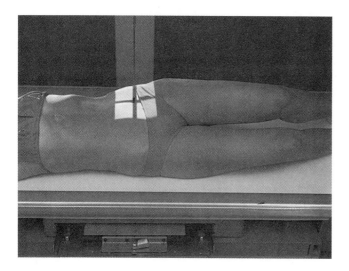

Figure 8-73

20. Fig. 8-73:

Exercise 8: Evaluating Radiographs of the Vertebral Column

Instructions: This exercise presents radiographs of the vertebral column to give you practice evaluating vertebral column positioning. These images are not from *Merrill's Atlas of Radiographic Positions and Radiologic Procedures.* Each radiograph shows at least one positioning error. Examine each image and answer the questions that follow by providing a short answer.

1. Fig. 8-74 shows an image of the AP projection (open mouth) with the patient incorrectly positioned. State the positioning error that produced this image.

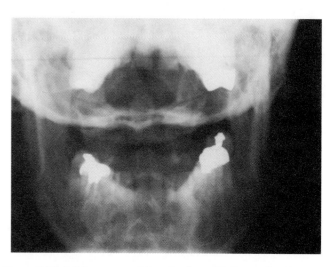

Figure 8-74 AP (open mouth) projection with the patient improperly positioned.

2. Fig. 8-75 shows an image of the AP projection (open mouth) with the patient incorrectly positioned. State the positioning error that produced this image.

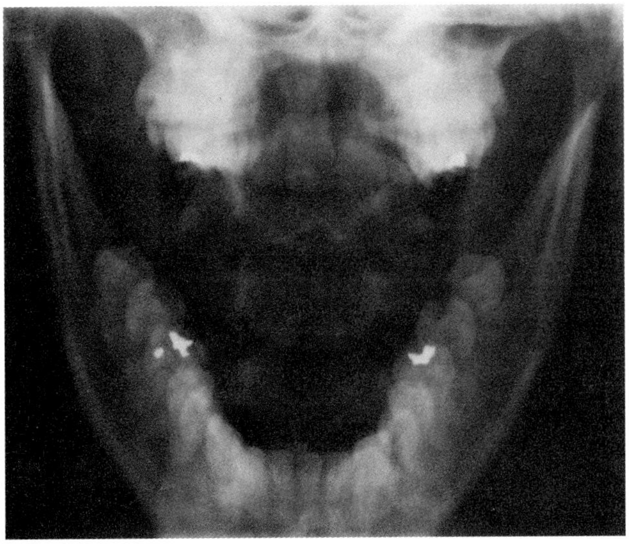

Figure 8-75 AP (open mouth) projection with the patient improperly positioned.

3. Fig. 8-76 shows an image of a lateral projection that does not meet all evaluation criteria for this projection. What evaluation criterion for this projection is not met?

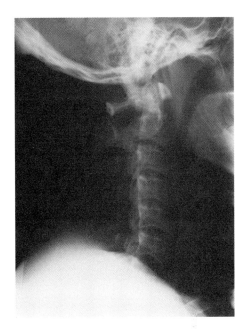

Figure 8-76 Lateral projection.

4. Fig. 8-77 shows an AP axial oblique projection radiograph. Examine the image and answer the questions that follow.

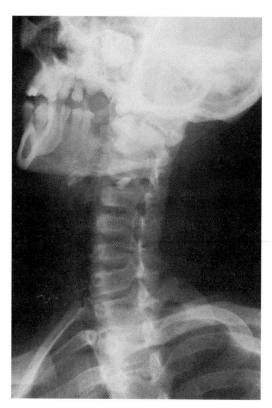

Figure 8-77 AP axial oblique projection.

a. In what body position was the patient placed?

b. List two evaluation criteria that this image does not meet.

c. List two ways the positioning of the patient could be improved to correct the errors seen in this image.

5. Fig. 8-78 shows a PA axial oblique projection radiograph of the left cervical intervertebral foramina demonstrated with the patient in the left anterior oblique (LAO) position. Examine the image and state why it is unacceptable.

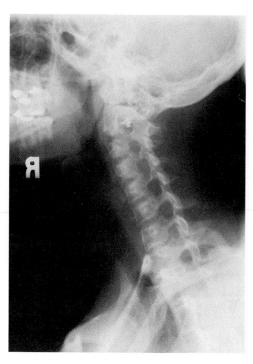

Figure 8-78 PA axial oblique projection demonstrating cervical intervertebral foramina.

6. Figs. 8-79 through 8-82 are lateral lumbar images that do not meet some of the evaluation criteria for the projection. Examine each image and describe in the space provided what type of error most likely occurred in the production of the image.

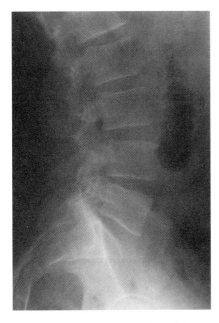

Figure 8-79 Rejected radiograph of the lateral position.

a. Fig. 8-79:

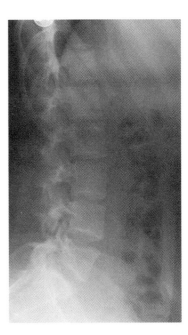

Figure 8-80 Rejected radiograph of the lateral position.

b. Fig. 8-80:

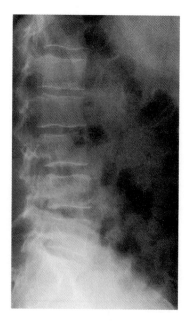

Figure 8-81 Rejected radiograph of the lateral position.

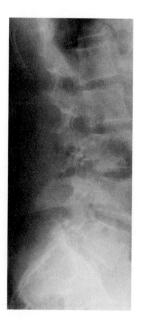

Figure 8-82 Rejected radiograph of the lateral position.

c. Fig. 8-81:

d. Fig. 8-82:

7. Fig. 8-83 shows an image of an AP oblique position with incorrect positioning of the patient. Examine the image and answer the questions that follow.

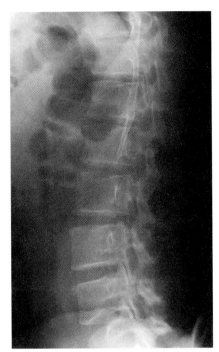

Figure 8-83 AP oblique image showing improper positioning of the patient.

a. What AP oblique position does the image represent?

b. Which side of the zygapophyseal joints should be best demonstrated?

c. Are the zygapophyseal joints well demonstrated?

d. Are the pedicles properly located within the "Scottie dog"? Explain.

e. What positioning error most likely caused the image to appear this way?

8. Fig. 8-84 shows an image of an AP oblique position with the patient incorrectly positioned. Examine the image and answer the questions that follow.

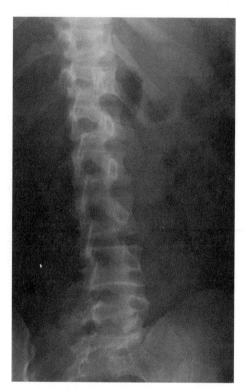

Figure 8-84 AP oblique image showing improper positioning of the patient.

a. Which AP oblique position does the image represent?

b. Which side of the zygapophyseal joints should be best demonstrated?

c. Are the zygapophyseal joints well demonstrated?

d. Are the pedicles properly located within the "Scottie dog"? Explain.

e. What positioning error most likely caused the image to appear this way?

Self-Test: Osteology, Arthrology, and Positioning of the Vertebral Column

Instructions: Answer the following questions by selecting the best choice.

1. Which two vertebral curvatures are anteriorly concave?

   a. Cervical and lumbar
   b. Cervical and pelvic
   c. Thoracic and lumbar
   d. Thoracic and pelvic

2. Which two vertebral curves are kyphotic curves?

   a. Cervical and lumbar
   b. Cervical and pelvic
   c. Thoracic and lumbar
   d. Thoracic and pelvic

3. Which two vertebral curves are lordotic curves?

   a. Cervical and lumbar
   b. Cervical and pelvic
   c. Thoracic and lumbar
   d. Thoracic and pelvic

4. Which two vertebral curves are primary curves?

   a. Cervical and lumbar
   b. Cervical and pelvic
   c. Thoracic and lumbar
   d. Thoracic and pelvic

5. Which spinal condition involves an excessive dorsal curvature of the thoracic vertebral column?

   a. Lordosis
   b. Scoliosis
   c. Kyphosis
   d. Spina bifida
   e. Spondylolisthesis

6. Which abnormal spinal condition involves any lateral curvature of the vertebral column?

   a. Lordosis
   b. Scoliosis
   c. Kyphosis
   d. Spina bifida
   e. Spondylolisthesis

7. What is the name of the short, thick bony processes that project posteriorly from the lateral and superior aspects of vertebral bodies of typical vertebrae?

   a. Laminae
   b. Pedicles
   c. Spinous processes
   d. Transverse processes

8. From the junction of which two vertebral structures do transverse processes originate in typical vertebrae?

   a. Pedicle and body
   b. Pedicle and lamina
   c. Spinous process and body
   d. Spinous process and lamina

9. Which vertebral structures unite at the origin of the spinous process of a typical vertebra?

   a. Both laminae
   b. Both pedicles
   c. Pedicle and body
   d. Pedicle and transverse process

10. Which structures of a typical vertebra are the zygapophyses?

    a. Vertebral foramen
    b. Articular processes
    c. Intervertebral disks
    d. Transverse processes
    e. Intervertebral foramina

11. On which structure is the dens located?

    a. C1
    b. C2
    c. Spinous process
    d. Transverse process

12. Which structure is known as the "atlas"?

    a. C1
    b. C2
    c. Dens
    d. Vertebra prominens

13. Which structure is known as the "axis"?

    a. C1
    b. C2
    c. Dens
    d. Vertebra prominens

14. On which structure is the dens located?

    a. Body of C1
    b. Body of C2
    c. Transverse process of C1
    d. Transverse process of C2

15. Which cervical vertebral structures are perforated with a foramen for the passage of the vertebral artery and vein?

    a. Body
    b. Laminae
    c. Pedicles
    d. Spinous processes
    e. Transverse processes

16. Which vertebral structures have bifid tips?

    a. Spinous processes of cervical vertebrae
    b. Spinous processes of thoracic vertebrae
    c. Transverse processes of cervical vertebrae
    d. Transverse processes of thoracic vertebrae

17. With reference to the midsagittal plane, how do zygapophyseal joints open in cervical vertebrae?

    a. 20 degrees anteriorly
    b. 20 degrees posteriorly
    c. 45 degrees anteriorly
    d. 45 degrees posteriorly
    e. 90 degrees laterally

18. With reference to the midsagittal plane, how do zygapophyseal joints open in thoracic vertebrae?

    a. 20 degrees anteriorly
    b. 20 degrees posteriorly
    c. 70 degrees anteriorly
    d. 70 degrees posteriorly
    e. 90 degrees laterally

19. Thoracic vertebrae differ from cervical and lumbar vertebrae because thoracic vertebrae have:

    a. Demifacets
    b. No transverse processes
    c. The largest spinous processes
    d. Bifid tips on the spinous processes

20. Which structures articulate with vertebral demifacets?

    a. Heads of ribs
    b. Tubercles of ribs
    c. Transverse processes
    d. Zygapophyseal joints

21. With reference to the midsagittal plane, how do zygapophyseal joints open in lumbar vertebrae?

    a. 20 degrees anteriorly
    b. 20 degrees posteriorly
    c. 30 to 50 degrees anteriorly
    d. 30 to 50 degrees posteriorly
    e. 90 degrees laterally

22. Lumbar vertebrae differ from cervical and thoracic vertebrae because lumbar vertebrae have:

    a. Demifacets
    b. Bifid spinous process tips
    c. Broad, large spinous processes
    d. Foramina through the transverse processes

23. Which parts of the sacrum form the joints with the ilia of the pelvis?

    a. Sacral cornua
    b. Auricular surfaces
    c. Sacral promontory
    d. Median sacral crest

24. The AP projection that demonstrates the dens using the Fuchs method differs from the AP projection (open mouth) because the Fuchs method:

    a. Directs the central ray to C4
    b. Angles the central ray 15 degrees cephalad
    c. Extends the chin and keeps the mouth closed
    d. Demonstrates intervertebral foramina of the upper vertebrae

25. The radiographer should not use the Fuchs method to obtain the AP projection of the dens if the patient is:

    a. Intoxicated
    b. Unable to suspend respiration
    c. Unable to depress both shoulders
    d. Suspected to have a fracture or degenerative disease

26. Which projection of the cervical vertebrae demonstrates the dens imaged within the foramen magnum?

    a. Lateral projection
    b. AP axial oblique projection
    c. AP projection (open mouth)
    d. AP projection (Fuchs method)

27. Which cervical structures are best demonstrated with the AP projection (open mouth)?

    a. C1 and C2
    b. Spinous processes
    c. Transverse processes
    d. Intervertebral disks
    e. Intervertebral foramina

28. How should the central ray be directed for the AP projection (open mouth)?

    a. Perpendicularly
    b. Caudally 15 degrees
    c. Cephalically 15 degrees
    d. Caudally 20 degrees
    e. Cephalically 20 degrees

29. How and where should the central ray be directed for the AP axial projection of the cervical vertebral column?

    a. Perpendicular to C4
    b. Perpendicular to C7
    c. 15 to 20 degrees cephalad to C4
    d. 15 to 20 degrees cephalad to C7

30. How should the IR be positioned for the AP axial projection of the cervical vertebral column?

    a. Centered to C4
    b. Centered to mastoid tips
    c. With the top border at the level of C4
    d. With the top border at the level of mastoid tips

31. For which projection of the cervical vertebrae should the central ray be angled 15 to 20 degrees cephalad?

    a. AP axial projection
    b. PA axial oblique projection
    c. AP projection (open mouth)
    d. AP projection (Fuchs method)

32. Which evaluation criterion does not apply to the AP axial projection of the cervical vertebral column?

    a. The intervertebral disk spaces should be open.
    b. The spinous processes should be equidistant to the pedicles.
    c. The mandibular angles should be equidistant to the vertebrae.
    d. C1 and C2 should be seen without mandibular superimpositioning.

33. Which projection of the cervical vertebral column requires a SID of 72 inches?

    a. AP projection
    b. Lateral projection
    c. PA axial oblique projection
    d. AP axial oblique projection

34. Which maneuver should be used to help obtain maximum depression of the shoulders in the lateral projection of the cervical vertebral column?

    a. Direct the central ray 15 degrees caudad.
    b. Direct the central ray 15 degrees cephalad.
    c. Direct a perpendicular central ray to C7.
    d. Suspend respiration after full inhalation.
    e. Suspend respiration after full expiration.

35. What should be done so that the magnified shoulder farthest from the IR is projected below the lower cervical vertebrae for the lateral projection of the cervical vertebrae?

    a. Direct a horizontal central ray to C4.
    b. Direct a horizontal central ray to C7.
    c. Angle the central ray 15 degrees caudad.
    d. Angle the central ray 15 degrees cephalad.

36. What should be done to prevent mandibular rami from superimposing cervical vertebrae in the lateral projection of the cervical vertebral column?

    a. Elevate the chin.
    b. Direct a horizontal central ray to C4.
    c. Direct a horizontal central ray to C7.
    d. Angle the central ray 15 degrees cephalad.
    e. Instruct the patient to hold weights in each hand.

37. What should be done to reduce the magnification caused by the increased object-to-image distance in lateral projections of the cervical vertebrae?

    a. Angle the central ray 15 degrees cephalad.
    b. Instruct the patient to hold weights in each hand.
    c. Take the exposure on suspended full expiration.
    d. Use a 40-inch SID.
    e. Use a 72-inch SID.

38. Which projection of the cervical vertebral column uses the same central ray direction and centering as hyperextension and hyperflexion studies of the cervical vertebrae?

    a. Lateral projection
    b. AP axial projection
    c. AP axial oblique projection
    d. AP (open mouth) projection

39. Which projection of the cervical vertebrae demonstrates the spinous processes elevated and widely separated?

    a. AP axial projection
    b. AP axial oblique projection
    c. Hyperflexion lateral projection
    d. Hyperextension lateral projection

40. Which projection of the cervical vertebrae demonstrates the spinous processes depressed and in close approximation?

    a. AP axial projection
    b. AP axial oblique projection
    c. Hyperflexion lateral projection
    d. Hyperextension lateral projection

41. Which projection of the cervical vertebrae should produce a radiographic image showing the patient's mandibular body nearly perpendicular to the lower border of the radiograph?

    a. AP projection (open mouth)
    b. AP axial oblique projection
    c. Hyperflexion lateral projection
    d. Hyperextension lateral projection

42. Which projection for cervical vertebrae must be exposed with a horizontal and perpendicular central ray?
    a. Lateral
    b. AP axial
    c. AP open mouth
    d. AP axial oblique

43. How should the central ray be directed for AP axial oblique projections of the cervical vertebral column?
    a. Horizontally
    b. Perpendicularly
    c. Caudally 15 to 20 degrees
    d. Cephalically 15 to 20 degrees

44. How should the central ray be directed for PA axial oblique projections of the cervical vertebral column?
    a. Vertically
    b. Perpendicularly
    c. Caudally 15 to 20 degrees
    d. Cephalically 15 to 20 degrees

45. Which projection of the cervical vertebral column best demonstrates the intervertebral foramina?
    a. Lateral projection
    b. AP axial projection
    c. AP axial oblique projection
    d. AP projection (open mouth)

46. Which position of the cervical vertebral column best demonstrates the left intervertebral foramina with the central ray angled 15 to 20 degrees cephalad?
    a. Left lateral
    b. Left anterior oblique (LAO)
    c. Left posterior oblique (LPO)
    d. Right anterior oblique (RAO)
    e. Right posterior oblique (RPO)

47. Which position of the cervical vertebral column best demonstrates the right intervertebral foramina with the central ray angled 15 to 20 degrees caudad?
    a. Right lateral
    b. LAO
    c. LPO
    d. RAO
    e. RPO

48. How many degrees from either the AP or the PA position should the entire body be rotated for oblique projections of the cervical column?
    a. 15 degrees
    b. 20 degrees
    c. 45 degrees
    d. 90 degrees

49. Which evaluation criterion pertains to the AP projection (Fuchs method) of the cervical vertebrae?
    a. The mandible rami should be superimposed.
    b. All seven cervical vertebrae should be demonstrated.
    c. The intervertebral foramina and disk spaces should be open.
    d. The entire dens should be seen through the foramen magnum.

50. Which evaluation criterion pertains to the AP axial projection of the cervical vertebral column?
    a. All seven cervical vertebrae should be demonstrated.
    b. The spinous processes should be equidistant to the pedicles.
    c. The intervertebral foramina should be open with those closest to the IR well demonstrated.
    d. The intervertebral foramina should be open with those farthest from the IR well demonstrated.

51. Which evaluation criterion pertains to the lateral projection of the cervical vertebral column?
    a. All seven cervical vertebrae should be demonstrated.
    b. The spinous processes should be equidistant to the pedicles.
    c. The intervertebral foramina should be open with those closest to the IR well demonstrated.
    d. The intervertebral foramina should be open with those farthest from the IR well demonstrated.

52. Which evaluation criterion pertains to the AP axial oblique projection of the cervical vertebral column?
    a. The rami of the mandible should be superimposed.
    b. The spinous processes should be equidistant to the pedicles.
    c. The intervertebral foramina should be open with those closest to the IR well demonstrated.
    d. The intervertebral foramina should be open with those farthest from the IR well demonstrated.

53. Which evaluation criterion pertains to PA axial oblique projections of the cervical vertebral column?
    a. The rami of the mandible should be superimposed.
    b. The spinous processes should be equidistant to the pedicles.
    c. The intervertebral foramina should be open with those closest to the IR well demonstrated.
    d. The intervertebral foramina should be open with those farthest from the IR well demonstrated.

54. Which projection should be included in a cervical series if the lateral projection does not demonstrate the C7 vertebra?

    a. AP axial oblique projection
    b. Lateral projection (Twining method)
    c. Lateral projection (dorsal decubitus position)
    d. AP projection, with a perpendicular central ray

55. For the lateral projection (Twining method) of the cervical vertebrae, how and where should the central ray be directed?

    a. Perpendicular to C4
    b. Perpendicular to the intervertebral disk space of C7 and T1
    c. Angled 15 degrees cephalad to C4
    d. Angled 15 degrees cephalad to the intervertebral disk space of C7 and T1

56. Which of the following structures are best demonstrated with the lateral projection (Twining method)?

    a. Lower cervical vertebrae
    b. Lower thoracic vertebrae
    c. Thoracic zygapophyseal joints
    d. Cervical intervertebral foramina

57. For the AP projection of the thoracic vertebral column, where should the central ray be directed on the anterior chest wall?

    a. To the sternal angle
    b. To the suprasternal notch
    c. Slightly above the sternal angle
    d. Slightly below the sternal angle

58. With reference to the patient, where should the top border of the IR be positioned for the AP projection of the thoracic vertebral column?

    a. To the level of T7
    b. Slightly below the sternal angle
    c. To the level of the manubrial notch
    d. $1\frac{1}{2}$ to 2 inches (3.8 to 5 cm) above the sternal angle
    e. $1\frac{1}{2}$ to 2 inches (3.8 to 5 cm) above the top of the shoulders

59. For the AP projection of the thoracic vertebral column with the patient in the supine position, why should the patient's hips and knees be flexed?

    a. To reduce dorsal kyphosis
    b. To increase dorsal kyphosis
    c. To depress the diaphragm to its lowest level
    d. To raise the diaphragm to its highest level
    e. To reduce part thickness and resultant scattered radiation

60. Which projection most requires usage of the anode heel effect to improve its image quality?

    a. AP projection of the lumbar vertebral column
    b. AP projection of the thoracic vertebral column
    c. AP axial projection of the cervical vertebral column
    d. AP projection of the cervical vertebrae (open mouth)

61. Which projection best demonstrates the intervertebral foramina of the thoracic vertebral column?

    a. AP projection
    b. Lateral projection
    c. From true lateral, patient rotated 20 degrees anteriorly
    d. From true lateral, patient rotated 20 degrees posteriorly

62. When performing the lateral projection for thoracic vertebrae, what is the preferred procedure that should be performed when the long axis of the vertebral column is not horizontal?

    a. Direct the central ray 10 to 15 degrees caudad.
    b. Direct the central ray 10 to 15 degrees cephalad.
    c. Extend the patient's left arm until it supports the patient's head.
    d. Elevate the lower or upper thoracic region with a radiolucent support.

63. To what level of the body should the central ray be directed for lateral projections of the thoracic vertebral column?

    a. Sternal angle
    b. Manubrial notch
    c. Xiphoid process
    d. Inferior angle of the scapula

64. What compensation should be made in the lateral projection of the thoracic vertebral column on a recumbent patient when the lower thoracic region is not parallel with the table?

    a. Place cushions under the patient's head.
    b. Direct the perpendicular central ray to T10.
    c. Angle the central ray 10 to 15 degrees caudad.
    d. Angle the central ray 10 to 15 degrees cephalad.

65. Which of the following structures are best demonstrated with the lateral position projection (Twining method)?

    a. Upper cervical vertebrae
    b. Upper thoracic vertebrae
    c. Thoracic zygapophyseal joints
    d. Cervical intervertebral foramina

66. Which projection of the vertebral column best demonstrates kyphosis?

    a. AP projection of the lumbar vertebral column
    b. AP projection of the thoracic vertebral column
    c. Lateral projection of the lumbar vertebral column
    d. Lateral projection of the thoracic vertebral column

67. Which projection of the vertebral column best demonstrates scoliosis?

    a. PA projection of the thoracic vertebral column
    b. Lateral projection of the lumbar vertebral column
    c. Lateral projection of the thoracic vertebral column
    d. AP projection of the cervical vertebrae (open mouth)

68. Which projection of the vertebral column best demonstrates lordosis?

    a. AP projection of the lumbar vertebral column
    b. AP projection of the thoracic vertebral column
    c. Lateral projection of the lumbar vertebral column
    d. Lateral projection of the thoracic vertebral column

69. Why should the patient flex the hips and knees for the AP projection of the lumbar vertebral column?

    a. To reduce the lordotic curvature
    b. To increase the lordotic curvature
    c. To raise the diaphragm to its highest level
    d. To depress the diaphragm to its lowest level

70. How should the IR be positioned for the AP projection of the lumbar vertebrae and sacrum?

    a. Centered on the xiphoid process
    b. Centered on the level of the iliac crests
    c. Centered on the level of the greater trochanters
    d. With the top border at the level of the iliac crests
    e. With the bottom border at the level of the iliac crests

71. Which positioning maneuver should be performed to reduce the normal lordotic curvature for the AP projection of the lumbar vertebral column?

    a. Fully extend the legs.
    b. Flex the hips and knees.
    c. Angle the central ray 5 to 8 degrees caudad.
    d. Place radiolucent cushions under the lumbar spine.

72. Which plane or line of the patient should be centered on the midline of the table for the AP projection of the lumbar vertebral column?

    a. Oblique
    b. Horizontal
    c. Midsagittal
    d. Midcoronal

73. Where should the central ray be directed for the AP projection of the lumbar vertebral column for a lumbosacral examination?

    a. L2
    b. L4
    c. 3 inches (7.6 cm) above the iliac crests
    d. 2 inches (5 cm) above the symphysis pubis

74. Which plane or line of the patient should be centered on the midline of the table for the lateral projection of the lumbar vertebral column?

    a. Oblique
    b. Horizontal
    c. Midsagittal
    d. Midcoronal

75. Which projection of the lumbar vertebral column best demonstrates intervertebral foramina?

    a. AP projection
    b. Lateral projection
    c. PA oblique projection
    d. AP oblique projection

76. How many degrees and in which direction should the central ray be directed for the lateral projection of the lumbar vertebral column when the vertebral column is parallel with the table?

    a. Perpendicular
    b. 5 degrees caudad
    c. 5 degrees cephalad
    d. 8 degrees caudad
    e. 8 degrees cephalad

77. How many degrees and in which direction should the central ray be directed for the lateral projection of the lumbar vertebral column when the lumbar vertebral column is not parallel with the table?

    a. Perpendicular for males, 8 degrees caudad for females
    b. Perpendicular for females, 5 degrees caudad for males
    c. 5 degrees caudad for males, 8 degrees caudad for females
    d. 5 degrees caudad for females, 8 degrees caudad for males

78. How many degrees and in which direction should the central ray be directed for the lateral projection of L5-S1 when the lumbar vertebral column is parallel with the table?

    a. Perpendicular
    b. 5 to 8 degrees caudad
    c. 5 to 8 degrees cephalad
    d. 10 to 15 degrees caudad

79. Which projection of the lumbar vertebral column best demonstrates zygapophyseal joints?

    a. AP projection
    b. Lateral projection
    c. AP oblique projection
    d. Lateral projection, L5-S1

80. Which vertebral structures are best demonstrated if a supine patient is rotated 45 degrees with the right side elevated and a perpendicular central ray is directed at the lumbar vertebrae?

    a. Intervertebral foramina
    b. Lumbar vertebral bodies in profile
    c. Zygapophyseal joints on the left side
    d. Zygapophyseal joints on the right side

81. Which vertebral structures are best demonstrated with the AP oblique projection of the lumbar vertebral column with the patient RPO?

    a. L5-S1 junction
    b. Intervertebral foramina
    c. Lumbar vertebral bodies in profile
    d. Zygapophyseal joints of the left side
    e. Zygapophyseal joints of the right side

82. Which vertebral structures are best demonstrated with the AP oblique projection of the lumbar vertebral column with the patient LPO?

    a. Intervertebral foramina
    b. Lumbar vertebral bodies in profile
    c. Zygapophyseal joints of the left side
    d. Zygapophyseal joints of the right side

83. Which positioning error most likely occurred if the zygapophyseal joints were not well demonstrated and the pedicle was quite anterior on the vertebral body in AP oblique projection radiographs of the lumbar vertebral column?

    a. The patient was rotated too much.
    b. The patient was not rotated enough.
    c. The spine was not parallel with the table.
    d. The central ray was not perpendicular to the IR.

84. Which positioning error most likely occurred if the zygapophyseal joints were not well demonstrated and the pedicle was quite posterior on the vertebral body AP oblique projection radiographs of the lumbar vertebral column?

    a. The patient was rotated too much.
    b. The patient was not rotated enough.
    c. The spine was not parallel with the table.
    d. The central ray was not perpendicular to the IR.

85. Which projection of the vertebral column demonstrates the "Scottie dog"?

    a. Lateral projection of the lumbar vertebral column
    b. Lateral projection of the thoracic vertebral column
    c. Oblique projection of the lumbar vertebral column
    d. Oblique projection of the cervical vertebral column

86. What is demonstrated if the "Scottie dog" is well visualized?

    a. Zygapophyseal joints of the lumbar vertebrae
    b. Zygapophyseal joints of the thoracic vertebrae
    c. Intervertebral foramina of the lumbar vertebrae
    d. Intervertebral foramina of the thoracic vertebrae

87. How many degrees of body rotation are necessary for the AP oblique projection of the lumbar vertebral column?

    a. 15 to 20 degrees
    b. 25 to 30 degrees
    c. 45 degrees
    d. 70 degrees

88. Which projection of the lumbar vertebral column places the midsagittal plane perpendicular to the IR?

    a. AP projection
    b. Lateral projection
    c. AP oblique projection
    d. Lateral projection, L5-S1

89. Which projection of the lumbar vertebral column places the midsagittal plane parallel with the IR?

    a. AP projection
    b. Lateral projection
    c. LPO projection
    d. RPO projection

90. How many degrees and in which direction should the central ray be directed for AP axial projections of the lumbosacral junction?

    a. Perpendicular
    b. 5 to 8 degrees caudad
    c. 5 to 8 degrees cephalad
    d. 30 to 35 degrees caudad
    e. 30 to 35 degrees cephalad

91. Which projection best demonstrates the right sacroiliac joint?

    a. AP projection with the patient supine
    b. Lateral projection with the patient right lateral recumbent
    c. PA oblique projection with the patient in the LAO position
    d. AP oblique projection with the patient in the LPO position
    e. AP oblique projection with the patient in the RPO position

92. Which projection best demonstrates the left sacroiliac joint?

    a. AP projection with the patient supine
    b. Lateral projection with the patient left lateral recumbent
    c. AP oblique projection with the patient in the LAO position
    d. PA oblique projection with the patient in the RAO position
    e. AP oblique projection with the patient in the RPO position

93. How many degrees of body rotation from the supine position are required for AP oblique projections of the sacroiliac joints?

    a. 15 to 20 degrees
    b. 25 to 30 degrees
    c. 35 to 45 degrees
    d. 45 to 55 degrees

94. How many degrees and in which direction should the central ray be directed for AP axial projections of the sacrum?

    a. Perpendicular
    b. 10 degrees caudad
    c. 10 degrees cephalad
    d. 15 degrees caudad
    e. 15 degrees cephalad

95. How many degrees and in which direction should the central ray be directed if it is necessary to have the patient prone for a PA axial projection of the sacrum?

    a. Perpendicular
    b. 10 degrees caudad
    c. 10 degrees cephalad
    d. 15 degrees caudad
    e. 15 degrees cephalad

96. How many degrees and in which direction should the central ray be directed for AP projections of the coccyx?

    a. Perpendicular
    b. 10 degrees caudad
    c. 10 degrees cephalad
    d. 15 degrees caudad
    e. 15 degrees cephalad

97. How many degrees and in which direction should the central ray be directed if it is necessary to have the patient prone for a PA projection of the coccyx?

    a. Perpendicular
    b. 10 degrees caudad
    c. 10 degrees cephalad
    d. 15 degrees caudad
    e. 15 degrees cephalad

98. How many degrees and in which direction should the central ray be directed for lateral projections of the sacrum?

    a. Perpendicular
    b. 10 degrees caudad
    c. 10 degrees cephalad
    d. 15 degrees caudad
    e. 15 degrees cephalad

99. How many degrees and in which direction should the central ray be directed for lateral projections of the coccyx?

    a. Perpendicular
    b. 10 degrees caudad
    c. 10 degrees cephalad
    d. 15 degrees caudad
    e. 15 degrees cephalad

100. Which projection of the Ferguson method should be performed to best evaluate scoliosis?

    a. Upright PA
    b. Upright AP
    c. Recumbent PA
    d. Recumbent AP

CHAPTER 9

Bony Thorax

SECTION 1

Osteology and Arthrology of the Bony Thorax

Exercise 1

Instructions: This exercise pertains to the bony thorax. Identify structures for each question.

1. Identify each lettered structure shown in Fig. 9-1.

   A. _____

   B. _____

   C. _____

   D. _____

   E. _____

   F. _____

   G. _____

   H. _____

   I. _____

   J. _____

   K. _____

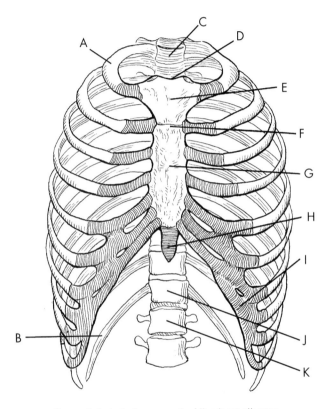

Figure 9-1 Anterior aspect of the bony thorax.

2. Identify each lettered structure of the sternum and the two types/groups of ribs shown in Fig. 9-2.

A. _____

B. _____

C. _____

D. _____

E. _____

F. _____

G. _____

3. Identify each lettered structure shown in Fig. 9-3.

A. _____

B. _____

C. _____

D. _____

E. _____

F. _____

G. _____

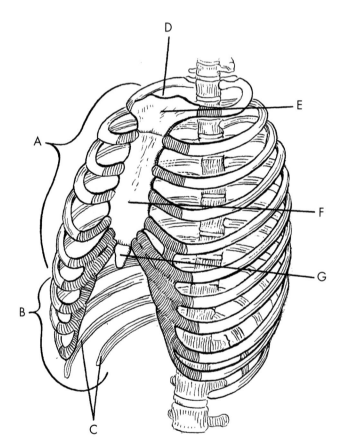

Figure 9-2 Anterolateral aspect of the bony thorax.

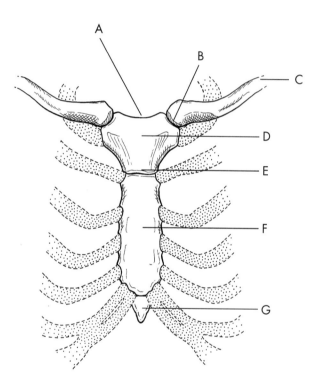

Figure 9-3 Anterior aspect of the sternum and sternoclavicular joints.

4. Identify each lettered rib or vertebra shown in Fig. 9-4.

A. _____

B. _____

C. _____

D. _____

E. _____

F. _____

5. Identify each lettered structure shown in Fig. 9-5.

A. _____

B. _____

C. _____

D. _____

E. _____

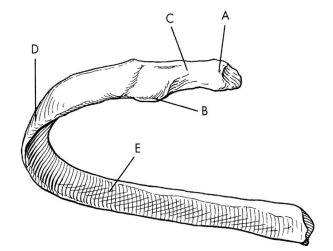

Figure 9-5 A typical rib viewed from the back.

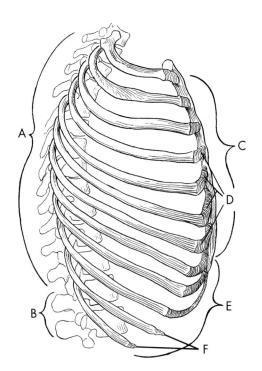

Figure 9-4 Lateral aspect of the bony thorax.

6. Identify each lettered structure or articulation shown in Fig. 9-6.

A. _____   F. _____

B. _____   G. _____

C. _____   H. _____

D. _____   I. _____

E. _____   J. _____

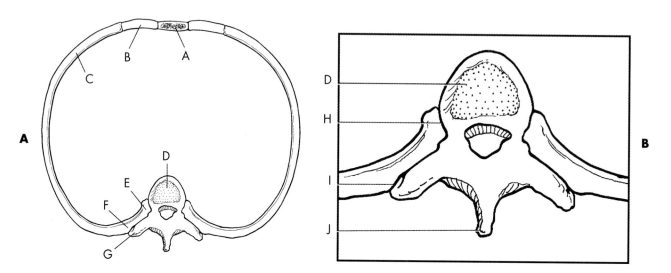

Figure 9-6 A, Superior aspect of ribs articulating with thoracic vertebra and sternum. **B,** Enlarged image of costovertebral articulations.

Exercise 2

Instructions: Use the following clues to complete the crossword puzzle. All answers refer to the bony thorax.

ACROSS

2. Both of these articulate with the manubrium
3. Ribs 8, 9, and 10
8. Twelve pairs of these are present in the thorax
10. Xiphoid process
12. Uppermost sternal joints
13. Rib classification

DOWN

1. _____ process
4. Rib joints with the sternum
5. Ribs without any anterior articulations
6. Superior sternal notch
7. The sternum
9. The breastbone
11. Superior part of sternum

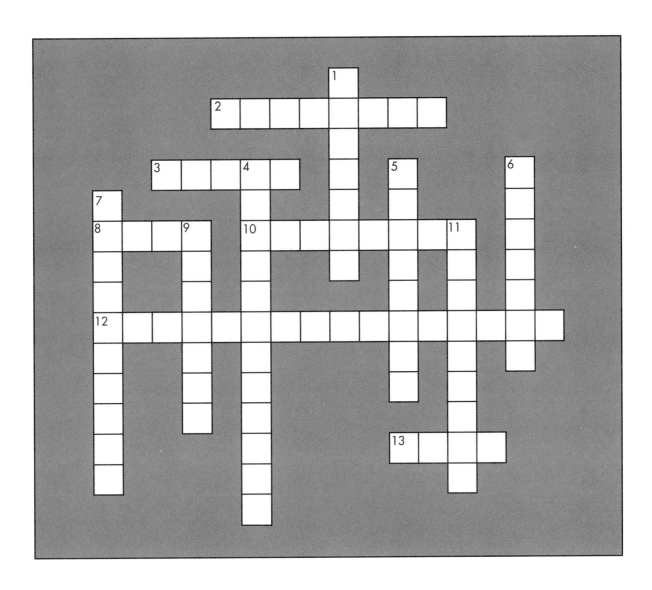

Exercise 3

Match the pathology terms in Column A with the appropriate definition in Column B. Not all choices from Column B should be selected.

Column A

_____ 1. Tumor

_____ 2. Fracture

_____ 3. Metastases

_____ 4. Osteoporosis

_____ 5. Osteopetrosis

_____ 6. Osteoarthritis

_____ 7. Osteomyelitis

_____ 8. Paget's disease

_____ 9. Chondrosarcoma

_____ 10. Multiple myeloma

Column B

a. Loss of bone density

b. Disruption of the continuity of bone

c. Benign tumor consisting of cartilage

d. Increased density of atypically soft bone

e. Malignant tumor arising from cartilage cells

f. Thick, soft bone marked by bowing and fractures

g. Inflammation of bone due to a pyogenic infection

h. Transfer of a cancerous lesion from one area to another

i. New tissue growth where cell proliferation is uncontrolled

j. Malignant neoplasm of plasma cells involving the bone marrow and causing destruction of bone

k. Form of arthritis marked by progressive cartilage deterioration in synovial joints and vertebrae

Exercise 4

Instructions: This exercise is a comprehensive review of the osteology and arthrology of the bony thorax. Provide a short answer, select the correct answer from a list, or choose true or false (explain any statement you believe to be false) for each item.

1. List the names and quantity of the structures that form the bony thorax.

2. What is the purpose of the bony thorax?

3. What is the formal name for the breastbone?

4. Name the parts of the sternum.

5. What is the approximate length of the sternum for the average adult?
   a. 2 inches (5 cm)
   b. 4 inches (10 cm)
   c. 6 inches (15 cm)

6. How many parts compose the sternum?

    a. 2
    b. 3
    c. 4

7. Which pairs of ribs attach their costal cartilage to the lateral borders of the sternum?

    a. The first seven pairs
    b. Pairs 8, 9, and 10
    c. Pairs 8, 9, 10, 11, and 12
    d. The last two pairs

8. Which part of the sternum supports the sternal ends of the clavicles?

    a. Body
    b. Manubrium
    c. Xiphoid process

9. What is the name for the most superior part of the sternum?

    a. Body
    b. Manubrium
    c. Xiphoid process

10. What is the name for the middle part of the sternum?

    a. Body
    b. Manubrium
    c. Xiphoid process

11. Which is the distal part of the sternum?

    a. Body
    b. Manubrium
    c. Xiphoid process

12. What is the name of the notch found on the superior border of the sternum?

    a. Sternal notch
    b. Jugular notch
    c. Manubrial notch

13. The jugular notch is found anterior to which precise location of the thoracic vertebral column?

    a. The disk space between C6 and C7
    b. The disk space between T2 and T3
    c. The disk space between T6 and T7

14. Where is the sternal angle located?

    a. At the junction of clavicles and manubrium
    b. At the junction of manubrium and sternal body
    c. At the junction of manubrium and xiphoid process

15. To which location of the thoracic column does the sternal angle correspond?

    a. The disk space between C7 and T1
    b. The disk space between T2 and T3
    c. The disk space between T4 and T5

16. To which location of the thoracic column does the xiphoid process correspond?

    a. T4
    b. T7
    c. T10

17. What determines whether a particular rib is a true rib or a false rib?

    a. Its anterior articulation
    b. Its posterior articulation
    c. Its articulations with costal tubercles

18. What pairs of ribs are classified as true ribs?

19. What pairs of ribs are classified as false ribs?

20. What pairs of ribs are referred to as "floating" ribs?

21. What structures form costovertebral joints?

22. With which structures do costal tubercles articulate?

24. True or False. The anterior end of a rib generally is located 3 to 5 inches (7.6 to 12.5 cm) below the level of its head.

25. True or False. Ribs increase in thickness the closer they are to the lumbar column.

23. What part of the sternum articulates with the anterior ends of the first pair of ribs to form the first sternocostal joints?

SECTION 2

Positioning of the Bony Thorax

Exercise 1: Positioning for the Sternum

Instructions: Most physicians require two views of the sternum to make an accurate diagnosis. In most cases, the projections of choice are the posteroanterior (PA) oblique projection (right anterior oblique [RAO] position) and the lateral projection. This exercise pertains to those projections. Identify structures, select the correct answer from a list, or choose true or false (explaining any statement you believe to be false) for each item.

Items 1 through 15 pertain to the *PA oblique projection (right anterior oblique [RAO] position)*. Examine Fig. 9-7, which shows a patient positioned for the right PA oblique projection, as you answer the following items.

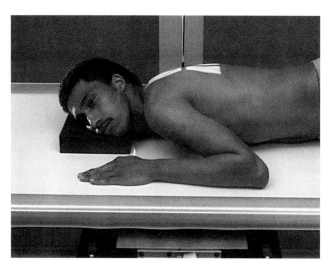

Figure 9-7 PA oblique sternum, RAO position.

1. Why should the patient be rotated into an oblique position instead of the positions used for AP or PA projections?
   a. To position the sternum parallel with the IR
   b. To prevent superimposition of the sternum with the heart
   c. To prevent superimposition of the sternum with the vertebral column

2. Why is an anterior oblique position preferred to a posterior oblique position?
   a. To reduce object-to-image receptor distance (OID) of the sternum
   b. To increase object-to-image receptor distance (OID) of the sternum
   c. To prevent superimposition of the sternum with the vertebral column

3. Why is the right anterior oblique projection, RAO position, preferred to the left anterior oblique projection (LAO) position?
   a. To use the heart shadow for background density
   b. To increase source-to-image receptor distance (SID) of the sternum
   c. To prevent superimposition of the sternum with the vertebral column

4. When the patient is positioned prone on the radiographic table, which side of the patient should be elevated away from the table?
   a. Right
   b. Left

5. Approximately how many degrees should the patient be rotated?
   a. 5 to 10
   b. 15 to 20
   c. 25 to 30
   d. 35 to 40

6. Which patient characteristic requires a greater amount of patient rotation to the RAO position?
   a. Deep chest
   b. Shallow chest

7. With reference to the patient, to what level should the top of the image receptor (IR) be placed?
   a. To $1\frac{1}{2}$ inches (3.8 cm) above the jugular notch
   b. To the jugular notch (T2-T3)
   c. To the midsternal area (T7)
   d. To the xiphoid process (T10)

8. From the following list, circle the two ways the patient's breathing should be controlled for the exposure.
   a. Breathe rapidly
   b. Breathe shallowly
   c. Suspend respiration after expiration
   d. Suspend respiration after inspiration

9. If a short exposure time is preferred, what breathing instructions should be given to the patient?
   a. Breathe rapidly
   b. Breathe shallowly
   c. Suspend respiration after expiration
   d. Suspend respiration after inspiration

10. How and where should the central ray be directed?
    a. Perpendicular to the xiphoid process
    b. Perpendicular to the elevated side of the posterior thorax at the level of T7
    c. 10 degrees cephalad to the xiphoid process
    d. 10 degrees cephalad to the elevated side of the posterior thorax at the level of T7

11. When the image made with the patient in the RAO position is properly viewed, where will the sternum appear with reference to the vertebral column?
    a. Toward the viewer's left and on the right side of the patient's thorax without vertebral superimposition
    b. Toward the viewer's right and on the left side of the patient's thorax without vertebral superimposition

12. True or False. The entire sternum should be seen without superimposition with vertebrae.

13. True or False. Pulmonary marking should be blurred when the patient is instructed to breathe slowly during the exposure.

14. True or False. The right sternoclavicular joint should be demonstrated superimposed with the vertebral column.

15. Identify each lettered structure shown in Fig. 9-8.

A. _____

B. _____

C. _____

D. _____

E. _____

F. _____

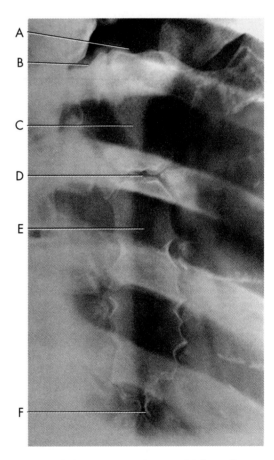

Figure 9-8 PA oblique sternum, RAO position.

Items 16 through 30 pertain to the *lateral projection*. Examine Fig. 9-9 as you answer the following items.

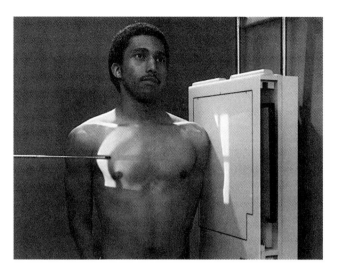

Figure 9-9 Lateral sternum.

16. How much SID is recommended for the lateral projection? Explain why.
    a. 40 inches; to blur overlying ribs
    b. 40 inches; to reduce magnification of the sternum
    c. 72 inches; to blur overlying ribs
    d. 72 inches; to reduce magnification of the sternum

17. With reference to the patient, where exactly should the IR be placed?
    a. The center of the IR should be at the level of the jugular notch
    b. The lower border of the IR should be at the level of the xiphoid process
    c. The upper border of the IR should be 1½ inches (3.8 cm) above the jugular notch

18. Describe how the patient's shoulders, arms, and hands should be positioned when the patient is in the upright position.

19. Describe how the patient's arms should be positioned when the patient is in the recumbent position.

20. For female patients with large breasts, what procedure should be done to prevent breast shadows from superimposing the sternum?

21. What breathing instructions should be given to the patient?

22. Why should the exposure be made with the patient following the required breathing instructions?

23. When the patient is in the lateral recumbent position, why should a support be placed under the lower thoracic region?

24. True or False. The midsagittal plane should be parallel with the plane of the image receptor.

25. True or False. The central ray should be directed perpendicular to the lateral border of the manubrium.

26. True or False. The patient should breathe slowly during the exposure in an effort to blur lung markings that may superimpose the sternum.

27. True or False. The sternum should be demonstrated in its entirety.

28. True or False. Patients who have experienced trauma may be positioned either upright, lateral recumbent, or supine, as their condition permits.

29. True or False. To help in determining that the sternum is positioned true lateral, the broad surface across the width of the sternum should be perpendicular to the plane of the image receptor.

30. Identify each lettered structure shown in Fig. 9-10.

   A. _____

   B. _____

   C. _____

   D. _____

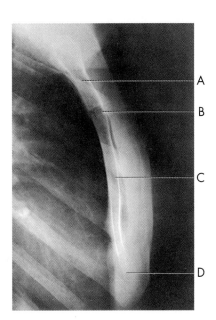

Figure 9-10 Lateral sternum.

Exercise 2: Positioning for Sternoclavicular Articulations

Instructions: Radiographs produced by the PA projection and PA oblique projections demonstrate the sternoclavicular (SC) joints. Provide a short answer, select the correct answer from a list, or choose true or false (explaining any statement you believe to be false) for each item. Items 1 through 8 pertain to the *PA projection.* Examine Fig. 9-11 as you answer the following items.

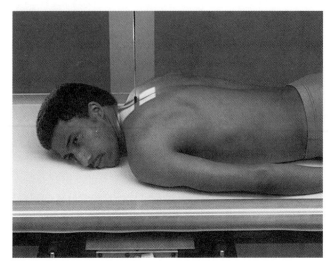

Figure 9-11 PA projection of left sternoclavicular articulation.

1. To what level of the patient's thoracic vertebral column should the image receptor be centered?

2. Describe how the patient's arms should be positioned when the patient is in the prone position.

3. For the bilateral procedure, how should the patient's head be positioned?

4. How does rotation of the patient's head to one side improve the demonstration of the affected sternoclavicular joint?

5. How and to where should the central ray be directed?

6. Which breathing instructions should be given to the patient?

   a. Breathe rapidly
   b. Breathe shallowly
   c. Suspend respiration after expiration
   d. Suspend respiration after inspiration

7. True or False. The clavicles should be demonstrated in their entirety.

8. True or False. Slight rotation of the vertebral column is permitted for the PA projection in bilateral examinations.

Items 9 through 15 pertain to the *PA oblique projection.* Examine Fig. 9-12 as you answer the following items.

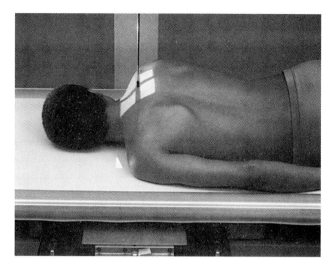

Figure 9-12 PA oblique projection of sternoclavicular articulation, LAO position.

9. Which SC joint—the affected side or the unaffected side—should be positioned closer to the IR for the body rotation method?

10. How many degrees should the patient be rotated for the body rotation method?

11. To what level of the patient should the IR be centered for the body rotation method?

12. How should the central ray be directed for the body rotation method?

    a. Perpendicularly
    b. 15 degrees caudad
    c. 15 degrees cephalad
    d. 15 degrees toward the midsagittal plane

13. Where should the IR be placed for the central ray (CR) angulation method when the patient is in the recumbent position?

    a. In the holder under the tabletop
    b. On top of the table and in contact with the patient

14. Describe how the central ray should be directed for the CR angulation method.

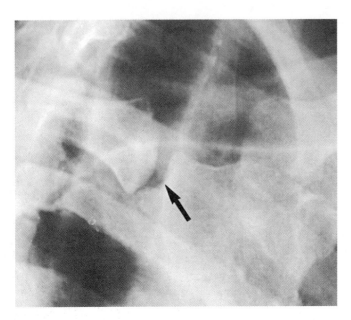

Fig. 9-13 Body rotation showing the sternoclavicular joint *(arrow)*.

15. Fig. 9-13 shows an image produced by the body rotation method. Examine the image and answer the questions that follow.

    a. How should the central ray be directed—angled or perpendicularly?

    _____

    b. Which body position—RAO or LAO—is represented in the image?

    _____

    c. Which sternoclavicular joint—right or left—is of primary interest?

    _____

Exercise 3: Positioning for the Ribs

Instructions: This exercise pertains to the projections used to demonstrate ribs. Provide a short answer, select from a list, or choose true or false (explaining any statement you believe to be false) for each question. Items 1 through 10 pertain to the *PA projection.* Examine Fig. 9-14 as you answer the following questions.

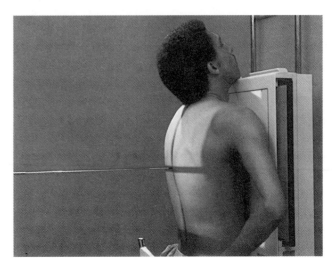

Figure 9-14 PA ribs.

1. Which ribs—above or below the diaphragm—are best demonstrated with the PA projection?

2. How should the patient be positioned—recumbent or upright—to best demonstrate ribs with the PA projection?

3. Why should the patient be positioned upright for the PA projection?

4. With reference to the patient, where should the top of the IR be positioned?

5. How should the patient's upper limbs (extremities) be placed to cause the scapulae to rotate laterally?

6. How should the patient's head be positioned if the patient is in the prone position?

7. What breathing instructions should be given to the patient? Explain why.

8. How and where should the central ray be directed?

9. Describe how the PA projection can be adjusted to better demonstrate the 7th, 8th, and 9th ribs when the diaphragm is in the way.

10. What pairs of ribs should be demonstrated in their entirety?

Items 11 through 18 pertain to AP projections for *demonstrating ribs above the diaphragm.* Examine Fig. 9-15 as you answer those items.

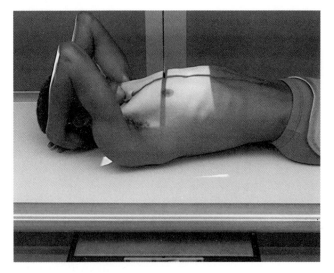

Figure 9-15 AP ribs above the diaphragm.

11. What is the preferred body position—supine or upright—for the patient? Explain why.

12. With reference to the patient, where should the top of the IR be positioned?

13. Why should a patient's shoulders be rotated forward?

14. What breathing instructions should be given to the patient? Explain why.

15. How and where should the central ray be directed?

16. Which ribs—anterior or posterior—are presented in best recorded detail?

17. What ribs should be demonstrated?

18. Suppose that a patient with injured posterior ribs numbers 5 and 6 needed proper radiographs. List (a) the body position in which the patient should be placed and (b) the recommended breathing instructions.

   a. _____

   b. _____

Items 19 through 25 pertain to AP projections for *demonstrating ribs below the diaphragm.* Examine Fig. 9-16 as you answer those items.

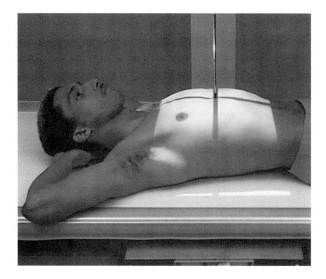

Figure 9-16 AP ribs below the diaphragm.

19. What size image receptor should be used for imaging the average adult?

20. What is the preferred body position—supine or upright—for the patient? Explain why.

21. If using the IR crosswise, to what level of the patient should the lower edge of the IR be aligned?

22. What breathing instructions should be given to the patient? Explain why.

23. How and where should the central ray be directed?

24. What pairs of ribs should be demonstrated?

25. Suppose that a patient with injured posterior ribs numbers 10 and 11 needed proper radiographs. List (a) the body position in which the patient should be placed and (b) the recommended breathing instructions.

a. _____

b. _____

Items 26 through 33 pertain to *AP oblique projections, RPO and LPO positions.* Examine Fig. 9-17 as you answer those items.

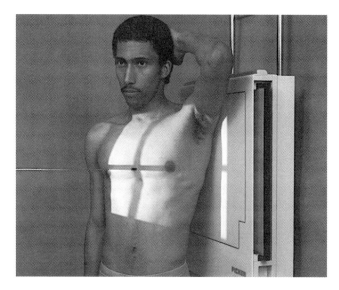

Figure 9-17 AP oblique ribs, LPO position.

26. True or False. AP oblique projections demonstrate posterior ribs better than anterior ribs.

27. True or False. The AP oblique projection with the patient LPO best demonstrates the posterior and axillary portions of the left ribs.

28. Which ribs—the affected side or the unaffected side—should be placed closer to the IR for best imaging with AP oblique projections?

29. How many degrees of body rotation are required to image the axillary portion of the ribs without self-superimposition?

30. With reference to the patient, where should the IR be placed for the following injured ribs?

    a. Ribs 5 and 6: _____

    b. Ribs 10 and 11: _____

31. What factor determines the breathing instructions that should be given to the patient?

32. What pairs of ribs above the diaphragm should be demonstrated?

33. What pairs of ribs below the diaphragm should be demonstrated?

34. Examine Fig. 9-18 and answer the following questions.

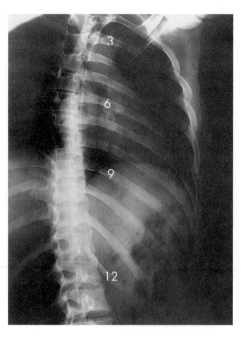

Figure 9-18 AP oblique ribs.

a. What radiographic position is represented in the image?

b. The ribs of which side are best demonstrated?

c. Which side of the patient is closest to the film?

Questions 35 through 40 pertain to *PA oblique projections, RAO and LAO positions.* Examine Fig. 9-19 as you answer those questions.

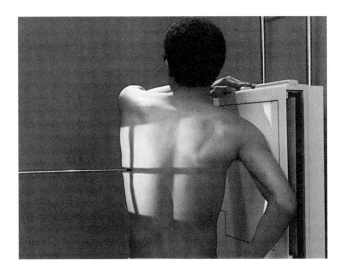

Figure 9-19 PA oblique ribs, RAO position.

35. With a patient in the upright position, which shoulder should be moved away from the IR if the ribs of the right side need to be demonstrated?

36. Which PA oblique projection—RAO or LAO—should be used to best demonstrate ribs of the left side?

37. Which ribs—those of the right side or those of the left side—are best demonstrated with the patient in the LAO position?

38. Which positioning factor could prevent using the recumbent position to demonstrate ribs below the diaphragm?
    a. Patient condition
    b. Image receptor size
    c. Source-to-image receptor distance

39. Examine Fig. 9-20 and answer the following questions.

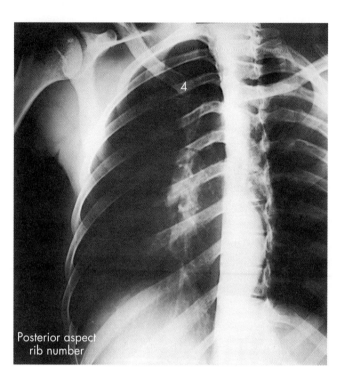

Figure 9-20 PA oblique ribs.

a. Which body position is represented in the image?

_____

b. Which ribs are best demonstrated?

_____

c. Which side of the patient is closest to the film?

_____

d. What breathing instructions should be given to the patient?

_____

40. From the following list, circle the five evaluation criteria indicating that the patient was properly positioned and imaged for AP oblique and PA oblique projections.

a. The trachea should be visible in the midline.

b. The 1st through 10th ribs should be seen above the diaphragm for upper ribs.

c. The axillary portion of the ribs should be demonstrated free of superimposition.

d. The 8th through 12th ribs should be seen below the diaphragm for lower ribs.

e. Both clavicles should be seen in a horizontal placement superior to the apices.

f. The ribs should be demonstrated clearly through the lungs or abdomen according to the region examined.

g. The distance from the vertebral column to the lateral border of the ribs should be equidistant on each side.

h. The distance between the vertebral column and the outer border of the ribs on the affected side should be approximately twice that of the unaffected side.

Self-Test: Osteology, Arthrology, and Positioning of the Bony Thorax

Instructions: Answer the following questions by selecting the best choice.

1. Which bone classification are ribs?

   a. Flat
   b. Long
   c. Short
   d. Irregular

2. What is the proper name for that structure commonly called the "breastbone"?

   a. Scapula
   b. Sternum
   c. Manubrium
   d. Xiphoid process

3. Which bone classification is the sternum?

   a. Flat
   b. Long
   c. Short
   d. Irregular

4. Which three bony parts compose the sternum?

   a. Head, body, and xiphoid process
   b. Head, body, and odontoid process
   c. Manubrium, body, and xiphoid process
   d. Manubrium, body, and odontoid process

5. Which part of the sternum is most superior?

   a. Head
   b. Body
   c. Manubrium
   d. Xiphoid process

6. Which of the following articulates with the articular facets located just lateral to the jugular notch?

   a. Ribs
   b. Clavicles
   c. Sternal body
   d. Xiphoid process

7. The junction of which structures creates the sternal angle?

   a. Ribs and sternal body
   b. Clavicles and manubrium
   c. Manubrium and sternal body
   d. Manubrium and xiphoid process

8. Which part of the sternum is the elongated central portion?

   a. Head
   b. Body
   c. Sternal angle
   d. Xiphoid process

9. Where on the sternum is the jugular notch located?

   a. Lateral border of the body
   b. Lateral border of the manubrium
   c. Superior border of the body
   d. Superior border of the manubrium

10. What is the smallest part of the sternum?

    a. Body
    b. Manubrium
    c. Xiphoid process

11. Which part of the sternum is located at the level of T10?

    a. Body
    b. Angle
    c. Manubrium
    d. Xiphoid process

12. With which part of the sternum does the first pair of ribs articulate?

    a. Lateral border of the manubrium
    b. Lateral border of the body
    c. Superior border of the manubrium
    d. Superior border of the body

13. Which classification refers to ribs that attach their costal cartilages directly to the sternum?

    a. True
    b. False
    c. Primary
    d. Floating

14. Which classification refers to ribs that have no anterior attachments?

    a. True
    b. Primary
    c. Floating
    d. Secondary

15. Which classification refers to the 11th and 12th pairs of ribs?

    a. True
    b. False
    c. Primary
    d. Secondary

16. Which pairs of ribs are classified as true ribs?

    a. The first seven pairs
    b. Pairs 8, 9, and 10
    c. Pairs 8, 9, 10, 11, and 12
    d. The last two pairs

17. How many pairs of ribs are classified as floating ribs?

    a. 1
    b. 2
    c. 7
    d. 10

18. Which articulation is formed in part with a head of a rib?

    a. Costosternal
    b. Costovertebral
    c. Costotransverse
    d. Sternoclavicular

19. With which structures do heads of ribs articulate?

    a. Cartilage of adjacent ribs
    b. Lateral borders of the sternum
    c. Demifacets of thoracic vertebrae
    d. Transverse processes of thoracic vertebrae

20. Which articulation involves the tubercle of a rib?

    a. Costosternal
    b. Costovertebral
    c. Costotransverse
    d. Sternoclavicular

21. Which radiographic position best demonstrates the sternum projected within the heart shadow?

    a. LAO
    b. LPO
    c. RAO
    d. RPO

22. For the oblique position that best demonstrates the sternum, how many degrees should the patient be rotated?

    a. 15 to 20 degrees
    b. 25 to 30 degrees
    c. 30 to 40 degrees
    d. 35 to 45 degrees

23. Which two projections generally compose the typical series demonstrating the sternum?

    a. PA and lateral
    b. PA and right PA oblique, RAO position
    c. Lateral and left PA oblique, LAO position
    d. Lateral and right PA oblique, RAO position

24. How should the central ray be directed for the oblique position to best demonstrate the sternum?

    a. Perpendicularly
    b. Caudally 15 degrees
    c. Cephalically 15 degrees
    d. Caudally 20 degrees

25. To best demonstrate the sternum, the patient should be rotated into the _____ position to image the sternum _____.

    a. LAO; within the heart shadow
    b. RAO; within the heart shadow
    c. LAO; without superimposing with the vertebral column
    d. RAO; without superimposing with the vertebral column

26. With reference to the patient, where should the top border of the IR be positioned for the lateral projection of the sternum?

    a. At the level of the clavicles
    b. At the level of the sternal angle
    c. $1^1/_2$ inches (3.8 cm) above the jugular notch
    d. $1^1/_2$ inches (3.8 cm) above the top of the shoulders

27. Which procedure should be performed for the lateral projection of the sternum?

    a. Rotate the shoulders forward.
    b. Ask the patient to take slow, shallow breaths.
    c. Raise both arms and rest forearms on top of the head.
    d. Increase the source-to-image receptor distance to 72 inches.

28. Which procedure should be performed to demonstrate only one sternoclavicular joint with the PA projection?

    a. Rest the patient's head on the chin.
    b. Direct the central ray 15 degrees medially.
    c. Turn the patient's head to face the affected side.
    d. Elevate the shoulder of the affected side 15 degrees.

29. Which procedure should be performed to demonstrate both sternoclavicular joints with the PA projection?

    a. Rest the patient's head on the chin.
    b. Direct the central ray 15 degrees medially.
    c. Have the patient breathe slowly with shallow breaths.
    d. Direct the central ray to enter the patient's back at T7.

30. How should the central ray be directed and centered for the PA projection for bilateral sternoclavicular joints?

    a. Perpendicular to T3
    b. Perpendicular to T7
    c. Angled medially 15 degrees, entering at T3
    d. Angled cephalically 15 degrees, entering at T7

31. To demonstrate bilateral sternoclavicular joints, which evaluation criterion indicates that the patient was properly positioned?

    a. Slight rotation of the affected side should be seen.
    b. The sternum should be demonstrated in its entirety.
    c. No rotation of the SC joints should be demonstrated.
    d. Both clavicles should be demonstrated in their entirety.

32. To most effectively demonstrate injured anterior ribs numbers 5 and 6 on the right side, which two projections should be included as part of the series?

    a. PA and PA oblique with the patient LAO
    b. PA and PA oblique with the patient RAO
    c. AP and AP oblique with the patient LPO
    d. AP and AP oblique with the patient RPO

33. To most effectively demonstrate injured anterior ribs numbers 6 and 7 on the left side, which two projections should be included as part of the series?

    a. PA and PA oblique with the patient LAO
    b. PA and PA oblique with the patient RAO
    c. AP and AP oblique with the patient LPO
    d. AP and AP oblique with the patient RPO

34. To most effectively demonstrate injured posterior ribs numbers 5 and 6 on the left side, which two projections should be included as part of the series?

    a. PA and PA oblique with the patient LAO
    b. PA and PA oblique with the patient RAO
    c. AP and AP oblique with the patient LPO
    d. AP and AP oblique with the patient RPO

35. To most effectively demonstrate injured posterior ribs numbers 6 and 7 on the right side, which two projections should be included as part of the series?

    a. PA and PA oblique with the patient LAO
    b. PA and PA oblique with the patient RAO
    c. AP and AP oblique with the patient LPO
    d. AP and AP oblique with the patient RPO

36. Which procedure should be used to obtain radiographs of injured anterior ribs numbers 5 and 6?

    a. Patient upright; exposure taken on suspended expiration
    b. Patient upright; exposure taken on suspended inspiration
    c. Patient recumbent; exposure taken on suspended expiration
    d. Patient recumbent; exposure taken on suspended inspiration

37. If the patient's condition permits, which procedure should be used to best demonstrate injured posterior ribs numbers 10, 11, and 12?

    a. Patient prone; exposure taken on suspended expiration
    b. Patient prone; exposure taken on suspended inspiration
    c. Patient supine; exposure taken on suspended expiration
    d. Patient supine; exposure taken on suspended inspiration

38. Which two projections best demonstrate injured posterior ribs numbers 10, 11, and 12 on the right side?

    a. AP and AP oblique with the patient LPO
    b. AP and AP oblique with the patient RPO
    c. PA and AP oblique with the patient LPO
    d. PA and AP oblique with the patient RPO

39. Which two projections best demonstrate injured posterior ribs numbers 10, 11, and 12 on the left side?

    a. PA and AP oblique with the patient LPO
    b. PA and AP oblique with the patient RPO
    c. AP and AP oblique with the patient LPO
    d. AP and AP oblique with the patient RPO

40. Which radiographic position best demonstrates the posterior 11th rib on the right side without vertebral superimposition?

    a. LAO
    b. LPO
    c. RAO
    d. RPO

41. Which radiographic position best demonstrates the posterior 10th rib on the left side without vertebral superimposition?

    a. LAO
    b. LPO
    c. RAO
    d. RPO

42. Which radiographic position best demonstrates the anterior 6th rib on the left side without vertebral superimposition?

    a. LAO
    b. LPO
    c. RAO
    d. RPO

43. Which radiographic position best demonstrates the anterior 5th rib on the right side without vertebral superimposition?

    a. LAO
    b. LPO
    c. RAO
    d. RPO

44. With reference to the patient, where should the top border of the IR be positioned for the PA projection to demonstrate ribs above the diaphragm?

    a. At the level of T7
    b. At the level of the clavicles
    c. $1\frac{1}{2}$ inches (3.8 cm) above the shoulders
    d. $1\frac{1}{2}$ inches (3.8 cm) above the sternal angle

45. For the AP projection demonstrating ribs above the diaphragm, when should respiration be suspended and what effect will that have on the diaphragm?

    a. On full inspiration; will depress the diaphragm
    b. On full inspiration; will elevate the diaphragm
    c. On full expiration; will depress the diaphragm
    d. On full expiration; will elevate the diaphragm

46. For the AP projection demonstrating ribs below the diaphragm, when should respiration be suspended and what effect will that have on the diaphragm?

    a. On full inspiration; will depress the diaphragm
    b. On full inspiration; will elevate the diaphragm
    c. On full expiration; will depress the diaphragm
    d. On full expiration; will elevate the diaphragm

47. When performing the AP projection to demonstrate ribs below the diaphragm, with reference to the patient, how should the image receptor be positioned?

    a. Center the image receptor at the level of L3
    b. Center the image receptor at the level of iliac crests
    c. Lower border of the image receptor at the level of L3
    d. Lower border of the image receptor at the level of iliac crests

48. Which projection best demonstrates the axillary portion of ribs?

    a. AP projection
    b. PA projection
    c. Lateral projection
    d. AP oblique projection

49. Which procedure can be performed to better demonstrate the 7th, 8th, and 9th ribs away from the shadow of the diaphragm?

    a. Central ray directed perpendicular to T7
    b. Rapid breathing to blur the diaphragm shadow
    c. Higher centering and caudal angulation of the central ray
    d. Higher centering and cephalad angulation of the central ray

50. Which of the following evaluation criteria pertains to the AP oblique projection for ribs?

    a. Trachea should be seen in the midline of the thorax.
    b. Heart and mediastinum should be seen in the center of the image.
    c. Axillary portion of the ribs of interest should be free of superimposition.
    d. Sternal ends of the clavicles should be equidistant from the vertebral column.

CHAPTER 10

Thoracic Viscera

SECTION 1

Anatomy of the Chest

Exercise 1

Instructions: This exercise pertains to the chest and thoracic viscera. Identify structures for each illustration.

1. Identify each lettered structure shown in Fig. 10-1.

    A. _____

    B. _____

    C. _____

    D. _____

    E. _____

    F. _____

    G. _____

2. Identify each lettered structure shown in Fig. 10-2.

    A. _____

    B. _____

    C. _____

    D. _____

    E. _____

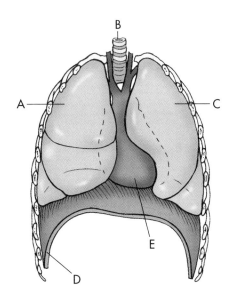

Figure 10-2 Thoracic cavity with anterior ribs removed.

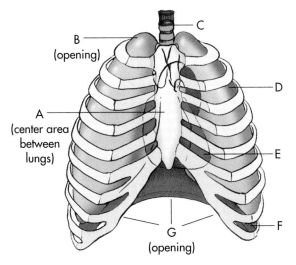

Figure 10-1 Thoracic cavity.

3. Identify each lettered structure shown in Fig. 10-3.

A. _____

B. _____

C. _____

D. _____

E. _____

F. _____

G. _____

H. _____

I. _____

J. _____

K. _____

L. _____

4. Identify each lettered structure shown in Fig. 10-4.

A. _____

B. _____

C. _____

D. _____

E. _____

F. _____

G. _____

H. _____

I. _____

J. _____

K. _____

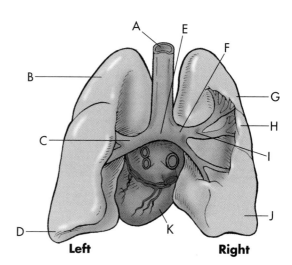

Figure 10-4 Posterior aspect of heart, lungs, trachea, and

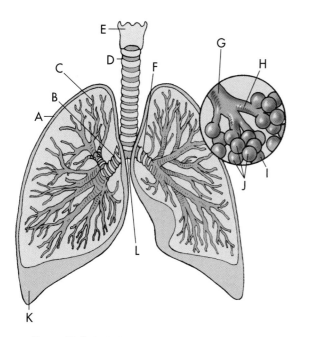

Figure 10-3 Anterior aspect of respiratory system.

5. Identify each lettered structure in Figure 10-5.

A. _____

B. _____

C. _____

D. _____

E. _____

F. _____

G. _____

H. _____

I. _____

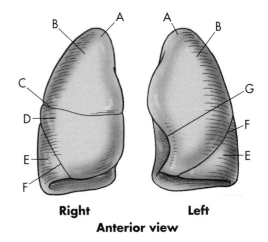

Right   **Left**

Anterior view

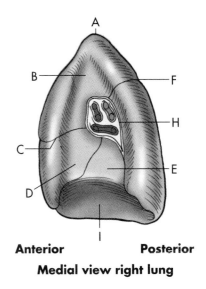

Anterior   **Posterior**

Medial view right lung

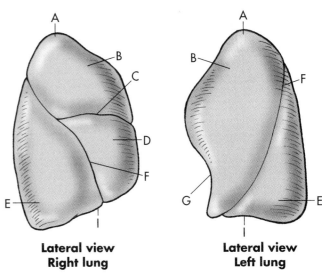

Lateral view   **Lateral view**
Right lung   **Left lung**

Figure 10-5 Three views of the lungs.

Exercise 2

Instructions: Use the following clues to complete the cross-word puzzle. All answers refer to the lungs and thoracic cavity.

ACROSS

1. Found in each lobe
3. Where vessels enter a lung
4. Superior portion of a lung
5. Inferior border of thoracic cavity
7. Respiratory organ
10. Major airway tube
13. Body type
14. Number of lobes in the right lung
16. Side of lung where vessels enter
17. Double-walled, serous membrane sac
18. Respiratory sacs

DOWN

1. Anterior bony wall of the mediastinum
2. Area between the lungs
3. Mediastinal organ
6. Mediastinal blood vessel
7. Major section of a lung
8. This lung has two lobes
9. Inferior part of a lung
11. Pertaining to the chest cavity
12. These branch from the trachea
15. Separates a lung into lobes

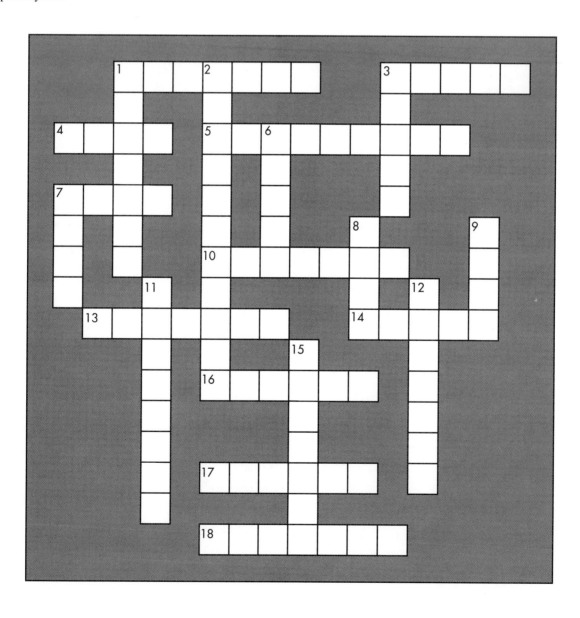

Exercise 3

Instructions: This exercise pertains to the anatomic structures found in the chest. Provide a short answer or select the correct answer from a list for each question.

1. Which cavity contains the heart and lungs?

   a. Thoracic
   b. Abdominal
   c. Mediastinum

2. Which structure separates the thoracic cavity from the abdominal cavity?

   a. Liver
   b. Heart
   c. Trachea
   d. Diaphragm

3. Which part of the thoracic cavity contains all thoracic organs except the lungs and pleurae?

   a. Mediastinum
   b. Pleural cavity
   c. Abdominal cavity

4. Which bony structure forms the anterior border of the mediastinum?

   a. Sternum
   b. Scapulae
   c. Thoracic vertebral column

5. What mediastinal structure consists of C-shaped cartilaginous rings?

   a. Trachea
   b. Diaphragm
   c. Esophagus

6. What area of the trachea divides into two lesser tubes?

   a. Carina
   b. Larynx
   c. Pharynx

7. Which structures branch from the distal end of the trachea?

   a. Tertiary bronchi
   b. Primary bronchi
   c. Secondary bronchi

8. Which primary bronchus is shorter and wider than the other?

   a. Left
   b. Right
   c. Inferior
   d. Superior

9. What thoracic structures are the organs of respiration?

   a. Lungs
   b. Bronchi
   c. Bronchiole

10. What is the name of the medial aspect of each lung in which the primary bronchus enters?

    a. Apex
    b. Hilum
    c. Pleural space

11. What is the name of the superior portion of each lung?

    a. Base
    b. Apex
    c. Hilum

12. Which structures are at the terminal end of the respiratory system?

    a. Alveoli
    b. Bronchi
    c. Bronchioles

13. How many lobes are found in the right lung? The left lung?

14. Which lung—right or left—is shorter and broader than the other? Explain why.

15. Name the three portions of the pleura.

   a. Inner layer:

   b. Outer layer:

   c. Space between layers:

Exercise 4

Match the pathology terms in Column A with the appropriate definition in Column B. Not all choices from Column B should be selected.

Column A

_____ 1. Atelectasis

_____ 2. Sarcoidosis

_____ 3. Emphysema

_____ 4. Tuberculosis

_____ 5. Pneumothorax

_____ 6. Pleural effusion

_____ 7. Pulmonary edema

_____ 8. Lobar (bacterial) pneumonia

_____ 9. Lobular (bronchopneumonia)

_____ 10. Hyaline membrane disease (respiratory distress syndrome)

a. A collapse of all or part of a lung

b. Collection of fluid in the pleural cavity

c. Pneumonia caused by aspiration of foreign particles

d. Underaeration of the lungs due to a lack of surfactant

e. Chronic infection of the lung due to the tubercle bacillus

f. Condition of the lung marked by formation of granulomas

g. Replacement of air with fluid in the lung interstitium and alveoli

h. Pneumonia involving the bronchi and scattered throughout the lung

i. Condition of unknown origin often associated with pulmonary fibrosis

j. Accumulation of air in the pleural cavity resulting in collapse of the lung

k. Pneumonia involving the alveoli of an entire lobe without involving the bronchi

l. Destructive and obstructive airway changes leading to an increased volume of air in the lungs

SECTION 2

Positioning of the Chest

Exercise 1: PA and Lateral Projections

Instructions: Various projections are used to obtain views of the heart and lungs. Usually only two views—the posteroanterior (PA) projection and the lateral projection—are necessary to adequately demonstrate thoracic viscera. This exercise pertains to those two projections. Identify structures, provide a short answer, or choose true or false (explaining any statement you believe to be false) for each item.

Items 1 through 17 pertain to the *PA projection.* Examine Fig. 10-6 as you answer the following items.

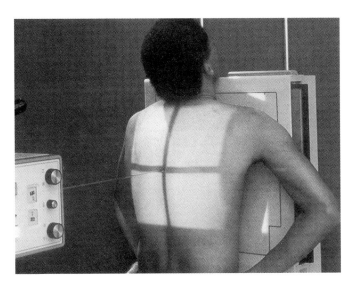

Figure 10-6 PA chest.

1. What is the recommended source-to-image receptor distance (SID)? Explain why.

2. Why is it preferable to have the patient upright?

3. Which body plane should be perpendicular and centered to the midline of the image receptor?

4. How should the patient's hands be positioned? Explain why.

5. With reference to the patient, where should the upper border of the image receptor (IR) be placed?
   a. At the level of the clavicles
   b. At the level of the acromion processes
   c. About $1\frac{1}{2}$ to 2 inches (3.8 to 5 cm) above the top of the shoulders

6. What is the purpose of depressing the shoulders?
   a. To move the scapulae laterally
   b. To keep the clavicles below the apices
   c. To place the midsagittal plane in a vertical position

7. Why should the shoulders be rotated forward?
   a. To keep the clavicles below the apices
   b. To place the diaphragm at its lowest point
   c. To move the scapulae laterally away from the lung fields

8. What special positioning instructions may be given to a woman with large, pendulous breasts to avoid superimposing the lower part of the lung fields?
   a. Instruct the patient to cross both arms above the head
   b. Instruct the patient to pull her breasts upward and laterally
   c. Instruct the patient to press her breasts directly in front of her against the vertical IR holder

9. Which is the most likely effect to the image if a patient were to remove one shoulder from contact with the grid device prior to the exposure of the radiograph?

   a. The clavicles would appear above the apices.

   b. The sternum would superimpose the vertebral column.

   c. The sternoclavicular joints would appear symmetrical.

   d. The sternal ends of the clavicles would no longer be equidistant from the vertebral column.

10. How and where should the central ray be directed?

   a. Angled caudally to the center of the image receptor at the level of T7

   b. Angled caudally to the center of the image receptor at the level of T10

   c. Perpendicular to the center of the image receptor and the midsagittal plane at the level of T7

   d. Perpendicular to the center of the image receptor and the midsagittal plane at the level of T10

11. What breathing instructions should be given to the patient? Explain why.

12. List two reasons why exposures can be made after both inspiration and expiration.

13. To demonstrate the heart, why should the exposure be made after normal inspiration rather than deep inspiration?

14. Figs. 10-7 and 10-8 are PA projection radiographs of the same patient, but with one difference in positioning. Examine the images and answer the questions that follow.

a. Which image was produced with the patient lifting and pulling her breasts laterally before the exposure?

b. Which aspect of the image helped you to determine that answer?

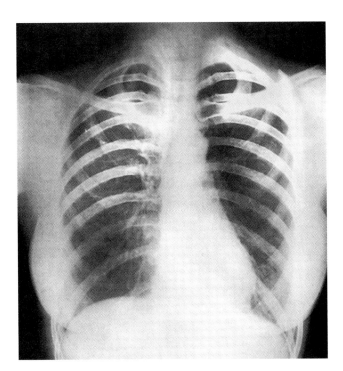

Figure 10-7 PA chest.

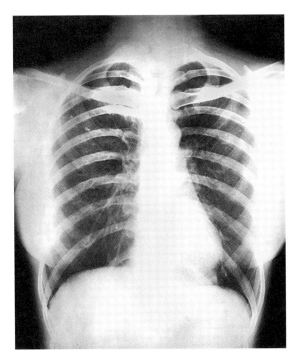

Figure 10-8 PA chest.

15. Figs. 10-9 and 10-10 are PA projection radiographs for which different breathing instructions were given to the patients. Examine the images and answer the questions that follow.

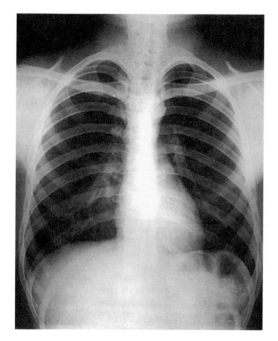

Figure 10-9 PA chest.

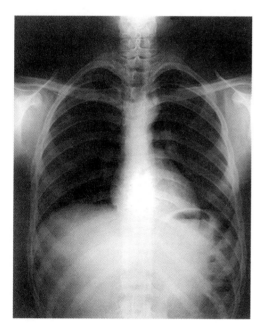

Figure 10-10 PA chest.

a. Which image was exposed with the patient suspending respiration on full inspiration?

b. Which aspect of the image helped you to determine that answer?

c. How many posterior ribs should be demonstrated above the diaphragm with proper full inspiration?

16. From the following list, circle eight evaluation criteria that indicate a patient was properly positioned for a PA projection.

    a. The trachea should be visible in the midline.
    b. The heart and diaphragm should show sharp outlines.
    c. The clavicles should be lying superiorly to the apices.
    d. Ten posterior ribs should be seen above the diaphragm.
    e. The scapulae should be projected outside the lung fields.
    f. The exposure should clearly demonstrate the lung fields.
    g. The ribs should be superimposed posterior to the vertebral column.
    h. The hilum should be seen in the approximate center of the radiograph.
    i. The entire lung fields from the apices to the costophrenic angles should be seen.
    j. No rotation; the sternal ends of the clavicles should be equidistant from the vertebral column.
    k. The clavicles should be lying horizontal with their medial ends overlapping the first or second ribs.
    l. A faint shadow of the ribs and superior thoracic vertebrae should be seen through the heart shadow.

17. Identify each lettered structure shown in Fig. 10-11.

    A. _____

    B. _____

    C. _____

    D. _____

    E. _____

    F. _____

    G. _____

    H. _____

    I. _____

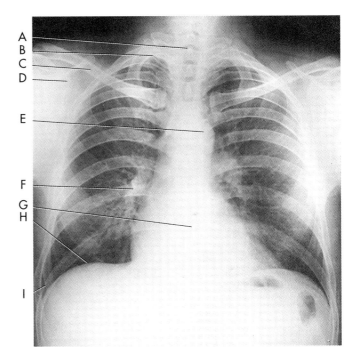

Figure 10-11 PA chest.

Items 18 through 30 pertain to the *lateral projection.* Examine Fig. 10-12 as you answer the following items.

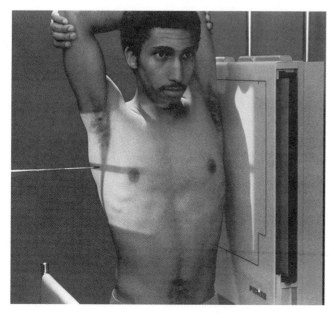

Figure 10-12 Lateral chest.

18. Which thoracic structures are of primary interest with the left lateral projection?

    a. Heart and left lung
    b. Heart and right lung
    c. Trachea and diaphragm
    d. Trachea and esophagus

19. Which thoracic structure is of primary interest with the right lateral projection?

    a. Heart
    b. Trachea
    c. Left lung
    d. Right lung

20. What body plane should be perpendicular and centered to the midline of the image receptor?

21. Describe how the patient's arms should be positioned.

22. What purpose might an IV stand serve when the patient is positioned?

23. How far above the top of the shoulders should the upper border of the IR be placed?

24. What breathing instructions should be given to the patient?

25. Describe how and where the central ray should be directed and centered.

26. True or False. The midsagittal plane should be placed perpendicular to the plane of the IR.

27. True or False. A lateral projection radiograph of the chest should be placed on an illuminator so that the side of the patient where the central ray entered is nearer the viewer.

28. True or False. The patient's heart will appear larger in the right lateral projection radiograph than in the left lateral projection radiograph.

29. From the following list, circle the nine evaluation criteria that indicate the patient was properly positioned for a lateral projection.

   a. The heart and diaphragm should be seen in sharp outline.
   b. The sternum should be seen in lateral view without rotation.
   c. Penetration of lung fields and heart should be clearly seen.
   d. The ribs should be superimposed posterior to the vertebral column.
   e. Neither the arm nor its soft tissues overlap the superior lung field.
   f. The hilum should be seen in the approximate center of the radiograph.
   g. The sternal ends of clavicles should be superimposed with the vertebral column.
   h. The sternal ends of clavicles should be seen equidistant from the vertebral column.
   i. The thoracic intervertebral spaces should be open (except in patients with scoliosis).
   j. The costophrenic angles and lower apices of lungs should be clearly demonstrated.
   k. A small amount of the heart should be seen on the right side of the vertebral column.
   l. The long axis of lung fields should be demonstrated in the vertical position without forward–backward leaning.

30. Identify each lettered structure shown in Fig. 10-13.

   A. _____

   B. _____

   C. _____

   D. _____

   E. _____

   F. _____

   G. _____

   H. _____

   I. _____

   J. _____

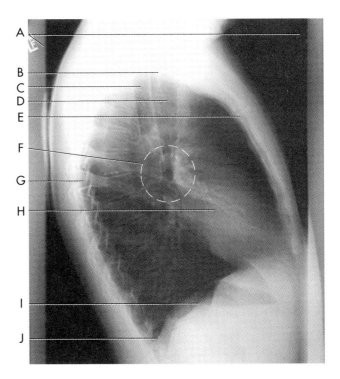

Figure 10-13 Lateral chest.

Exercise 2: PA Oblique Projections—Right Anterior Oblique (RAO) and Left Anterior Oblique (LAO) Positions

Instructions: PA oblique projections are sometimes used to supplement the standard PA and lateral views. This exercise pertains to PA oblique projections. Identify structures, provide a short answer, or choose true or false (explaining any statement you believe to be false) for each item.

Examine Figs. 10-14 and 10-15 as you answer the following items.

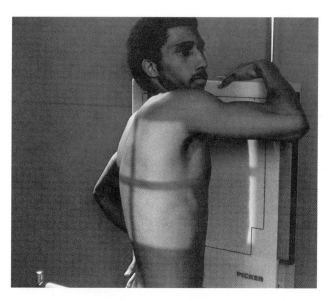

Figure 10-14 PA oblique chest, LAO position.

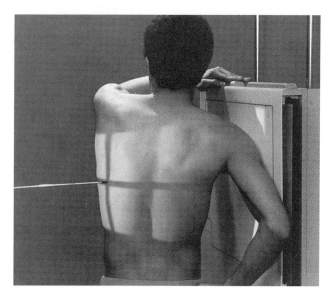

Figure 10-15 PA oblique chest, RAO position.

1. Which side—the one closer to or the one farther from the IR—is generally the side of interest?

2. Which side of the chest—right or left—is of primary interest with the right PA oblique projection (RAO position)?

3. With reference to the patient, where should the upper border of the IR be placed?

4. When performing the right PA oblique projection (RAO position), how many degrees should be patient be rotated?

5. What determines how many degrees the patient should be rotated for the left PA oblique projection (LAO position)?

6. When performing the left PA oblique projection (LAO position) to demonstrate lungs, how many degrees should the patient be rotated?

7. When performing the left PA oblique projection (LAO position) to demonstrate the heart and great vessels, how many degrees should the patient be rotated?

8. With reference to patient respiration, when should the exposure be made?

9. To what level of the patient should the central ray be directed?

10. Which PA oblique projection provides the best view of the left atrium and the entire left branch of the bronchial tree?

11. True or False. When viewing PA oblique projection radiographs, the patient's left side should be toward the viewer's right side.

12. True or False. When viewing left PA oblique projection radiographs (LAO position), the left lung should be partially superimposed by the spine.

13. True or False. The heart and mediastinal structures should be clearly demonstrated within the lung field of the elevated side in oblique images of 45 degrees of body rotation.

14. Figs. 10-16 and 10-17 are PA oblique projection radiographs. Examine the images and answer the questions that follow.

a. Which image represents the RAO position?

b. Which image represents the LAO position?

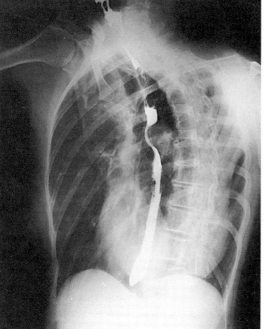

c. Assuming the patient was properly rotated, which image was produced with the patient rotated 45 degrees?

Figure 10-16 PA oblique chest with barium-filled esophagus.

d. Assuming the patient was properly rotated, which image was produced with the patient rotated 55 to 60 degrees?

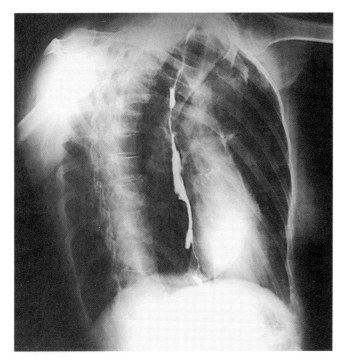

e. Which image demonstrates the maximum area of the left lung?

Figure 10-17 PA oblique chest with barium-filled esophagus.

15. Identify each lettered structure shown in Fig. 10-18.

A. _____

B. _____

C. _____

D. _____

E. _____

F. _____

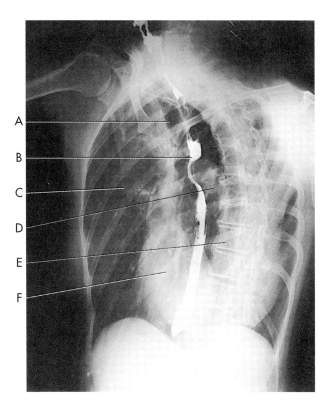

Figure 10-18 PA oblique chest with barium-filled esophagus.

Exercise 3: AP Oblique Projections—Right Posterior Oblique (RPO) and Left Posterior Oblique (LPO) Positions

Instructions: Anteroposterior (AP) oblique projections are sometimes used when supplementary positions are needed and the patient is unable to turn to the PA position. This exercise pertains to AP oblique projections. Identify structures, select the correct choice, or provide a short answer for each item.

Examine Figs. 10-19 and 10-20 as you answer the following items.

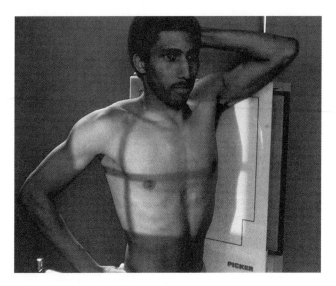

Figure 10-19 Upright AP oblique chest, LPO position.

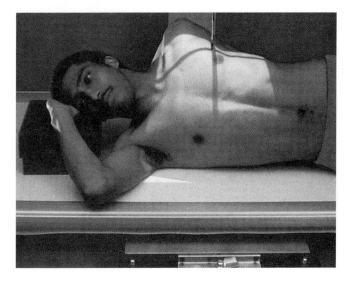

Figure 10-20 Recumbent AP oblique chest, RPO position.

1. Which side—the one closer to or the one farther from the IR—is generally the side of interest?

2. Which AP oblique image—right AP oblique (RPO position) or left AP oblique (LPO position)—demonstrates the maximum area of the left lung?

3. What is the minimum recommended SID?

4. Which AP oblique projection produces an image very similar to that produced by the right PA oblique projection (RAO position)?
   a. Left AP oblique projections (LPO position)
   b. Right AP oblique projections (RPO position)

5. How many degrees should the patient be rotated?
   a. 25 degrees
   b. 35 degrees
   c. 45 degrees
   d. 55 degrees

6. How far above the top of the shoulders should the upper border of the IR be placed?

7. What breathing instructions should be given to the patient?

8. To what level of the patient should the central ray be directed?

9. Identify each lettered structure shown in Fig. 10-21.

    A. _____

    B. _____

    C. _____

    D. _____

    E. _____

10. Examine Fig. 10-21 and answer the questions that follow.

    a. Which projection is represented in the image?

    b. Which radiographic position is the patient in?

    c. Which side of the patient is closer to the film?

    d. Which lung should be seen in its maximum extent?

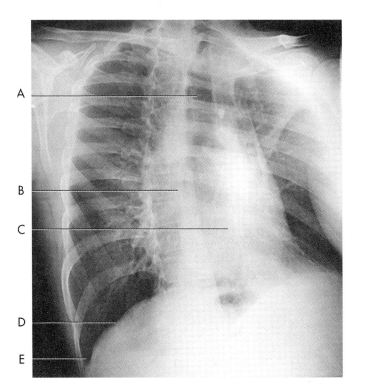

Figure 10-21 AP oblique chest.

Exercise 4: The AP Projection

Instructions: The AP projection is used when the patient is too ill to turn to the prone position or to sit for a PA projection, and it is often used for bedridden patients. This exercise pertains to the AP projection. Identify structures, select choices from a list, and provide a short answer for each question.

Examine Fig. 10-22 as you answer the following items.

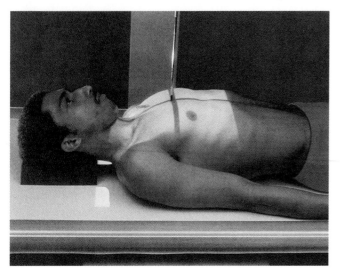

Figure 10-22 AP chest.

1. What is the recommended SID?

2. What body plane should be centered to the midline of the image receptor?

3. With reference to the patient, where should the IR be placed?

4. If the patient's condition permits, how should the arms and shoulders be positioned? Explain why.

5. What breathing instructions should be given to the patient?

6. Why should the patient perform the recommended breathing instructions?

7. To what level of the patient should the central ray be directed?

8. Describe how the following structures appear in the AP projection image compared with how they appear in the PA projection image.

   a. Heart and great vessels: _____

   b. Lungs: _____

   c. Clavicles: _____

   d. Ribs: _____

9. From the following list, circle the six evaluation criteria that indicate the patient was properly positioned for an AP projection.

   a. The trachea should be seen in the midline.
   b. The sternum should be lateral without rotation.
   c. The ribs should be superimposed posterior to the vertebral column.
   d. The hilum should be seen in the approximate center of the radiograph.
   e. The lung fields should be seen from the apices to the costophrenic angles.
   f. The medial portion of the clavicles should be equidistant from the vertebral column.
   g. A faint image of the ribs and thoracic vertebrae should be seen through the heart shadow.
   h. The clavicles will lie more horizontal and will obscure more of the apices than in PA projections.
   i. The distance from the vertebral column to the lateral border of the ribs should be equidistant on both sides.
   j. Approximately twice as much distance should be seen between the vertebral column and the outer margin of the ribs on the dependent side compared with the remote side.

10. Identify each thoracic structure shown in Fig. 10-23.

    A. _____

    B. _____

    C. _____

    D. _____

    E. _____

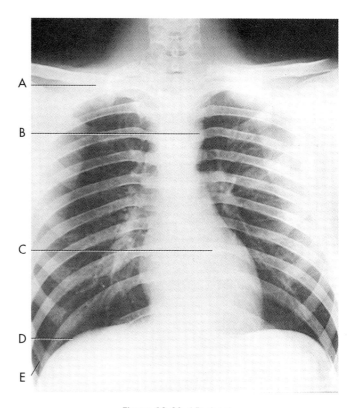

Figure 10-23 AP chest.

Exercise 5: The AP Axial Projection (Lordotic Position)

Instructions: The AP axial projection is sometimes used to demonstrate interlobar effusions. This exercise pertains to the AP axial projection. Provide a short answer or select the correct choice from a list for each item.

Examine Fig. 10-24 as you answer the following items.

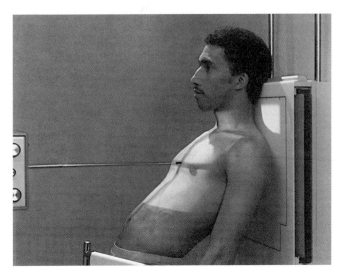

Figure 10-24 AP axial projection, lordotic position.

1. Which portion of the lung is generally the area of primary interest?
   a. Base
   b. Apex
   c. Hilum

2. Describe how the patient should be positioned.

3. What breathing instructions should be given to the patient?

4. Where should the central ray enter the patient?

5. From the following list, circle the five evaluation criteria that indicate the patient was properly positioned for an AP axial projection (lordotic position).
   a. The clavicles should lie superior to the apices.
   b. The sternum should be lateral without rotation.
   c. The apices and lungs should be included in their entirety.
   d. The ribs should be superimposed posterior to the vertebral column.
   e. Approximately 2 inches of lung apex should be seen above the clavicles.
   f. The sternal ends of the clavicles should be equidistant from the vertebral column.
   g. The ribs should appear distorted with their anterior and posterior portions somewhat superimposed.
   h. The clavicles should be lying horizontal with their medial ends overlapping only the first or second ribs.

Exercise 6: Lateral Decubitus Positions

Instructions: This exercise pertains to lateral decubitus positions of the chest. Fill in missing words, provide a short answer, select from a list, or choose true or false (explaining any statement you believe to be false) for each item.

Examine Fig. 10-25 as you answer the following items.

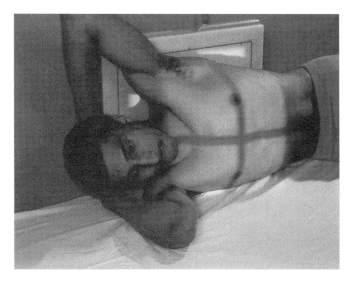

Figure 10-25 AP projection, right lateral decubitus position.

1. What is the general purpose for using a lateral decubitus position?

2. True or False. The patient can be positioned upright in a lateral decubitus position.

3. True or False. The image receptor must be placed vertically against a patient.

4. True or False. The projection may be either AP or PA.

5. True or False. The central ray must be directed horizontally.

6. True or False. The affected side should be up to demonstrate a fluid level.

7. True or False. Both sides should be seen in their entirety.

8. If fluid in the right side of the thorax needs to be demonstrated with a lateral decubitus position, in which body position should the patient be placed?

   a. Left lateral upright
   b. Left lateral recumbent
   c. Right lateral upright
   d. Right lateral recumbent

9. Which side of the thorax—right or left—will best demonstrate free air when the patient is in the left lateral decubitus position?

10. To demonstrate free air in the thorax with a lateral decubitus position, why is it preferable to position the patient with the affected side up instead of with the affected side down?

11. To demonstrate a fluid level in the thorax with a lateral decubitus position, why is it preferable to position the patient with the affected side down instead of with the affected side up?

12. What breathing instructions should be given to the patient?

13. Fig. 10-26 is an image of the right lateral decubitus position. Examine the image and answer the following items.

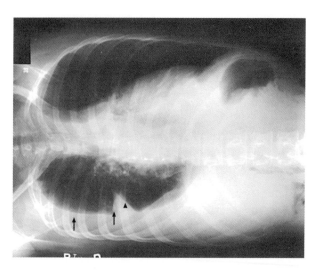

Figure 10-26 AP projection, right lateral decubitus position.

a. This position should be used to demonstrate an air level

in the _____ side of the thorax.

b. This position should be used to demonstrate a fluid

level in the _____ side of the thorax.

c. Which level—air or fluid—are the arrows pointing to in the image?

14. Fig. 10-27 is an image of the left lateral decubitus position. Examine the image and complete the statements that follow.

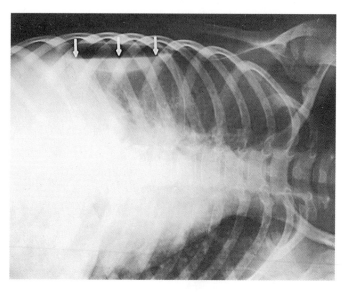

Figure 10-27 AP projection, left lateral decubitus position.

a. The arrows in the image are pointing to an air/fluid level

in the _____ (right or left) side of the thorax.

b. In this image the affected side is _____ (up or down).

15. From the following list, circle the five evaluation criteria that indicate a patient is properly positioned for a lateral decubitus position projection.

a. The apices should be included.
b. The clavicles should lie superior to the apices.
c. The affected side should be included in its entirety.
d. The patient should not be rotated from a true frontal position.
e. The patient's arms should be removed from the field of interest.
f. The ribs should be superimposed posterior to the vertebral column.
g. Proper identification should be visible to indicate that the decubitus position was used.
h. The clavicles should be lying horizontal with their medial ends overlapping only the first or second ribs.

Exercise 7: Ventral and Dorsal Decubitus Positions

Instructions: Sometimes it is necessary to demonstrate an air or fluid level while the patient is in the supine or prone position. This is accomplished through lateral projections using the ventral and dorsal decubitus positions. This exercise pertains to those two positions. Fill in missing words, select from a list, or provide a short answer for each item.

Examine Fig. 10-28 as you answer the following items.

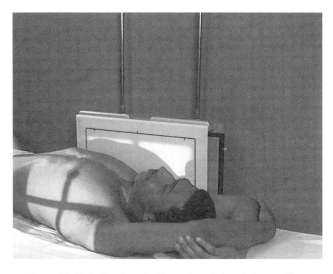

Figure 10-28 Lateral projection, dorsal decubitus position.

1. For the dorsal decubitus position projection, the patient

   must be placed in the _____ position.

2. For the ventral decubitus position projection, the patient

   must be placed in the _____ position.

3. In addition to being perpendicular to the IR, the central ray

   must also be directed _____.

4. How much should the thorax be elevated?

5. How long should a patient remain in position? Why?

6. Describe how the patient's arms should be positioned.

7. With reference to the patient, how and where should the IR be placed?

8. Concerning respiration, when should the exposure be made?

9. Where should the central ray enter the patient?

10. From the following list, circle the four evaluation criteria that indicate the patient was properly positioned for the dorsal decubitus or ventral decubitus position.

   a. The arms should not obscure the upper lung field.
   b. The thorax should not be rotated from a true lateral position.
   c. The medial portion of the clavicles should be equidistant from the vertebral column.
   d. A small amount of the heart should be seen on the right side of the vertebral column.
   e. Proper identification should be visible to indicate that the decubitus position was used.
   f. The entire lung fields, including the anterior and posterior surfaces, should be demonstrated.
   g. The distance from the vertebral column to the lateral border of the ribs should be equidistant on both sides.

Exercise 8: Evaluating Radiographs of the Chest

Instructions: This exercise consists of using radiographs of the chest to give you practice evaluating chest positioning. These images are not from *Merrill's Atlas of Radiographic Positions and Radiologic Procedures*. Each radiograph shows at least one positioning error. Examine each image and answer the questions that follow by providing a short answer.

1. Fig. 10-29 shows a PA projection radiograph that does not meet all evaluation criteria for this type of projection. Examine the image and identify the evaluation criterion that this image does not meet.

2. Fig. 10-30 shows a lateral projection radiograph with the patient incorrectly positioned. Examine the image and list the three evaluation criteria that it does not meet.

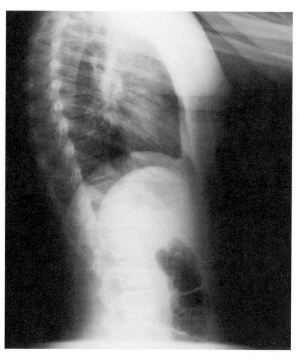

Figure 10-30 Lateral chest showing improper positioning.

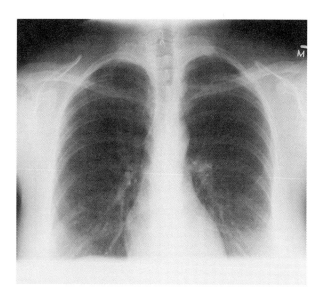

Figure 10-29 PA chest showing improper positioning.

3. Examine Fig. 10-31 and answer the following questions.

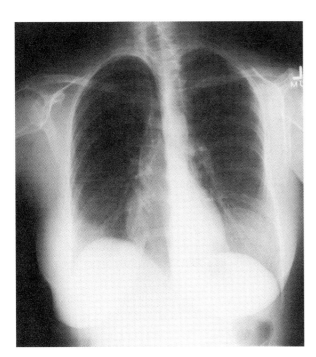

Figure 10-31 AP chest showing improper positioning.

a. State the major positioning error that necessitates repetition of the examination.

b. Describe how patient positioning should be adjusted to produce a more acceptable image with a subsequent projection.

Self-Test: Anatomy and Positioning of the Chest

Instructions: Answer the following questions by selecting the best choice.

1. What is the name of the area between the two pleural cavities?

   a. Hilum
   b. Mediastinum
   c. Pleural space
   d. Thoracic cavity

2. Which structure is not demonstrated within the mediastinum in PA projections of the chest?

   a. Heart
   b. Trachea
   c. Diaphragm
   d. Esophagus

3. Which pathologic condition of the lung involves the replacement of air with fluid in the lung interstitium and alveoli?

   a. Atelectasis
   b. Tuberculosis
   c. Pneumothorax
   d. Pulmonary edema

4. Why should chest radiographs be performed with a 72-inch SID?

   a. To blur involuntary heart motion
   b. To minimize magnification of the heart
   c. To maximize magnification of the heart
   d. To project the clavicles above the apices

5. Why should chest radiographs be performed after the patient has suspended respiration after the second inspiration?

   a. To blur rib markings
   b. To better expand the lungs
   c. To demonstrate a collapsed lung
   d. To calm the heart and reduce cardiac motion

6. With reference to the IR, how are the midsagittal plane and the midcoronal plane positioned for the PA projection of the chest?

   a. Midsagittal: parallel; midcoronal: parallel
   b. Midsagittal: parallel; midcoronal: perpendicular
   c. Midsagittal: perpendicular; midcoronal: parallel
   d. Midsagittal: perpendicular; midcoronal: perpendicular

7. For the PA projection of the chest, which positioning maneuver should be performed to best remove scapulae from lung fields?

   a. Place the hands on the hips.
   b. Rotate the shoulders forward.
   c. Cross both arms over the head.
   d. Place the hands behind the back.

8. Why would the chest most likely be demonstrated using two PA projections (in which the patient is seen in suspended inspiration and suspended expiration)?

   a. To demonstrate pneumothorax
   b. To evaluate the heart and great vessels
   c. To measure the width of the mediastinum
   d. To demonstrate movement of the diaphragm

9. Which of the following is an effective way to detect rotation of the patient with the PA projection radiograph of the chest?

   a. The number of ribs demonstrated above the diaphragm
   b. The asymmetrical appearance of the sternoclavicular joints
   c. The amount of apical area demonstrated above the clavicles
   d. The appearance of the lateral border of the scapulae outside the lung fields

10. For which projection of the chest should the midsagittal plane be parallel with the image receptor?

    a. PA projection
    b. Lateral projection
    c. AP projection (left lateral decubitus position)
    d. AP axial projection (lordotic position; Lindblom method)

11. With reference to the IR, how are the midcoronal plane and the midsagittal plane positioned for the lateral projection of the chest?

    a. Midcoronal: parallel; midsagittal: parallel
    b. Midcoronal: parallel; midsagittal: perpendicular
    c. Midcoronal: perpendicular; midsagittal: parallel
    d. Midcoronal: perpendicular; midsagittal: perpendicular

12. Which projection of the chest best demonstrates lung apices free from superimposition with the clavicles?

    a. PA projection
    b. Left lateral projection
    c. AP projection (left lateral decubitus position)
    d. AP axial projection (lordotic position; Lindblom method)

13. How many degrees should the patient be rotated for PA oblique projections of the chest to evaluate the heart and great vessels?

    a. RAO: 45 degrees; LAO: 45 degrees
    b. RAO: 45 degrees; LAO: 55 to 60 degrees
    c. RAO: 55 to 60 degrees; LAO: 45 degrees
    d. RAO: 55 to 60 degrees; LAO: 55 to 60 degrees

14. How many degrees should the patient be rotated for PA oblique projections of the chest to evaluate the lungs?

    a. RAO: 45 degrees; LAO: 45 degrees
    b. RAO: 45 degrees; LAO: 55 to 60 degrees
    c. RAO: 55 to 60 degrees; LAO: 45 degrees
    d. RAO: 55 to 60 degrees; LAO: 55 to 60 degrees

15. Using a lateral decubitus position for patients who are unable to stand upright best demonstrates which of the following pathologic conditions of the chest?

    a. Rib fractures
    b. Cardiomegaly
    c. Collapsed lung
    d. Air or fluid levels

16. With reference to the IR, how are the midsagittal plane and the midcoronal plane positioned for the AP chest (left lateral decubitus position)?

    a. Midsagittal: parallel; midcoronal: parallel
    b. Midsagittal: parallel; midcoronal: perpendicular
    c. Midsagittal: perpendicular; midcoronal: parallel
    d. Midsagittal: perpendicular; midcoronal: perpendicular

17. Which pathologic condition of the lungs is best demonstrated with the AP chest (left lateral decubitus position)?

    a. Free air in both sides of the chest
    b. Fluid levels in both sides of the chest
    c. Free air in the left side or fluid levels in the right side
    d. Fluid levels in the left side or free air in the right side

18. Which pathologic condition of the lungs is best demonstrated with the AP chest (right lateral decubitus position)?

    a. Free air in both sides of the chest
    b. Fluid levels in both sides of the chest
    c. Free air in the left side or fluid levels in the right side
    d. Fluid levels in the left side or free air in the right side

19. Which radiographic position requires that the patient be placed supine with the IR placed vertically against the patient's right side and a horizontal central ray directed to the center of the image receptor?

    a. Ventral decubitus
    b. Dorsal decubitus
    c. Right lateral decubitus
    d. Left lateral decubitus

20. Which radiographic position requires that the patient be placed prone?

    a. Left lateral decubitus
    b. Right lateral decubitus
    c. Dorsal decubitus
    d. Ventral decubitus

21. Which evaluation criterion pertains to the PA projection radiograph of the chest?

    a. The ribs should appear distorted.
    b. The sternum should be lateral, not rotated.
    c. Ten posterior ribs should be visible above the diaphragm.
    d. The ribs posterior to the vertebral column should be superimposed.

22. Which evaluation criterion pertains to the PA projection radiograph of the chest?

    a. The ribs should appear distorted.
    b. The clavicles should lie superior to the apices.
    c. The scapulae should be projected outside the lung fields.
    d. The ribs posterior to the vertebral column should be superimposed.

23. Which evaluation criterion pertains to the lateral projection radiograph of the chest?

    a. A small amount of the heart should be seen on the right side.
    b. The ribs posterior to the vertebral column should be superimposed.
    c. A faint shadow of superior thoracic vertebrae should be seen through the heart shadow.
    d. The distance from the vertebral column to the lateral border of the ribs should be equidistant on both sides.

24. Which evaluation criterion pertains to the AP axial projection (lordotic position) radiograph of the chest?

    a. The ribs should appear distorted.
    b. The clavicles should lie below the apices.
    c. The sternum should be lateral, not rotated.
    d. The thoracic intervertebral disk spaces should be open.

25. Which evaluation criterion pertains to the AP axial projection (lordotic position) radiograph of the chest?

    a. The clavicles should lie superior to the apices.
    b. The thoracic intervertebral disk spaces should be open.
    c. The ribs posterior to the vertebral column should be superimposed.
    d. Two inches (5 cm) of lung apices should be seen above the clavicles.

CHAPTER 11

Long Bone Measurement

Review

Instructions: This exercise pertains to radiographic measurement of long bones. Provide a short answer for each item.

1. Define orthoroentgenography.

2. What area of the body is more frequently radiographed for long bone measurement?

3. How many exposures should be made of each limb?

4. Why might movement by the patient cause the examination to be repeated?

5. What type of projection should be performed?

6. With reference to the affected lower limb, where should the metal ruler be placed when only one limb is imaged?

7. What procedure should be performed to the normal knee when the abnormal knee cannot be fully extended?

8. If the right side is shorter than the left side, which side should be radiographed?

9. Identify the centering point for each of the following joints:

   a. Shoulder: _____

   b. Elbow: _____

   c. Wrist: _____

   d. Hip: _____

   e. Knee: _____

   f. Ankle: _____

10. Why is the image of a limb made by a single x-ray exposure larger than the actual limb?

11. What two steps can the radiographer take to reduce the magnification produced when a single exposure is used to image a limb?

12. Why does orthoroentgenography produce more accurate long bone measurements than single-exposure examinations?

13. How is bone length determined with orthoroentgenography?

14. For simultaneous bilateral projections of lower limbs, where should the central ray be directed for each exposure?

15. Describe how the lower limbs should be adjusted for simultaneous bilateral projections of the lower limbs.

16. What body plane of the patient should be centered on the table for simultaneous bilateral projections of the lower limbs?

17. With reference to the lower limbs, where should the metal ruler be placed when both lower limbs are simultaneously imaged?

18. How many times should the patient be positioned when simultaneous bilateral projections of the lower limbs are made?

20. List two advantages that obtaining long bone measurements with computed tomography has over the conventional radiographic approach.

19. For simultaneous bilateral projections of the lower limbs, what procedure should be performed to correct an examination when bones of different lengths cause bilateral distortion?

Self-Test: Long Bone Measurement

Instructions: Answer the following questions by selecting the best choice.

1. What is the purpose of orthoroentgenography?
   a. To measure the length of long bones
   b. To identify the location of a foreign body
   c. To measure the calcium content of long bones
   d. To measure the length of the vertebral column

2. Into which body position should the patient be placed when an examination to measure long bones is performed?
   a. Prone
   b. Supine
   c. Upright
   d. Lateral

3. Which parameters should be moved when exposures for long bone measurement are made?
   a. X-ray tube and patient
   b. X-ray tube and image receptor
   c. Metal ruler and patient
   d. Metal ruler and image receptor

4. Which special device must be used for long bone measurement examinations?
   a. Leg brace
   b. Metal ruler
   c. Wedge filter
   d. Upright image receptor holder

5. For exposures made at the knee joint, the central ray should be directed to which of the following levels?
   a. Tibial tuberosity
   b. Base of the patella
   c. Widest point of the femoral epicondyles
   d. Depression between the femoral and tibial condyles

6. For orthoroentgenography, how many exposures should be made of each limb?
   a. One
   b. Two
   c. Three
   d. Four

7. For simultaneous bilateral projections of the lower limbs, how many exposures should be made?
   a. Two
   b. Three
   c. Four
   d. Six

8. Which procedure must be performed to ensure accuracy in long bone measurement examinations?
   a. Use the smaller focal spot size.
   b. Do not move the limb between exposures.
   c. Make all exposures with the patient upright.
   d. Use a source-to-image receptor distance (SID) of 72 inches.

9. For long bone measurement of the lower limbs, which procedure should be performed when the patient's right leg is noticeably shorter than the left leg?
   a. Radiograph both legs.
   b. Radiograph the left leg only.
   c. Radiograph the right leg only.

10. How should the lower limbs be positioned for bilateral projections of the lower limbs?
    a. In a lateral position with full extension
    b. In a lateral position with partial flexion
    c. In the anatomic position with slight medial rotation
    d. In the anatomic position with slight lateral rotation

CHAPTER 12

Contrast Arthrography

Review

Instructions: Contrast arthrography is a procedure that greatly enhances the visibility of joint structures when compared to plain-image radiography. A significant number of these procedures are still performed annually, even though other imaging modalities are reducing the need for contrast arthrography. This exercise pertains to contrast arthrography. Fill in missing words, provide a short answer, or choose true or false (explaining any statement you believe to be false) for each item.

1. Define arthrography.

2. What imaging modality has significantly reduced the number of arthrograms performed in radiography departments?

3. List four soft-tissue structures of joints that are often demonstrated with arthrographic examinations.

4. Identify the type of contrast media used for each of the following examinations.

   a. Opaque arthrography: _____

   _____

   _____

   b. Pneumoarthrography: _____

   _____

   _____

   c. Double-contrast arthrography: _____

   _____

   _____

5. The joint that is demonstrated by contrast arthrography more often than any other joint is the _____.

6. True or False. Contrast arthrography is usually performed with a local anesthetic.

7. True or False. The radiographer injects the contrast medium under carefully maintained aseptic conditions.

8. Who should manipulate the joint to ensure good distribution of the contrast medium?

9. For arthrography of the knee, what is the purpose of a stress device?

10. For arthrography of the knee, what is the purpose of "opening up" the side of the joint space being examined?

11. For the vertical-ray method of knee arthrography, what five conventional projections are made to complement fluoroscopy?

12. Hip arthrography is most often performed on children to evaluate congenital _____

_____ .

13. Give two reasons why hip arthrography is frequently performed on adults.

14. List the conventional projections that compose a shoulder arthrogram.

15. In addition to conventional radiography, what imaging modality is frequently used to demonstrate the shoulder after a double-contrast arthrogram?

16. What two imaging modalities have greatly reduced the demand for temporomandibular joint (TMJ) arthrography?

17. Contrast arthrography of the TMJ is particularly useful in diagnosing abnormalities of the articular

_____ .

18. Where is the injection site for TMJ arthrography?

19. What radiographic procedure is usually performed on the patient before injection of the contrast medium for TMJ arthrography?

20. For TMJ arthrography, in what positions should the patient hold his or her mouth for radiographs taken after injection of the contrast medium?

Self-Test: Contrast Arthrography

Instructions: Answer the following questions by selecting the best choice.

1. Which examination demonstrates joint structures after the introduction of only a water-soluble, iodinated contrast medium?

   a. Pneumoarthrography
   b. Opaque arthrography
   c. Double-contrast arthrography

2. Which examination combines radiopaque and radiolucent contrast media in a joint to demonstrate soft-tissue structures?

   a. Pneumoarthrography
   b. Opaque arthrography
   c. Single-contrast arthrography
   d. Double-contrast arthrography

3. Which examination room should be used for contrast arthrography?

   a. Surgical
   b. Sonographic
   c. Urologic-radiographic
   d. Fluoroscopic-radiographic

4. Which arthrogram would most likely include subtraction technique images with conventional radiography?

   a. Shoulder arthrography for rotator cuff tear
   b. Wrist arthrography for carpal tunnel syndrome
   c. Hip arthrography for congenital hip dislocation
   d. Hip arthrography to detect a loose hip prosthesis

5. Which articulation is examined by contrast arthrography more often than any other joint?

   a. Hip
   b. Knee
   c. Wrist
   d. Shoulder

6. What is the most common reason for performing hip arthrography on children?

   a. Child abuse
   b. Automobile accidents
   c. Long bone measurement
   d. Congenital hip dislocation

7. What is one of the two most common reasons for performing hip arthrography on adults?

   a. Automobile accidents
   b. Long bone measurement
   c. Congenital hip dislocation
   d. Detection of a loose hip prosthesis

8. Which two imaging modalities have greatly reduced the demand for TMJ arthrography?

   a. Computed tomography and sonography
   b. Computed tomography and magnetic resonance imaging
   c. Orthoroentgenography and sonography
   d. Orthoroentgenography and magnetic resonance imaging

9. Which structures are demonstrated with contrast arthrography?

   a. Bursae
   b. Tendons
   c. Ventricles
   d. Intervertebral disks

10. What are the two methods for performing contrast arthrography of a knee?

    a. Immediate and delayed
    b. Invasive and noninvasive
    c. Vertical ray and horizontal ray
    d. Perpendicular ray and angled ray

CHAPTER 13

Trauma Radiography

Review

Instructions: The condition of some trauma patients sometimes requires a radiographer to alter procedures associated with routine radiographic examinations. All radiographers must be competent in performing trauma radiography. This exercise pertains to trauma radiography. Provide a short answer for each of the following questions.

1. Define *trauma*. *Trauma is defined as sudden, unexpected, dramatic or violent event, such as: blunt force trauma, falls, assault, and motor vehicle accidents.*

2. How does a Level I trauma center differ from a Level IV trauma center?
Level I: Usually a university based center, research facility, or large medical center. (most comprehensive.) Level IV: differs in that it is not a research or teaching hospital.

3. Within how many feet from the x-ray tube should appropriate shielding be provided to patients on nearby stretchers when performing mobile radiography? *no less than 6ft.*

4. List five symptoms of shock that can be readily observed by a radiographer. *cool, clammy skin, slurred speech, diaphoresis. agitation or confusion.*

5. Concerning providing information to key personnel, what procedure should a radiographer perform if it is necessary to deviate from the routine projections? *perform additional projections within the scope of the ordered examination to aid in proper diagnosis.*

6. What should be the first projection performed for a trauma patient with a cervical injury? *Cervical spine, dorsal decubitus position, (crosstable lat.)*

7. When is it necessary to perform the lateral projection for the cervicothoracic region? *should be performed if the entire c-spine, including C7 and the inter-space between T 1 is not demonstrated in the dorsal decubitus lateral projection*

8. What condition must be met before attempting to move the patient's arms for the lateral projection of the cervicothoracic region, dorsal decubitus position? *the PT must be able to move his arms, Do not move the PTs arms w/o the attending phys, permission.*

9. When performing the lateral projection for the cervicothoracic region, dorsal decubitus position, when may the central ray (CR) be caudally angled? *when the pt. Can not depress the tube side shoulder*

10. When performing the lateral projection of the cervicothoracic region, dorsal decubitus position, what is the purpose for using a long exposure time with the patient breathing normally? *to blur the rib shadow.*

11. When performing the anteroposterior (AP) axial projection on a patient who is not on a backboard or x-ray table, who should lift the patient's head and neck so that a radiographer can position the image receptor (IR) under the patient? *The attending phys. should be the one to lift the PTs head & neck,*

12. When performing the AP axial oblique projection for cervical vertebrae, why should you *not* use a grid IR? *because the compound central ray angle will result in grid cut-off.*

13. When performing the AP axial oblique projection for cervical vertebrae on a supine trauma patient, how should the central ray be directed with a nongrid IR? *use a 45 degree angle.*

14. When performing the AP axial oblique projection for cervical vertebrae on a supine trauma patient, where should the CR enter the patient? *The CR is positioned 45 degrees mediolaterally, and if possible, 15 to 20 degrees cephalad,*

15. When demonstrating lumbar vertebrae on a trauma patient who is supine on a backboard, what should be the first projection performed? *always use the dorsal decubitus projection.*

16. When performing the lateral projection for thoracic vertebrae on a trauma patient who is supine on a backboard, how should the CR be directed? *Central ray is horizontal, perpendicular to the center of the IR.*

17. When performing the AP projection of the abdomen on a trauma patient, what should be obtained before moving the patient to the radiographic table? *Verify transfer with the attending phys.*

18. When performing the AP projection of the abdomen on a trauma patient, what procedure should the radiographer do if the patient's abdomen becomes increasingly distended and firm to the touch? *Do a cross-table lateral.*

19. When performing the AP projection of the abdomen on a trauma patient on a gurney, why must the grid IR be perfectly horizontal and the CR directed perpendicularly to the IR? *to avoid grid cut off.*

20. When performing the AP projection of the abdomen, left lateral decubitus position, why should the patient be placed in the left lateral recumbent position for at least 5 minutes before making the exposure? *to allow for separation of air & water.*

21. What emergency medical conditions are of primary concern with pelvic fractures? *internal hemorrhage, & shock*

22. What action should a radiographer initiate if a head trauma patient has unequal pupils or experiences a decrease in the level of consciousness? *Should inform the attending phys.*

23. When performing the acanthioparietal projection, Reverse Waters method, for facial bones on a supine trauma patient, how should the infraorbitomeatal line (IOML) be positioned with reference to the IR? the IOML should be approx. perpendicular to the IR.

24. What is the general rule concerning demonstrating adjacent joints when radiographing long bones on trauma patients? get views of both ends (Joints)

25. What is the general rule concerning immobilization devices when radiographing upper and lower limbs on trauma patients? do not remove before procedure or until you know that it safe to do so.

Self-Test: Trauma Radiography

Instructions: Answer the following questions by selecting the best choice.

1. Which of the following is an example of *blunt trauma*?
   a. Frostbite
   b. Gunshot wound
   c. Impalement injury
   d. Motor vehicle accident

2. Which procedure should be performed when taking radiographs to localize a penetrating foreign object?
   a. Reduce kVp to produce short-scale contrast.
   b. Mark entrance and/or exit wounds with a radiopaque marker.
   c. Provide a written description of the location of the entrance wound.
   d. Use twice the usual source-to-image distance (SID) to increase detail of structures.

3. Which procedure should a radiographer perform if a trauma patient begins to experience a seizure?
   a. Provide a drink of water.
   b. Roll the patient onto the side.
   c. Inform the attending physician.
   d. Cover the patient with a blanket.

4. Which of the following symptoms is associated with stroke injuries?
   a. Slurred speech
   b. Cool, clammy skin
   c. Excessive sweating
   d. Increased drowsiness

5. Which of the following statements is *not* an appropriate rule for trauma radiographers?
   a. Always make at least three radiographs for each area of injury.
   b. Never leave a trauma patient unattended during imaging procedures.
   c. Never remove any immobilization device without physician's orders.
   d. Always ask the attending physician before giving a trauma patient anything to eat or drink.

6. Which of the following projections should be the first one performed for a multiple-trauma patient?
   a. AP lumbar spine
   b. Lateral lumbar spine, dorsal decubitus position
   c. AP cervical spine
   d. Lateral cervical spine, dorsal decubitus position

7. When performing the AP axial oblique projection for cervical vertebrae on a supine trauma patient, how should the CR be directed if only one angle is used?
   a. 15 degrees cephalad
   b. 45 degrees cephalad
   c. 15 degrees lateromedially
   d. 45 degrees lateromedially

8. When performing the AP projection of the abdomen on a trauma patient, what should be obtained before moving the patient to the radiographic table?
   a. Vital signs
   b. Written consent from the patient
   c. Permission from the attending physician
   d. Lateral cervical vertebrae, dorsal decubitus position

9. Which of the following procedures should the radiographer perform if a trauma patient has bleeding wounds?
   a. Protect the IR with plastic.
   b. Enclose the IR inside a pillowcase.
   c. Provide fluids to the patient by mouth or intravenously.
   d. Have emergency room personnel assist with the procedure.

10. Why should the left lateral decubitus position be used for demonstrating free air within the abdominal cavity?
    a. Free air will collect under the left hemidiaphragm.
    b. Fluid levels will collect under the right hemidiaphragm.
    c. The density of the liver provides good contrast for free air.
    d. The density of the stomach provides good contrast for free air.

11. How should a radiographer determine if an AP projection of the abdomen, left lateral decubitus position, is being requested for demonstrating free air or fluid levels?
    a. Ask the patient.
    b. Ask the attending physician.
    c. Examine for penetrating wounds.
    d. Examine for distended or firm abdomen.

12. When performing the AP projection of the abdomen, left lateral decubitus position, which of the following procedures should be performed when fluid levels are of primary interest?
    a. Ensure the entire left side is demonstrated.
    b. Ensure the entire right side is demonstrated.
    c. Center the IR 4 inches above the iliac crests to include the diaphragm.
    d. Have the patient drink one full glass of water before making the radiograph.

13. Which projection of the abdomen should be performed to demonstrate air or fluid levels when a trauma patient is unable to be positioned either upright or in the lateral recumbent position?

    a. AP
    b. Left AP oblique
    c. Right AP oblique
    d. Lateral, dorsal decubitus position

14. When performing the AP projection for the pelvis with a trauma patient, which of the following procedures should *not* be performed?

    a. Use a grid IR directly under the patient.
    b. Rotate the femurs 15 degrees medially.
    c. Transfer the patient to a radiographic table.
    d. Center the IR to a level of 2 inches inferior to the anterosuperior iliac spine (ASIS).

15. Which action should a radiographer perform if a semiconscious head trauma patient begins vomiting during radiographic procedures?

    a. Obtain vital signs.
    b. Give the patient a plastic bag.
    c. Move the patient to a sitting position.
    d. Logroll the patient to the lateral recumbent position.

16. Which of the following procedures should a radiographer perform if a trauma patient with a head injury displays unequal pupils?

    a. Give the patient a drink of water.
    b. Remove restrictive immobilization devices.
    c. Immediately inform the attending physician.
    d. Logroll the patient into a lateral recumbent position.

17. Which of the following projections of the cranium would best demonstrate a suspected fracture of the posterior cranium?

    a. AP
    b. PA
    c. AP axial, Towne method
    d. Lateral, dorsal decubitus position

18. Which positioning line of the head should be nearly perpendicular to the IR when performing the acanthioparietal projection, Reverse Waters method, for facial bones on a supine trauma patient?

    a. Mentomeatal
    b. Orbitomeatal
    c. Glabellomeatal
    d. Infraorbitomeatal

19. How should the central ray be directed when performing the acanthioparietal projection, Reverse Waters method, for facial bones on a supine trauma patient?

    a. 37 degrees cephalad
    b. Perpendicular to the IR
    c. Parallel with the mentomeatal line
    d. Parallel with the infraorbitomeatal line

20. Which of the following general rules should be followed when radiographing upper and lower limbs on trauma patients?

    a. Always obtain two radiographs, 90 degrees apart.
    b. Always position for true AP and lateral projections.
    c. When demonstrating long bones, always remove immobilization devices.
    d. When demonstrating long bones, always transfer the patient to the radiographic table.

Answers to Exercises

CHAPTER 1 Preliminary Steps in Radiography

Review

1. a. The degree of image blackening
   b. The difference in density of any two areas on a radiograph
   c. The ability to visualize small structures
   d. The misrepresentation of the size or shape of any anatomical structure
2. a, b, f
3. a. Insufficient density
   b. Proper density
4. Kilovoltage peak (kVp)
5. a. Long scale (low contrast)
   b. Short scale (high contrast)
6. a, b, c, d, f, g
7. a. Sharp image
   b. Unsharp image
8. d, e
9. True
10. Image A
11. a, b, c, d, e
12. As though the patient were standing in the anatomical position, face-to-face with the viewer
13. Image A
14. As though the viewer sees the patient from the perspective of the x-ray tube (Display the radiograph so that the side of the patient closer to the IR during the procedure is also the side of the image closer to the viewbox.)
15. Image A
16. With the digits pointing upward and as viewed from the perspective of the x-ray tube
17. Image A
18. Image A
19. (1) with the patient in the anatomical position, and (2) in the manner in which the IR was positioned when the exposure was made
20. a. Right lateral decubitus
    b. Left lateral decubitus
21. The radiographer
22. Washing the hands
23. Pathogenic microorganisms
24. Gloves
25. Place them in a puncture-proof container
26. a. A chemical substance that kills pathogenic bacteria
    b. A chemical substance that inhibits the growth of pathogenic microorganisms without necessarily killing them
    c. The destruction of all microorganisms
    d. The process of killing only pathogenic microorganisms
27. Antiseptic

28. An outline of each procedure, the number of staff required, duties of each member of the team, and a listing of the required sterile and nonsterile items
29. Limited diet, laxatives, and enemas
30. Smooth, involuntary (peristalsis); cardiac, involuntary (systole); and striated, voluntary
31. Peristalsis
32. Exposure time
33. Central nervous system
34. c, d, e, g, h
35. To prevent confusing shadows
36. Dentures, removable bridgework, earrings, necklaces, hairpins, and eyeglasses
37. Give an explanation of the procedure to be performed.
38. Four
39. Inspiration and expiration
40. Inspiration
41. Slow, deep breathing
42.
1. b	4. a	7. a	10. b
2. b	5. a	8. b	11. b
3. a	6. b	9. a	12. a
43. a, c, d, f
44. a. The level of the fulcrum
    b. The cumulative time following the introduction of contrast medium
45.
1. c	3. c	5. a	7. d	9. d
2. a	4. d	6. a	8. f	10. g
46. Increase the SID.
47. To avoid the superimposition of overlying or underlying structures, to avoid stacking a curved structure on itself, to project through angled joints, and to project through angled structures without foreshortening or elongation
48. Radiographic contrast is increased because scatter radiation is reduced, thereby producing a shorter scale of contrast.
49. When the gonads are in close proximity to the primary x-ray field (about 5 cm); when the clinical objective of the examination is not compromised; and when the patient has a reasonable reproductive potential
50. The imaging plate contains special image-storage phosphors that acquire the latent image for later processing into a digital format by computer technology.

Self-Test: Preliminary Steps in Radiography

1. c	6. a	11. c	16. c	21. c
2. b	7. a	12. c	17. c	22. d
3. a	8. d	13. b	18. c	23. d
4. d	9. b	14. c	19. c	24. c
5. d	10. d	15. d	20. b	25. c

CHAPTER 2 **Radiation Protection**

Review

1. b, d, f
2. a, b
3. False (Late genetic effects have not been measured in humans.)
4. False (A whole-body exposure of at least 25,000 mrads is necessary to produce a measurable hematologic depression.)
5. Radiation protection procedures have been improved.
6. Leukemia
7. b
8. a. roentgen (R); C/kg
   b. rad; gray (Gy)
   c. rem; sievert (Sv)
   d. curie (Ci); becquerel (Bq)
9. a. 1000; 0.01; 10
   b. 0.5; 0.005; 5
   c. 10; 10,000; 100
   d. 25; 25,000; 0.25
10. c
11. d
12. c
13. c
14. a, b, f
15. c
16. b
17. c
18. b
19. The higher the total filtration, the lower the patient dose.
20. The smaller the area of irradiated tissue (the greater the collimation), the lower the patient dose.
21. The higher the kilovoltage peak (kVp), the lower the patient dose.
22. When the patient is of reproductive age, when the gonads lie in the path of or near the useful (primary) beam, and when the use of such shielding will not compromise the required information
23. Decrease
24. To maintain density, a large reduction in mAs must accompany an appreciable increase in kVp
25. a. Any barrier that intercepts the useful (primary) beam
    b. Any barrier that intercepts only leakage and secondary radiation
26. a. Primary barrier
    b. Primary barrier
    c. Secondary barrier
    d. Secondary barriers
27. a. Any area adjacent to an exposure room that is occupied only by radiation workers and patients
    b. Any area adjacent to an exposure room that is occupied by persons in the general population
28. Controlled
29. a. The fraction of percent of time that the useful (primary) beam is directed to a barrier
    b. An expression of the extent to which the area being protected is occupied
30. Time, distance, and shielding
31. Ensure that the 5-minute fluoroscopic reset timer is functioning and is properly used; remain positioned away from the edge of the x-ray table; and wear protective lead apparel.
32. 5 minutes
33. Pocket ionization chamber, film badge, and thermoluminescent dosimeter (TLD)
34. Outside the protective apron, unshielded, at the collar level
35. Nearly 100%

Self-Test: Radiation Protection

1. b	6. b	11. b	16. b	21. d
2. b	7. d	12. d	17. c	22. d
3. c	8. d	13. b	18. b	23. b
4. c	9. a	14. c	19. d	24. d
5. a	10. d	15. a	20. b	25. a

CHAPTER 3 **General Anatomy and Radiographic Positioning Terminology**

Review

1. a. The science of the structure of the body
   b. The study of the function of the body organs
   c. The detailed study of the body of knowledge relating to the bones of the body
2. The body standing erect, face and eyes directed forward, arms extended by the sides with the palms of the hands facing forward, heels together, and the toes pointing anteriorly with the great toes touching
3. Sagittal, coronal, horizontal, and oblique
4. Sagittal
5. Coronal
6. Midcoronal (also referred to as the midaxillary plane)
7. Midsagittal
8. Horizontal (also referred to as a transverse or axial plane)
9. A. Sagittal plane
   B. Coronal plane
   C. Horizontal plane
   D. Oblique plane
10. Thoracic and abdominal
11.

1. b	7. b	13. a
2. a	8. a	14. b
3. a	9. c	15. b
4. c	10. b	16. a
5. b	11. b	17. c
6. c	12. b	

12. A. Thoracic
    B. Abdominal
    C. Pleural
    D. Pericardial
    E. Pelvic
13. A. Right upper quadrant
    B. Left upper quadrant
    C. Right lower quadrant
    D. Left lower quadrant
14. A. Right hypochondrium
    B. Epigastrium
    C. Left hypochondrium
    D. Right lateral (lumbar)
    E. Umbilical
    F. Left lateral (lumbar)
    G. Right inguinal
    H. Hypogastrium
    I. Left inguinal

15. 1. b 6. n 11. f
2. a 7. h 12. l
3. c 8. g 13. k
4. d 9. j 14. m
5. e 10. i

16. A. Gonion
B. Mastoid tip
C. Vertebra prominens

17. A. C5 and thyroid cartilage
B. T1
C. T2, T3, and jugular notch
D. T4, T5, and sternal angle
E. T7 and inferior angle scapula
F. T9, T10, and xiphoid process
G. L2, L3, and inferior costal margin
H. L4, L5, and crest of ilium
I. S1 and anterior superior iliac spine
J. Coccyx, pubic symphysis, and greater trochanters

18. Sthenic, asthenic, hyposthenic, and hypersthenic

19. a. Hypersthenic
b. Sthenic
c. Hyposthenic
d. Asthenic

20. 206

21. Appendicular and axial

22. b, c, e, f

23. a, b, c, d

24. 1. c
2. b
3. d
4. a

25. a, b, c, f

26. 1. b 6. d 11. a
2. c 7. a 12. d
3. b 8. c 13. d
4. d 9. a 14. c
5. d 10. b 15. c

27. a. Long bones consist of a body and two articular ends.
b. Short bones consist mainly of spongy tissue and have only a thin outer layer of compact bone.
c. Flat bones consist mainly of compact bone in the form of two plates that enclose a layer of spongy tissue.
d. Irregular bones, because of their peculiar shape, cannot be classified as long, short, or flat bones.
e. Sesamoid bones are small oval bones that develop in and near tendons and function to protect tendons from excessive wear.

28. Synarthroses, amphiarthroses, and diarthroses

29. 1. b
2. a
3. c

30. Fibrous, cartilaginous, and synovial

31. 1. b
2. a
3. c

32. a. Diarthrodial; synovial
b. Synarthrodial; fibrous
c. Amphiarthrodial; cartilaginous

33. 1. f
2. e
3. d
4. c
5. a
6. b

34. 1. a, b
2. c, d
3. e
4. c, d, f, g, h
5. c, d, f, g, h
6. c, d, e, f, g, h

35. 1. f 5. f 8. d
2. d 6. c 9. e
3. d 7. b 10. a
4. e

36. 1. j 6. g 11. e
2. i 7. k 12. o
3. d 8. m 13. l
4. n 9. f 14. h
5. a 10. c 15. b

37. 1. b
2. d
3. e
4. c
5. a
6. f

38.

39. 1. d 6. l 11. f 16. o 21. i
2. t 7. q 12. m 17. g 22. p
3. v 8. k 13. u 18. s 23. e
4. j 9. b 14. c 19. h 24. n
5. r 10. a 15. q 20. j

40.

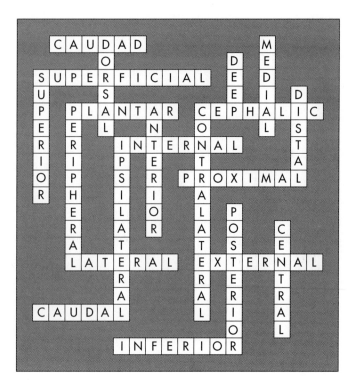

41. a. Refers to the path of the central ray
   b. As a noun: a specific patient body position (e.g., body position or radiographic position); as a verb: the act of placing a patient in the appropriate position
   c. The body part as it is seen from the perspective of an x-ray film or other recording media (restricted to the discussion of the radiograph or image)
   d. Denotes the originator of a particular radiographic procedure, or additionally specifies placement of the IR and central ray

42. a. P   f. B   k. P
    b. B   g. P   l. B
    c. B   h. P   m. P
    d. P   i. P   n. R
    e. R   j. R   o. R

43. 1. c
    2. a
    3. b
    4. d
    5. e
    6. f

44. a. Anteroposterior (AP) projections
    b. Posteroanterior (PA) projections
    c. Axial projections
    d. Tangential projections
    e. Lateral projections
    f. Oblique projections

45. 1. e
    2. f
    3. c
    4. a
    5. d
    6. b

46. a. Supine (dorsal recumbent)
    b. Prone (ventral recumbent)
    c. Right lateral recumbent
47. a. Left lateral
    b. Right lateral
    c. Right anterior oblique (RAO)
    d. Left anterior oblique (LAO)
    e. Left posterior oblique (LPO)
    f. Right posterior oblique (RPO)
    g. Left lateral decubitus
    h. Right dorsal decubitus
    i. Ventral decubitus
48. 1. n
    2. a
    3. m
    4. h
    5. k
    6. g
    7. f
    8. b
    9. j
    10. l
    11. i
    12. e
    13. c
    14. d
49. a. A. abduction; B. adduction
    b. A. flexion; B. extension
    c. A. eversion; B. inversion
    d. Pronation
    e. Supination
    f. Tilt
50. a. Alae
    b. Alveoli
    c. Appendices
    d. Calculi
    e. Diagnoses
    f. Diverticula
    g. Ganglia
    h. Ilia
    i. Laminae
    j. Metastases

Self-Test: General Anatomy and Radiographic Positioning Terminology

1. c	9. d	17. c	24. d
2. a	10. b	18. c	25. a
3. c	11. a	19. a	26. d
4. d	12. a	20. a	27. d
5. b	13. b	21. c	28. b
6. b	14. d	22. d	29. c
7. b	15. c	23. b	30. b
8. c	16. a		

CHAPTER 4 **Upper Limb**
SECTION 1 **Osteology and Arthrology of the Upper Limb**

Exercise 1

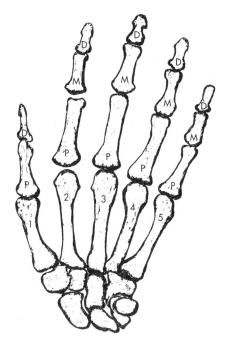

Exercise 2

A. First metacarpal
B. Proximal phalanx of the first digit (thumb)
C. Proximal interphalangeal joint of the second digit
D. Middle phalanx of the third digit
E. Distal interphalangeal joint of the fourth digit
F. Distal phalanx of the fifth digit
G. Fifth metacarpophalangeal joint
H. Fifth metacarpal

Exercise 3

A. Scaphoid
B. Lunate
C. Triquetrum
D. Pisiform

Exercise 4

A. Trapezium
B. Trapezoid
C. Capitate
D. Hamate

Exercise 5

A. Triquetrum
B. Pisiform
C. Hamate
D. Capitate
E. Trapezoid
F. Trapezium

Exercise 6

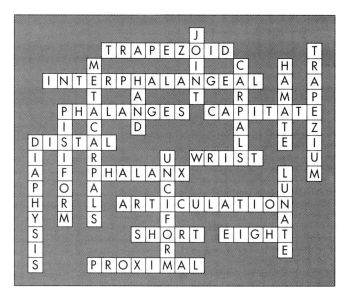

Exercise 7

A. Olecranon process
B. Trochlear notch
C. Coronoid process
D. Body
E. Head
F. Styloid process

Exercise 8

A. Head
B. Tubercle
C. Body
D. Styloid process

Exercise 9

A. Humeroulnar
B. Proximal radioulnar
C. Humeroradial
D. Distal radioulnar
E. Radiocarpal

Exercise 10

A. Coronoid fossa
B. Medial epicondyle
C. Trochlea
D. Capitulum
E. Lateral epicondyle
F. Olecranon fossa
G. Body of the humerus

Exercise 11

A. Humerus
B. Radius
C. Ulna
D. Olecranon process
E. Medial epicondyle
F. Trochlea
G. Lateral epicondyle
H. Capitulum

Exercise 12

A. Head
B. Greater tubercle
C. Lesser tubercle
D. Body
E. Medial epicondyle
F. Trochlea
G. Coronoid fossa
H. Lateral epicondyle
I. Capitulum

Exercise 13

1. c
2. a
3. d
4. e
5. b

Exercise 14

1. D
2. D
3. D
4. P
5. P
6. P
7. D
8. P
9. P
10. D
11. P
12. P
13. D
14. D
15. D

Exercise 15

1. R, U, H
2. H
3. H
4. U
5. H
6. H
7. R, U
8. H
9. U
10. H
11. R
12. U
13. U
14. H
15. H

Exercise 16

1. a
2. b, c, d, e, f
3. b, c
4. b, c, d, e, f
5. g
6. g
7. b, c

Exercise 17

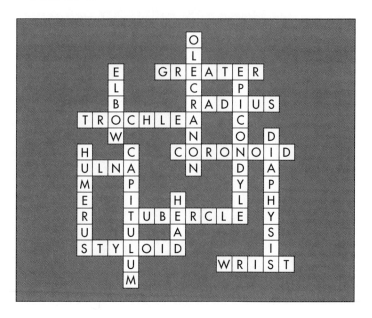

Exercise 18

1. m
2. b
3. h
4. f
5. q
6. j
7. r
8. c
9. n
10. l
11. p
12. o
13. e
14. d
15. i

Exercise 19

1. Phalanges, 14; metacarpals, 5; and carpals, 8
2. b
3. c
4. c
5. Carpals
6. Head
7. b
8. c
9. a
10. a. 5
    b. 4
    c. 5
11. b
12. b

13. a. Scaphoid; navicular (P)
    b. Lunate; semilunar (P)
    c. Triquetrum; triquetral; cuneiform; triangular (P)
    d. Pisiform (P)
    e. Trapezium; greater multangular (D)
    f. Trapezoid; lesser multangular (D)
    g. Capitate; os magnum; capitatum (D)
    h. Hamate; unciform (D)
14. Wrist joint proper
15. Radius (lateral) and ulna (medial)
16. Distal
17. Proximal
18. Distal
19. Proximal
20. d
21. c
22. a
23. d
24. c
25. b
26. a
27. b, c, f
28. b
29. Humeroulnar, humeroradial, and scapulohumeral
30. Coronoid fossa (anterior surface); olecranon fossa (posterior surface)

SECTION 2 Positioning of the Upper Limb

Exercise 1: Positioning for the Fingers

1. A. Distal phalanx
   B. Distal interphalangeal joint
   C. Middle phalanx
   D. Proximal interphalangeal joint
   E. Proximal phalanx
   F. Metacarpophalangeal joint
   G. Head of metacarpal
2. PA
3. c
4. a
5. From the prone position, the second digit was internally rotated 90 degrees to place it in a lateral position
6. a
7. To accurately demonstrate the bones and joints
8. 45 degrees
9. To place the part closer to the IR and to improve its recorded detail
10. The wedge supports the digits in a position parallel with the plane of the image receptor so that the interphalangeal joint spaces will be open.

Exercise 2: Positioning for the Thumb

1. Internal rotation
2. Metacarpophalangeal
3. Oblique
4. b
5. c

6. A. Distal phalanx
   B. Interphalangeal joint
   C. Proximal phalanx
   D. Metacarpophalangeal joint
   E. First metacarpal
   F. Carpometacarpal joint

Exercise 3: Positioning for the Hand

1. Palmar
2. Metacarpophalangeal
3. c
4. A. Distal phalanx of the second digit
   B. Middle phalanx of the second digit
   C. Proximal phalanx of the second digit
   D. Second metacarpophalangeal joint
   E. Radius
   F. Ulna
   G. Distal interphalangeal joint of the third digit
   H. Proximal interphalangeal joint of the third digit
   I. Phalanges
   J. Metacarpals
   K. Carpals
5. Fig. 4-16 (The digits are parallel with the plane of the image receptor.)
6. Fig. 4-18 demonstrates open interphalangeal joints because the digits are parallel with the plane of the IR. In Fig. 4-19 the digits are not parallel with the IR; therefore, they appear foreshortened and their interphalangeal joints are closed on most digits.
7. b
8. c
9. b
10. A. Phalanges
    B. Metacarpals
    C. Carpals
    D. Distal phalanx of the thumb
    E. Proximal phalanx of the thumb
    F. First metacarpal
    G. Radius
    H. Ulna

Exercise 4: Positioning for the Wrist

1. Anterior
2. To place the wrist in close contact with the image receptor
3. Midcarpal
4. A. Pisiform
   B. Triquetrum
   C. Hamate
   D. Lunate
   E. Capitate
   F. Scaphoid
   G. Trapezoid
   H. Trapezium
5. c
6. a
7. A. First metacarpal
   B. Trapezium
   C. Scaphoid
   D. Capitate
   E. Lunate
   F. Radius
   G. Ulna

8. Radius and ulna
9. Anterior
10. c
11. Ulna
12. A. First metacarpal
    B. Trapezium
    C. Trapezoid
    D. Scaphoid
    E. Lunate
    F. Radius
    G. Ulna
13. d
14. a
15. c
16. Anterior
17. c
18. b
19. a
20. c
21. Parallel
22. Hyperextended
23. b
24. c
25. A. Lunate
    B. Trapezoid
    C. Trapezium
    D. Scaphoid
    E. Triquetrum
    F. Capitate
    G. Hamulus of hamate
    H. Pisiform

Exercise 5: Positioning for the Forearm

1. d
2. a
3. False (The hand should be supinated. Pronation of the hand for the AP projection of the forearm will cause radial crossover to occur.)
4. True
5. A. Medial epicondyle
   B. Lateral epicondyle
   C. Radial head
   D. Radial neck
   E. Radial tubercle
   F. Ulnar body
   G. Radial body
   H. Epiphysis
   I. Radial styloid process
6. c
7. b
8. False (The hand should be in the lateral position with the thumb side up.)
9. True
10. A. Olecranon process
    B. Humeral epicondyle
    C. Coronoid process
    D. Radial head
    E. Ulnar body
    F. Radial body
    G. Ulnar styloid process

Exercise 6: Positioning for the Elbow

1. Supinated
2. To prevent rotation of the bones of the forearm
3. a
4. a
5. A. Medial epicondyle
   B. Lateral epicondyle
   C. Capitulum
   D. Trochlea
   E. Proximal ulna
   F. Radial head
   G. Radial neck
   H. Radial tuberosity
6. b
7. c
8. 90 degrees
9. Superimposed
10. A. Humeral epicondyles
    B. Olecranon process
    C. Coronoid process
    D. Radial head
    E. Radial neck
11. c
12. a
13. Medial rotation
14. A. Olecranon process
    B. Medial epicondyle
    C. Trochlea
    D. Coronoid process
15. A. Capitulum
    B. Radial head
    C. Radial neck
    D. Radial tuberosity
16. a. Fig. 4-33
    b. Fig. 4-32
    c. Fig. 4-33
    d. Fig. 4-32
    e. Fig. 4-32
17. a. Fig. 4-34
    b. Fig. 4-35
    c. Fig. 4-35
    d. Distal humerus
    e. Proximal radius and ulna
    f. Radius and ulna
    g. Distal humerus
18. 1. f
    2. c
    3. e
    4. b
    5. a

Exercise 7: Positioning for the Humerus

1. Upper margin of the IR should be $1\frac{1}{2}$ inches (3.8 cm) above the humeral head
2. b
3. a
4. Supine
5. To place the affected arm in contact with the IR or table
6. b, d, f

7. A. Acromion process
   B. Greater tubercle
   C. Glenoid cavity
   D. Lesser tubercle
   E. Body
   F. Medial epicondyle
   G. Capitulum
   H. Trochlea
   I. Ulna
   J. Radius
8. Upper margin of the IR should be $1^1/_2$ inches (3.8 cm) above the humeral head
9. Internally rotate the arm, flex the elbow approximately 90 degrees, and place the patient's hand on the hip.
10. Perpendicular
11. The elbow joint may appear partially closed.
12. Epicondyles
13. The proximal portion (including the humeral head), the lesser tubercle, and the greater tubercle
14. a, c, e
15. A. Clavicle
    B. Acromion process
    C. Lesser tubercle
    D. Superimposed epicondyle

Exercise 8: Positioning of the Upper Limb

1. First metacarpophalangeal joint
2. AP projection
3. Proximal interphalangeal joint of the third digit
4. To minimize object-to-image receptor distance (OID)
5. Distal and proximal phalanges of the thumb and the first metacarpal
6. Second (index finger) and fifth (little finger)
7. Perpendicular to the third metacarpophalangeal joint
8. Anterior (palmar or ventral)
9. 45; 90
10. Elevated from the IR and parallel with the plane of the IR
11. Metacarpals
12. Phalanges
13. To place the anterior surface of the wrist in contact with the IR
14. Perpendicular to the midcarpal area
15. Distal radius, distal ulna, and proximal metacarpals
16. 45
17. Lateral
18. Ulnar (medial)
19. Lateral
20. Lateral (radial)
21. Scaphoid and trapezium
22. Scaphoid
23. The IR is inclined toward the elbow at an angle of 20 degrees.
24. The radius crosses over the ulna, which results in an oblique image of the forearm.
25. Supinated
26. Styloid process
27. Superimposed over each other
28. True lateral, thumb side up
29. The hand was not supinated.
30. To help adjust the humeral epicondyles and the anterior surface of the forearm parallel with the plane of the IR
31. Head, neck, and tuberosity

32. True lateral with the thumb side up (to keep the radial head from rotating from its lateral position)
33. AP medial oblique
34. Laterally (externally)
35. Two
36. For one exposure the humerus is parallel and in contact with the IR; for the other exposure the forearm is parallel and in contact with the IR.
37. About $1^1/_2$ inches (4 cm) above the head of the humerus
38. Epicondyles
39. AP
40. Place the IR between the humerus and the thorax.

Exercise 9: Identifying Projections of the Upper Limb

1. PA third digit
2. PA oblique first digit (thumb)
3. PA hand
4. PA wrist
5. Lateral wrist
6. PA wrist in ulnar deviation
7. PA axial wrist (Stecher method) for scaphoid
8. Tangential (inferosuperior) (Gaynor-Hart method) for carpal canal
9. AP forearm
10. AP elbow
11. AP oblique elbow, medial rotation
12. AP oblique elbow, lateral rotation
13. AP elbow, partial flexion
14. AP humerus
15. Lateral humerus

Exercise 10: Evaluating Radiographs of the Upper Limb

1. The proximal and distal interphalangeal joints are not well demonstrated because of overlapping ends of the phalanges. Apparently this finger was slightly flexed and not entirely in contact with the image receptor.
2. The first metacarpal and the trapezium are not seen.
3. Radial crossover is demonstrated because the hand was pronated.
4. a
5. c
6. b
7. b
8. b

Self-Test: Osteology, Arthrology, and Positioning of the Upper Limb

1. b	16. c	31. b	45. b	59. b	73. c	87. c
2. a	17. a	32. d	46. d	60. b	74. d	88. c
3. d	18. a	33. a	47. c	61. b	75. c	89. b
4. d	19. d	34. d	48. a	62. c	76. b	90. c
5. b	20. b	35. a	49. a	63. c	77. b	91. d
6. a	21. d	36. a	50. c	64. c	78. c	92. a
7. b	22. c	37. d	51. c	65. d	79. b	93. b
8. a	23. c	38. d	52. d	66. c	80. c	94. d
9. b	24. c	39. c	53. a	67. a	81. a	95. b
10. c	25. a	40. d	54. c	68. b	82. a	96. c
11. d	26. c	41. c	55. b	69. d	83. b	97. d
12. d	27. b	42. c	56. b	70. d	84. b	98. b
13. b	28. d	43. b	57. a	71. c	85. b	99. d
14. b	29. c	44. a	58. a	72. d	86. a	100. a
15. d	30. b					

CHAPTER 5 **Shoulder Girdle**
SECTION 1 **Osteology and Arthrology of the Shoulder Girdle**

Exercise 1

1. A. Acromial extremity
   B. Body
   C. Sternal extremity
2. Long
3. Sternal
4. Acromial
5. Lateral
6. Medial
7. Just above the first rib
8. a
9. b
10. Males

Exercise 2

A. Glenoid cavity
B. Acromion
C. Coracoid process
D. Scapular notch
E. Superior border
F. Superior angle
G. Medial border
H. Inferior angle
I. Lateral border
J. Subscapular fossa

Exercise 3

A. Superior angle
B. Crest of spine
C. Medial border
D. Inferior angle
E. Infraspinatus fossa
F. Supraspinatus fossa
G. Superior border
H. Scapular notch
I. Coracoid process
J. Acromion
K. Spine
L. Glenoid cavity
M. Lateral border

Exercise 4

A. Acromion
B. Spine
C. Dorsal (posterior) surface
D. Lateral border
E. Inferior angle
F. Superior angle
G. Coracoid process
H. Glenoid cavity
I. Costal (anterior) surface

Exercise 5

1. d
2. e
3. n
4. f
5. c
6. a
7. j
8. h
9. m
10. g
11. o
12. i
13. k
14. l

Exercise 6

A Lesser tubercle
B. Anatomic neck
C. Head
D. Greater tubercle
E. Intertubercular groove
F. Surgical neck
G. Body

Exercise 7

1. g
2. d
3. c
4. h
5. e
6. b

Exercise 8

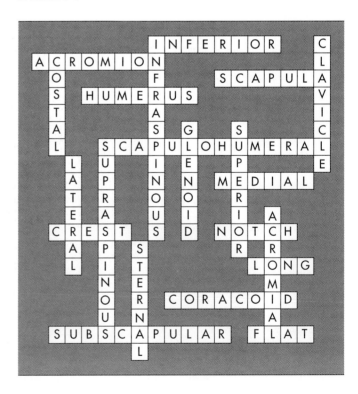

Exercise 9

1. l
2. b
3. c
4. k
5. f
6. a
7. m
8. e
9. g
10. i

Exercise 10

1. Flat
2. a. Two
   b. Three
   c. Three
3. Anterior
4. Supraspinatus and infraspinatus
5. Scapular spine
6. Acromion
7. Near the lateral end of the superior border
8. Coracoid process
9. Superior, medial, and lateral
10. Superior, inferior, and lateral
11. Clavicle
12. Subscapularis
13. Anatomic
14. Bursae
15. Three
16. Scapulohumeral, acromioclavicular, and sternoclavicular
17. Ball and socket for the scapulohumeral articulation; gliding for the acromioclavicular and sternoclavicular articulations
18. Humerus
19. Sternum
20. Acromion

SECTION 2 Positioning of the Shoulder Girdle

Exercise 1: Positioning for the Shoulder

1. Perpendicular to a point 1 inch (2.5 cm) inferior to the coracoid process
2. Rotation of the arm
3. Suspended
4. a. Rotation and placement of the humerus
   b. Fig. 5-6
   c. Fig. 5-8
   d. Fig. 5-7
   e. Fig. 5-6
   f. Fig. 5-7
   g. Fig. 5-8
   h. Fig. 5-6
   i. Fig. 5-8
   j. Fig. 5-6

5. A. Clavicle
   B. Acromioclavicular joint
   C. Acromion
   D. Head of the humerus
   E. Lesser tubercle
   F. Glenoid cavity
6. b
7. b
8. b
9. a
10. A. Scapula
    B. Sternum
    C. Clavicle
    D. Acromion
    E. Humeral head
    F. Lateral border of the scapula
11. False (The IR should be placed on edge against the top of the shoulder and as close as possible to the neck.)
12. True
13. True
14. As close as possible to right angles
15. c
16. a
17. b
18. The degree of abduction of the affected arm
19. b, c, d, g
20. True
21. True
22. Stop breathing for the exposure.
23. d
24. c
25. A. Acromion
    B. Coracoid process
    C. Body of scapula
    D. Inferior angle
    E. Humerus
26. a. Fully extend the affected limb with the hand supinated.
    b. Vertically place against the superior surface of the shoulder.
    c. Angle 10 to 15 degrees posteriorly (downward from horizontal) to the long axis of the humerus.
27. Forearm
28. 10, 15
29. c
30. A. Intertubercular groove
    B. Greater tubercle
    C. Lesser tubercle
    D. Coracoid process

Exercise 2: Positioning for the Acromioclavicular Articulations

1. False (To best demonstrate acromioclavicular joints, the patient should be in the upright position because dislocations of the AC joint tend to reduce themselves in the recumbent position.)
2. True
3. False (The central ray should be directed to the midline of the body at the level of the acromioclavicular joints.)
4. Two image receptors should be used and exposed simultaneously.
5. The weights enable better demonstration of a separation of an acromioclavicular joint.

Exercise 3: Positioning for the Clavicle

1. 24 × 30 cm (10 × 12 inch) crosswise
2. Suspend respiration after expiration
3. PA (because of decreased OID)
4. True
5. False (Although the entire clavicle should be imaged, the medial half of the clavicle should be demonstrated superimposed over the thorax.)
6. A. Acromion
   B. Acromioclavicular articulation
   C. Clavicle
   D. Coracoid process
   E. Sternoclavicular articulation
7. a. 15 to 30 degrees cephalad
   b. 15 to 30 degrees caudad
8. AP axial
9. The size of the patient (thickness of the thorax)
10. 0 to 15 degrees cephalad
11. False (Although the entire clavicle should be imaged, the medial end will superimpose the first or second ribs.)
12. False (Respiration should be suspended after full inspiration.)

Exercise 4: Positioning for the Scapula

1. Coracoid process
2. a
3. a
4. a
5. True
6. True
7. False (Rotation of the patient toward the affected side offsets the effect of drawing the scapula laterally.)
8. A. Acromion
   B. Coracoid process
   C. Glenoid cavity
   D. Lateral border
   E. Medial border
   F. Inferior angle
9. The placement of the arm determines what part of the scapula is demonstrated in superimposition with the humerus.
10. Perpendicular to the medial border of the affected scapula
11. Instruct the patient to flex the elbow and place the hand on the posterior thorax.
12. True
13. True
14. True
15. A. Acromion
    B. Coracoid process
    C. Humerus
    D. Body of the scapula
    E. Inferior angle

Exercise 5: Identifying Projections of the Shoulder Girdle

1. AP axial clavicle, lordotic position
2. Bilateral AP acromioclavicular articulations
3. AP shoulder, neutral rotation humerus
4. AP shoulder, external rotation humerus
5. AP shoulder, internal rotation humerus
6. AP scapula
7. Inferosuperior axial shoulder joint, Lawrence method

8. Supine tangential intertubercular groove
9. Upright transthoracic lateral shoulder, Lawrence method
10. PA oblique shoulder joint
11. Lateral scapula, RAO body position
12. Standing tangential intertubercular groove, Fisk modification

Self-Test: Osteology, Arthrology, and Positioning of the Shoulder Girdle

1. a	7. c	13. c	19. c	25. c	31. d
2. b	8. b	14. b	20. c	26. d	32. a
3. a	9. a	15. a	21. d	27. a	33. d
4. b	10. c	16. b	22. b	28. b	34. c
5. b	11. d	17. d	23. d	29. a	35. d
6. b	12. b	18. d	24. d	30. c	

CHAPTER 6 Lower Limb
SECTION 1 Osteology and Arthrology of the Lower Limb

Exercise 1

A. Phalanges
B. Metatarsals
C. Tarsals
D. Medial cuneiform
E. Intermediate cuneiform
F. Lateral cuneiform
G. Navicular
H. Cuboid
I. Talus
J. Calcaneus
K. Distal phalanx (of the fifth digit)
L. Middle phalanx (of the fifth digit)
M. Proximal phalanx (of the fifth digit)
N. Fifth metatarsal

Exercise 2

A. Tibia
B. Calcaneus
C. Cuboid
D. Fifth metatarsal
E. Fibula
F. Lateral malleolus
G. Navicular
H. Lateral cuneiform
I. Metatarsals
J. Phalanges

Exercise 3

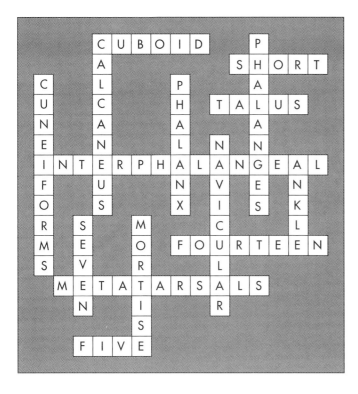

Exercise 4

A. Apex
B. Fibular head
C. Lateral condyle
D. Intercondylar eminence
E. Medial condyle
F. Tuberosity
G. Fibular body
H. Tibial body
I. Lateral malleolus
J. Medial malleolus

Exercise 5

A. Tuberosity
B. Anterior crest
C. Tibial body
D. Lateral condyle
E. Apex
F. Head of the fibula
G. Fibular body
H. Medial malleolus
I. Lateral malleolus

Exercise 6

1. f   5. h   8. b
2. d   6. i   9. g
3. c   7. k   10. j
4. a

Exercise 7

A. Neck
B. Lesser trochanter
C. Body
D. Medial epicondyle
E. Medial condyle
F. Head
G. Greater trochanter
H. Lateral epicondyle
I. Lateral condyle
J. Patellar surface

Exercise 8

A. Greater trochanter
B. Head
C. Neck
D. Lesser trochanter
E. Body
F. Lateral epicondyle
G. Lateral condyle
H. Medial epicondyle
I. Medial condyle
J. Intercondylar fossa

Exercise 9

A. Anterior cruciate ligament
B. Lateral meniscus
C. Fibular collateral ligament
D. Patellar surface
E. Posterior cruciate ligament
F. Medial meniscus
G. Tibial collateral ligament
H. Fibula

Exercise 10

A. Medial meniscus
B. Anterior cruciate ligament
C. Articular cartilage
D. Posterior cruciate ligament
E. Lateral meniscus
F. Femur
G. Synovial fluid
H. Meniscus
I. Patella
J. Tibia

Exercise 11

1. d
2. c
3. e
4. h
5. g
6. a

Exercise 12

1. P	4. P	7. P	10. D	13. D
2. P	5. P	8. D	11. D	14. D
3. P	6. P	9. P	12. D	15. P

Exercise 13

1. c	6. a
2. a, c	7. b
3. a, b	8. c
4. b	9. a
5. a	10. b

Exercise 14

1. b, c
2. b, c
3. a
4. b, c
5. b, c, d, e
6. h
7. a
8. b, c, d, e

Exercise 15

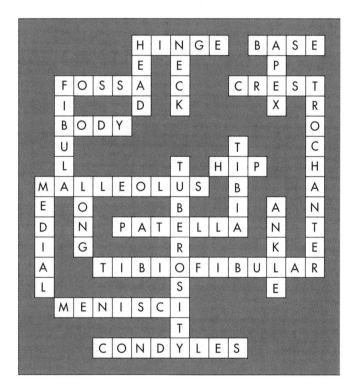

Exercise 16

1. j	6. i
2. c	7. e
3. k	8. g
4. d	9. f
5. b	10. h

Exercise 17

1. 30
2. Phalanges, 14; metatarsals, 5; tarsals, 7
3. Nine
4. Flexion and extension
5. Hinge
6. Proximal phalanges
7. Numbered 1 through 5 from the medial side (great toe) to the lateral side (small toe)
8. a. Metatarsals and phalanges
   b. Cuneiforms, cuboid, and navicular
   c. Talus and calcaneus
9. The fifth metatarsal
10. Medial cuneiform, intermediate cuneiform, lateral cuneiform, navicular, cuboid, talus, and calcaneus
11. Calcaneus
12. Calcaneus
13. Talus
14. Cuboid
15. Cuboid
16. Navicular
17. Cuneiforms and cuboid
18. Talus
19. Tibia and fibula
20. Fibula
21. Fibula
22. Intercondylar eminence
23. Lateral
24. On the anterior surface of the tibia, just inferior from the condyles
25. Medial malleolus
26. Talus
27. Femorotibial, proximal tibiofibular, distal tibiofibular, and tibiotalar
28. Femur
29. At the distal end of the femur, posteriorly between the condyles
30. a. Patella
    b. Sesamoid

SECTION 2 Positioning of the Lower Limb

Exercise 1: Positioning for the Toes

1. At the third metatarsophalangeal joint
2. c
3. a
4. a
5. a. Fig. 6-10
   b. Fig. 6-10
   c. Fig. 6-9
   d. Fig. 6-10
6. A. Phalanges
   B. Sesamoid
   C. Metatarsals
   D. Distal interphalangeal joint
   E. Distal phalanx
   F. Middle phalanx
   G. Proximal interphalangeal joint
   H. Proximal phalanx
   I. Metatarsophalangeal joint

7. Medially
8. 30 to 45 degrees
9. Fourth and fifth (and sometimes, third)
10. Distal
11. Perpendicular
12. Third metatarsophalangeal
13. False (The distal end [head] of metatarsals should be seen.)
14. True
15. Tape all toes above the affected toe into a flexed position.
16. Perpendicular
17. Metatarsalphalangeal
18. Proximal interphalangeal
19. True
20. True

Exercise 2: Positioning for the Foot

1. c
2. Plantar
3. To the base of the third metatarsal
4. Perpendicular and 10 degrees posteriorly (toward the heel)
5. 10 degrees posteriorly (toward the heel)
6. a
7. A. First metatarsophalangeal joint
   B. First tarsometatarsal joint
   C. Medial cuneiform
   D. Navicular
   E. Phalanges
   F. Metatarsals
   G. Tarsals
   H. Cuboid
8. Medially
9. d
10. c
11. c
12. The base of the third metatarsal
13. First and second
14. A. Medial cuneiform
    B. Intermediate cuneiform
    C. Metatarsals
    D. Tuberosity (of the fifth metatarsal)
    E. Lateral cuneiform
    F. Cuboid
    G. Calcaneus
    H. Navicular
    I. Talus
    J. Sinus tarsi
15. Lateral
16. Dorsiflex the foot to form a 90-degree angle with the lower leg
17. Perpendicular
18. The base of the third metatarsal
19. The distal fibula should overlap the posterior portion of the tibia.
20. A. Phalanges
    B. Metatarsals
    C. Fibula
    D. Tibia
    E. Tibiotalar joint (mortise joint)
    F. Navicular
    G. Talus
    H. Sinus tarsi
    I. Calcaneus
    J. Tarsals

Exercise 3: Positioning for the Calcaneus

1. Axial
2. Perpendicular
3. 40 degrees cephalad
4. The base of the third metatarsal
5. Two images should be performed to completely demonstrate the entire calcaneus.
6. False (The heel should be in contact with the IR; the plantar surface should be perpendicular to the IR.)
7. False (The central ray should enter the plantar surface.)
8. A. Sustentaculum tali
   B. Trochlear process
   C. Lateral process
   D. Tuberosity
9. True
10. At the midportion of the calcaneus (1 inch distal to the medial malleolus)
11. Lateral
12. A. Tibiotalar joint (mortise joint)
    B. Sinus tarsi
    C. Tuberosity
    D. Talus
    E. Navicular
    F. Sustentaculum tali

Exercise 4: Positioning for the Ankle

1. With the leg extended, rest the heel of the foot on the IR with the foot dorsiflexed enough to place the long axis of the foot perpendicular to the IR.
2. At a point midway between the malleoli on the anterior surface of the ankle
3. True
4. True
5. False (Some overlapping of the distal fibula with the talus and tibia is expected.)
6. True
7. A. Fibula
   B. Tibiotalar joint
   C. Lateral malleolus
   D. Tibia
   E. Medial malleolus
   F. Talus
8. To prevent lateral rotation of the ankle
9. At the medial malleolus
10. Perpendicularly
11. True
12. False (The distal fibula will appear superimposed with the talus.)
13. A. Tibia
    B. Fibula
    C. Tibiotalar joint
    D. Talus
    E. Navicular
    F. Cuboid
    G. Calcaneus
14. Supine with the affected limb fully extended
15. Centered to the ankle joint midway between the malleoli so that its long axis is parallel with the long axis of the leg
16. 45 degrees medially
17. Midway between the malleoli
18. a, d, e, f

19. 15 to 20 degrees
20. The intermalleolar plane should be parallel with the image receptor.
21. Malleoli
22. Perpendicular
23. True
24. False (The foot should be dorsiflexed to place the long axis of the foot perpendicular to the image receptor.)
25. True
26. A. Fibula
    B. Lateral malleolus
    C. Tibia
    D. Medial malleolus
    E. Mortise joint
    F. Talus
27. To verify the presence of a ligamentous tear
28. Keeping the ankle in the AP position, the foot is forcibly turned into inversion, or eversion, and the exposure is made. (Sometimes both movements are required to complete the study.)
29. The patient may be instructed to pull on a strip of bandage that is looped around the foot.
30. An increase in the joint space on the side of the injury indicates a torn ligament.

Exercise 5: Positioning for the Leg

1. a
2. a
3. a
4. False (Proximal and distal articulations of tibia and fibula should have moderate overlapping.)
5. A. Femur
    B. Knee joint
    C. Head of the fibula
    D. Fibula
    E. Tibia
    F. Lateral malleolus
6. Perpendicular
7. Perform a cross-table lateral projection by placing an image receptor vertically between the patient's legs and directing a horizontal central ray to the leg.
8. The natural divergence of the beam may prevent the femoral condyles from appearing superimposed.
9. True
10. A. Patella
    B. Femoral condyles
    C. Tibia
    D. Fibula

Exercise 6: Positioning for the Knee

1. The size of the patient's knee, the preference of the radiologist, and the preference of the radiographer
2. c
3. d
4. 1. b
    2. a
    3. c
5. a
6. c
7. True
8. True

9. A. Femur
    B. Patella
    C. Lateral epicondyle
    D. Lateral condyle
    E. Lateral tibial plateau
    F. Intercondylar eminence
    G. Head of fibula
    H. Fibula
    I. Medial epicondyle
    J. Medial condyle
    K. Medial tibial plateau
    L. Tibia
10. i. b
    ii. The angulation of the central ray was different.
    iii. It was probably angled 3 to 5 degrees cephalad; the femorotibial joint space is demonstrated open.
    iv. It was directed perpendicularly or some angulation other than 3 to 5 degrees cephalad; the femorotibial joint space is not well demonstrated open.
    v. Fig. 6-22
11. Perpendicular
12. 20 to 30 degrees
13. 10 degrees
14. The fracture may separate, causing a fragment to be displaced.
15. 5 to 7 degrees cephalad
16. To prevent the joint space from being obscured by the magnified shadow of the femoral condyle
17. Medial epicondyle
18. b
19. True
20. False (The femoropatellar space should be open.)
21. A. Femur
    B. Femoral condyles
    C. Patella
    D. Tibial plateau
    E. Tibia
    F. Fibula
22. a
23. 35 × 43 cm; crosswise
24. To $1/_2$ inch below the level of the patellar apices
25. Horizontal and perpendicular to the center of the IR at a point $1/_2$ inch below the level of the apices of the patellae
26. False (The patient should stand straight with both knees fully extended and weight equally distributed on the feet.)
27. True
28. c
29. b
30. a
31. c
32. a
33. a. B
    b. B
    c. B
    d. L
    e. M
    f. L
    g. M
    h. B
    i. L
    j. M

34. A. Femur
    B. Patella
    C. Medial femoral condyle
    D. Lateral femoral condyle
    E. Lateral tibial plateau
    F. Medial tibial plateau
    G. Medial tibial condyle
    H. Fibula
    I. Tibia
35. A. Patella
    B. Medial femoral condyle
    C. Lateral femoral condyle
    D. Medial tibial plateau
    E. Lateral tibial plateau
    F. Medial tibial condyle
    G. Lateral tibial condyle
    H. Tibiofibular articulation
    I. Fibula
    J. Tibia

Exercise 7: Positioning for the Intercondylar Fossa

1. Kneeling
2. The patient can be standing with the affected knee flexed and resting on a horizontally oriented image receptor that is placed on a stool; the patient can be standing with the affected knee flexed and placed in contact with a vertically oriented image receptor; the patient can be kneeling on the radiographic table with the affected knee over the image receptor.
3. Against the anterior surface of the knee and centered to the patellar apex
4. Perpendicular to the center of the IR, entering the posterior surface of the knee
5. 70 degrees
6. The intercondylar fossa is primarily demonstrated, but the intercondylar tubercles, the femoral condyles, and the tibial plateaus can also be seen.
7. A. Patella
   B. Lateral femoral condyle
   C. Intercondylar fossa
   D. Medial femoral condyle
   E. Medial tibial spine
   F. Lateral tibial spine
   G. Tibia
   H. Fibula
8. a
9. b
10. Rest the patient's foot on a support.
11. Leg (tibia)
12. 40 degrees caudad (when the knee is flexed 40 degrees) or 50 degrees caudad (when the knee is flexed 50 degrees)
13. The amount of knee flexion
14. Intercondylar fossa
15. c, d, e, f, g, h, i

Exercise 8: Positioning for the Patella

1. Prone
2. Parallel
3. PA projections provide better recorded detail because of a closer object-to-image distance (OID) than the AP projection.
4. Use supports under the patient's thigh and leg to remove pressure from the patella.

5. Rotate the heel 5 to 10 degrees laterally
6. Perpendicularly to the midpopliteal area, exiting the patella
7. True
8. 10 degrees
9. A reduction in the femoropatellar joint space
10. Directed perpendicular to the knee, entering at the mid-patellofemoral joint
11. The patient can be placed in the prone position with the knee flexed and centered over the IR; the patient can be lateral recumbent with a vertically oriented IR placed against the anterior surface of the distal thigh; the patient can be sitting with his or her feet off the radiographic table and a horizontally oriented IR placed against the anterior surface of the distal thigh, or can be sitting with both feet on the radiographic table with the affected knee flexed and holding a IR against the anterior surface of the lower thigh.
12. The knee can usually be flexed to a greater degree, and immobilization is easier.
13. Lateral (to rule out a transverse fracture)
14. Instruct the patient to hold over his or her shoulder the ends of a long strip of bandage that is looped around the ankle or foot.
15. Perpendicular to the patellofemoral joint space (CR angulation will typically be 15 to 20 degrees.)
16. The degree of flexion of the knee
17. False (The patellofemoral articulation should be open.)
18. True
19. True
20. A. Patella
    B. Patellofemoral articulation
    C. Lateral femoral condyle
    D. Medial femoral condyle
    E. Fibula

Exercise 9: Positioning for the Femur

1. b
2. b
3. To place it in true anatomic profile and to place the femoral neck in profile
4. Perpendicular to the midfemur
5. The site of injury or pathology (The joint nearest the site of injury or pathology should be demonstrated.)
6. Use two image receptors to ensure that the entire femur is demonstrated.
7. Not foreshortened (in profile)
8. The lesser trochanter should not be seen beyond the medial border of the femur, or only a very small portion of the lesser trochanter should be seen.
9. The entire orthopedic appliance should be demonstrated.
10. False (Gonadal shielding can be positioned without superimposing the femur.)
11. A. Acetabulum
    B. Femoral head
    C. Greater trochanter
    D. Femoral neck
    E. Lesser trochanter
    F. Femoral body
12. c
13. a
14. (a) At the level of the ASIS; (b) 2 inches (5 cm) below the knee
15. (a) Posterior to the affected thigh; (b) anterior to the affected thigh
16. 45

17. Perpendicular to the midthigh
18. The IR should be placed vertically along the medial or lateral side of the thigh and knee.
19. a, c, e, f
20. A. Femoral head
    B. Femoral neck
    C. Lesser trochanter
    D. Ischial tuberosity
    E. Femoral body

Exercise 10: Evaluating Radiographs of the Lower Limb

1. The toes are not separated from each other.
2. a. Moderate overlapping of the talus with the distal tibia has occurred, which obscures the tibiotalar joint, and some overlap of the medial talomalleolar articulation has occurred.
   b. The foot was plantar-flexed rather than dorsiflexed, as evidenced by the appearance of the tarsals and the bases of the metatarsals.
3. The talofibular joint is not open, probably resulting from too much internal rotation of the lower leg.
4. i. a, b, e
   ii. Perpendicular (The magnified shadow of the medial femoral condyle obscures the femorotibial joint space.)

Self-Test: Osteology, Arthrology, and Positioning of the Lower Limb

1. a	26. c	51. b	76. d
2. c	27. c	52. a	77. d
3. b	28. b	53. d	78. a
4. d	29. d	54. b	79. a
5. a	30. d	55. d	80. c
6. d	31. b	56. d	81. a
7. b	32. a	57. d	82. b
8. c	33. c	58. b	83. a
9. d	34. b	59. c	84. d
10. d	35. d	60. d	85. b
11. b	36. b	61. c	86. d
12. b	37. d	62. b	87. a
13. c	38. d	63. b	88. b
14. c	39. b	64. b	89. c
15. a	40. a	65. d	90. d
16. d	41. d	66. b	91. a
17. c	42. d	67. a	92. c
18. b	43. c	68. a	93. b
19. b	44. b	69. d	94. a
20. c	45. c	70. b	95. c
21. a	46. b	71. a	96. d
22. a	47. b	72. c	97. d
23. b	48. d	73. d	98. a
24. b	49. b	74. c	99. d
25. c	50. b	75. a	100. a

CHAPTER 7 Pelvis and Upper Femora
SECTION 1 Osteology and Arthrology of the Pelvis and Upper Femora

Exercise 1

A. Iliac crest
B. Anterior superior iliac spine
C. Anterior inferior iliac spine
D. Acetabulum
E. Ischium
F. Obturator foramen
G. Ilium (or the ala of the ilium)
H. Auricular surface
I. Posterior superior iliac spine
J. Posterior inferior iliac spine
K. Ischial spine
L. Pubis

Exercise 2

A. Posterior superior iliac spine
B. Posterior inferior iliac spine
C. Greater sciatic notch
D. Ischial spine
E. Lesser sciatic notch
F. Ischial tuberosity
G. Ischium
H. Ischial ramus
I. Ilium (or the ala of the ilium)
J. Iliac crest
K. Anterior superior iliac spine
L. Anterior inferior iliac spine
M. Acetabulum
N. Superior ramus of the pubis
O. Obturator foramen
P. Pubis
Q. Inferior ramus of the pubis

Exercise 3

A. Greater trochanter
B. Neck
C. Head
D. Lesser trochanter
E. Body
F. Fovea capitis
G. Intertrochanteric crest

Exercise 4

A. Iliac crest
B. Anterior superior iliac spine
C. Ala
D. Sacroiliac joint
E. Sacrum
F. Acetabulum (or hip joint)
G. Greater trochanter
H. Lesser trochanter
I. Ischial ramus
J. Ischial spine
K. Obturator foramen
L. Pubic symphysis
M. Coccyx
N. Inferior ramus of the pubis

Exercise 5

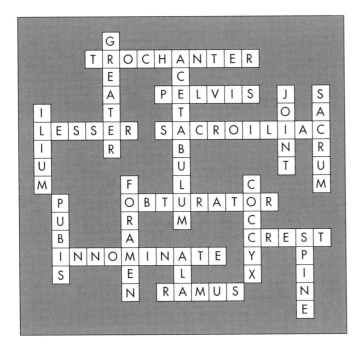

Exercise 6

1. a
2. c
3. j
4. e
5. d
6. i
7. k
8. g
9. h
10. f

Exercise 7

1. Pelvis
2. c
3. d
4. b
5. c
6. c
7. Ilium
8. Ischium and pubis
9. Acetabulum
10. Sacrum and coccyx
11. Greater (false) pelvis and lesser (true) pelvis
12. a. Above
    b. Below
13. Pelvic cavity
14. Female
15. Female
16. d
17. d
18. Femoral neck and intertrochanteric crest
19. Anteriorly
20. One pubic symphysis, two hip joints (femoral head and acetabulum), and two sacroiliac joints

21. Anterior superior iliac spine and superior margin of the pubic symphysis
22. Make a line from the anterior superior iliac spine to the upper margin of the pubic symphysis. At the midpoint of that line, extend a second line at a right angle and inferolaterally toward the femur. The long axis of the femoral neck lies parallel with the second line.
23. False (The greater sciatic notch extends from just below the posterior inferior iliac spine to the ischial spine.)
24. True
25. True

SECTION 2 Positioning of the Pelvis and Upper Femora

Exercise 1: Positioning for the Pelvis

1. Extend and rotate the lower limbs medially 15 to 20 degrees.
2. To place the femoral necks parallel with the plane of the IR
3. c
4. b
5. Midway between the ASIS and the pubic symphysis (approximately 2 inches [5 cm] above the pubic symphysis)
6. 1 to 1½ inches (2.5 to 3.8 cm) above the iliac crest
7. Perpendicular to the midpoint of the IR (approximately 2 inches [5 cm] above the pubic symphysis)
8. a. The proximal femora (greater and lesser trochanters and femoral neck)
   b. Fig. 7-5 (The lesser trochanters are minimally seen on the medial border of the femora; the greater trochanters are fully demonstrated; and the femoral necks are demonstrated in their full extent without anteversion.)
   c. Fully extended and rotated medially 15 to 20 degrees
   d. Fully extended with the feet rotated laterally into a naturally relaxed position
9. a, b, c, d, e, f, g, h, i, k, n
10. A. Iliac crest
    B. Ala of the ilium
    C. Anterior superior iliac spine (ASIS)
    D. Sacroiliac (SI) joint
    E. Anterior inferior iliac spine (AIIS)
    F. Femoral head
    G. Greater trochanter
    H. Obturator foramen
    I. Pubic symphysis
    J. Lesser trochanter

Exercise 2: AP Oblique Projection (Modified Cleaves Method)

1. Bilateral frogleg
2. As much as possible to get the femurs to a near-vertical position
3. 45 degrees
4. To place the long axis of the femoral necks parallel with the plane of the image receptor
5. Stop breathing (suspend respiration) during the exposure.
6. Perpendicular to a point on the midline of the patient about 1 inch (2.5 cm) above the pubic symphysis
7. c
8. False (The patient must be supine.)
9. False (The gonads should be carefully shielded to ensure that the shield does not superimpose the hip.)

10. True
11. False (The IR should be placed in the Bucky tray of the table.)
12. True
13. True
14. False (The greater trochanter can be minimally seen on the medial edge of the femur.)
15. True

Exercise 3: Projections for Demonstrating the Hip

1. a
2. d
3. c
4. Locate a point about 2½ inches (6 cm) distal on a line drawn perpendicular to the midpoint of a line between the ASIS and the pubic symphysis.
5. To the central ray (to a point about 2½ inches (6 cm) distal on a line drawn perpendicular to the midpoint of a line between the ASIS and the pubic symphysis)
6. Lesser
7. True
8. False (The patient should suspend breathing.)
9. True
10. A. Ilium
    B. Acetabulum
    C. Femoral head
    D. Greater trochanter
    E. Femoral neck
    F. Pubic symphysis
    G. Lesser trochanter
    H. Femoral body
11. a
12. Flex the affected knee and draw the thigh up to a nearly right-angle position relative to the affected hip centered to the midline of the table.
13. The unaffected leg should be extended and supported at the level of the hip.
14. To the hip joint, which is located midway between the ASIS and the pubic symphysis
15. a
16. d
17. A. Acetabulum
    B. Femoral head
    C. Femoral neck
    D. Lesser trochanter
    E. Ischial tuberosity
18. First, draw a line from the ASIS to the superior border of the pubic symphysis. Then draw another line from a point 1 inch (2.5 cm) inferior of the greater trochanter to the midpoint of the first line. The femoral neck runs parallel with this second line.
19. To elevate the pelvis and provide better centering of the hip to the image receptor
20. Flex the knee and hip of the unaffected side to elevate the thigh in a vertical position, then it can be rested on some support.
21. The IR should be placed in a vertical position with its upper border in the crease above the iliac crest and its lower border should be angled away from the body so that the IR is parallel with the long axis of the femoral neck.
22. Perpendicular to the long axis of the femoral neck, entering the patient on the medial aspect of the affected thigh near the groin, and centered to the image receptor

23. a
24. b
25. a
26. False (The pelvis should be adjusted so no rotation exists.)
27. False (The foot should be rotated medially if the patient's condition permits the maneuver.)
28. False (Only a small amount of the lesser trochanter should be seen on the posterior surface of the femur.)
29. False (No part of the unaffected thigh should superimpose the affected femur.)
30. A. Acetabulum
    B. Femoral head
    C. Femoral neck
    D. Greater trochanter
    E. Lesser trochanter

Self-Test: Osteology, Arthrology, and Positioning of the Pelvis and Upper Femora

1. a	5. c	9. a	13. a	17. c
2. d	6. a	10. d	14. c	18. d
3. a	7. a	11. b	15. b	19. d
4. b	8. b	12. b	16. c	20. d

CHAPTER 8 Vertebral Column
SECTION 1 Osteology and Arthrology of the Vertebral Column

Exercise 1

1. b, c, e
2. a, d, f
3. b, c, e
4. a, d, f

Exercise 2

1. A. Scoliosis
   B. Kyphosis
   C. Lordosis

Exercise 3

1. A. Transverse foramen
   B. Lateral mass
   C. Anterior arch
   D. Posterior arch
   E. Transverse process
   F. Superior articular process
2. A. Dens (odontoid process)
   B. Superior articular process
   C. Inferior articular process
   D. Transverse process
   E. Body
3. A. Dens (odontoid process)
   B. Superior articular process
   C. Spinous process
   D. Inferior articular process
   E. Transverse process
   F. Transverse foramen
   G. Body

4. A. Spinous process with bifid tips
   B. Superior articular process and facet
   C. Pedicle
   D. Transverse foramen
   E. Body
   F. Transverse process
   G. Vertebral foramen
   H. Lamina
5. A. Superior articular process
   B. Lamina
   C. Spinous process
   D. Inferior articular process
   E. Transverse process
   F. Body

Exercise 4

1. A. Spinous process
   B. Lamina
   C. Costal facet
   D. Superior articular facet
   E. Pedicle
   F. Body
   G. Transverse process
   H. Superior costal facet
   I. Vertebral foramen
2. A. Superior articular process
   B. Facet for costal tubercle
   C. Transverse process
   D. Lamina
   E. Spinous process
   F. Inferior articular processes
   G. Pedicle
   H. Superior costal facet
   I. Body
   J. Inferior costal facet
   K. Inferior vertebral notch

Exercise 5

1. A. Superior articular facet
   B. Accessory process
   C. Vertebral foramen
   D. Spinous process
   E. Lamina
   F. Mamillary process
   G. Transverse process
   H. Pedicle
   I. Body
2. A. Superior articular process
   B. Transverse process
   C. Lamina
   D. Spinous process
   E. Inferior articular process
   F. Pedicle
   G. Inferior vertebral notch
   H. Body
   I. Superior vertebral notch

Exercise 6

1. A. Sacrum
   B. Coccyx
   C. Ala
   D. Base
   E. Promontory
   F. Pubic (anterior) sacral foramina
2. A. Ala
   B. Superior articular process
   C. Sacral canal
   D. Body

Exercise 7

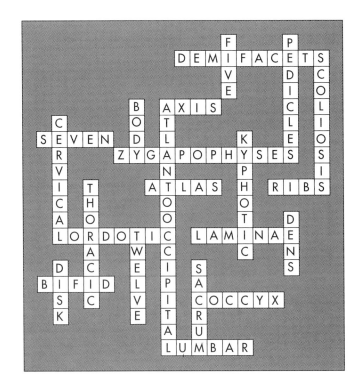

Exercise 8

1. e
2. f
3. a
4. d
5. b
6. c

Exercise 9

1. n   5. m   9. a   13. s   17. o
2. e   6. k   10. b 14. v   18. d
3. h   7. c   11. j 15. l   19. u
4. p   8. q   12. f 16. t   20. r

Exercise 10

1. The vertebral column encloses and protects the spinal cord; acts as a support for the trunk; supports the skull; and provides attachments for the ribs.
2. Cervical, thoracic, lumbar, and pelvic

3. Primary curves are formed before birth; secondary curves are formed after birth.
4. Thoracic and pelvic
5. Cervical and lumbar
6. Vertebral foramen
7. Atlas
8. Axis
9. Vertebra prominens
10. Body and spinous process
11. The transverse processes are perforated with a transverse foramen.
12. Axis (C2)
13. Odontoid process
14. Seven
15. 90 degrees
16. 45 degrees anteriorly
17. Thoracic
18. Thoracic
19. Ribs
20. 70 degrees anteriorly
21. 90 degrees
22. 30 to 50 degrees posteriorly
23. 90 degrees
24. Sacrum
25. 25 to 30 degrees anteriorly

SECTION 2 **Positioning of the Vertebral Column**

Exercise 1: Positioning for the Cervical Spine

1. The tip of the mastoid process
2. With the patient supine and the midsagittal plane centered to the midline of the table, extend the chin until the tip of the chin and the tip of the mastoid process are vertical.
3. Perpendicular to pass just below the tip of the chin, through the neck on the midsagittal plane, to the center of the image receptor
4. False (An attempt to use this position on a trauma patient may worsen the patient's condition.)
5. True
6. A. Anterior arch of the atlas
   B. Dens
   C. Foramen magnum
   D. Body of the axis
   E. Posterior arch of C1
   F. Occipital bone
7. b
8. Instruct the patient to open the mouth as wide as possible, then adjust the head so that a line from the lower edge of the upper incisors to the tip of the mastoid process (occlusal plane) is perpendicular to the image receptor.
9. Perpendicular to the center of the open mouth
10. To keep the tongue in the floor of the mouth
11. a
12. b
13. c
14. A. Occipital base
   B. Dens (odontoid process)
   C. Lateral mass of the atlas
   D. Inferior articular process of the atlas
   E. Spinous process of the axis

15. Extend the neck enough to lift the chin.
16. The occlusal plane should be perpendicular to the tabletop.
17. 15 to 20 degrees cephalad
18. C4
19. At or just inferior to the most prominent point of the thyroid cartilage
20. C1 and C2
21. d
22. a, b
23. All seven
24. C4
25. One inch (2.5 cm) above the EAM
26. Slightly elevate the patient's chin
27. Stop breathing after full expiration
28. Use an SID of at least 60 inches (150 cm) (72 inches [180 cm] is preferable).
29. Obtain a separate radiograph of the cervicothoracic region, usually by performing a "swimmer's lateral" (Twining method).
30. A. Mandibular rami
   B. Body of C3
   C. Inferior articular process
   D. Superior articular process
   E. Intervertebral disk
   F. Zygapophyseal joint
   G. Vertebra prominens (spinous process of C7)
31. Two inches (5 cm) above the EAM
32. The patient should drop the head forward and then draw the chin as close as possible to the chest.
33. The patient should elevate the chin as much as possible.
34. The body of the mandible should be almost vertical.
35. The body of the mandible should be almost horizontal.
36. All seven
37. a. All cervical spinous processes should be clearly demonstrated, elevated, and separated.
   b. All cervical spinous processes should be clearly demonstrated, depressed, and in close approximation.
38. b
39. 45 degrees
40. To C3
41. To prevent the mandible from superimposing the vertebrae
42. The superior vertebrae become rotated.
43. C4
44. 15 to 20 degrees cephalad
45. So that the beam coincides with the angle of the foramina and passes through the foramina openings
46. No
47. To keep the vertebral column horizontally aligned and parallel with the plane of the image receptor
48. Stop breathing for the exposure
49. b
50. a, c, d, e, g
51. a. RPO
   b. Left
   c. The ones farthest from the image receptor
52. Right
53. b
54. c
55. a
56. b
57. b
58. True

59. True
60. a. LAO
    b. Left
    c. Closer to

Exercise 2: Positioning for the Cervicothoracic Region

1. Swimmer's
2. Midcoronal
3. C7–T1
4. Elevate the arm closer to the IR, flex the elbow, and rest the forearm on the patient's head. The other arm should be extended along the side of the patient to depress the shoulder.
5. The shoulder closer to the IR should be rotated posteriorly, and the other shoulder should be depressed and rotated anteriorly.
6. The patient can be instructed to either stop breathing or take shallow breaths.
7. a
8. Lateral recumbent
9. Midcoronal
10. Head and lower thorax
11. c
12. a
13. False (The remote shoulder should be depressed and adjusted anteriorly or posteriorly to separate the shoulder shadows.)
14. a, b, c, d
15. A. Elevated humerus
    B. Elevated clavicle
    C. Depressed clavicle
    D. Depressed humerus

Exercise 3: Positioning for the Thoracic Vertebrae

1. c
2. a
3. c
4. Midway between the jugular notch and the xiphoid process
5. Approximately $1^1/_2$ to 2 inches (3.8 to 5 cm) above the upper border of the shoulders
6. Respiration should be stopped after full expiration to obtain a more uniform density.
7. The anode (so that the greatest percentage of the radiation beam is projected toward the thickest region of the thoracic vertebrae)
8. To avoid accentuating the thoracic kyphosis
9. Two radiographs should be taken (one for the upper vertebrae and one for the lower vertebrae), each with the appropriate exposure factors.
10. True
11. True
12. a. Fig. 8-32
    b. Fig. 8-32
    c. Fig. 8-32
    d. Fig. 8-31
13. b, d, e, f, h
14. A. 1st rib
    B. Clavicle
    C. T3 spinous process
    D. Vertebral body (T6)
    E. Transverse process
    F. Intervertebral disk
15. To place the heart closer to the IR, which minimizes overlapping of the vertebrae and heart

16. To keep the long axis of the vertebral column horizontal
17. $1^1/_2$ to 2 inches (3.8 to 5 cm) above the shoulders
18. Inferior angle of the scapulae
19. Place at right angles to the long axis of the body without drawing them too far forward.
20. Place a support of correct height under the foot of the shorter side.
21. To keep the long axis of the vertebral column horizontal with the plane of the image receptor
22. An average of 10 degrees cephalad for females and 15 degrees cephalad for males
23. Because men usually have a greater shoulder width than women
24. If the patient's condition permits, during quiet breathing, or if breathing is labored, at the end of expiration
25. To improve radiographic quality by preventing much scatter radiation from reaching the image receptor
26. The ribs should be superimposed posteriorly.
27. Swimmer's lateral
28. Perpendicularly
29. True
30. True
31. False (A breathing technique serves to blur lung markings; it has no effect on reducing scatter radiation.)
32. True
33. True
34. True
35. b, c, d, f, g, h

Exercise 4: Positioning for the Lumbar Vertebrae

1. A filled urinary bladder may produce an unwanted shadow on the radiograph and create secondary radiation.
2. 48 inches (122 cm); to reduce distortion, more completely open the intervertebral joint spaces, and improve the overall quality of the examination.
3. Midsagittal
4. Flex the patient's elbows and place the hands on the chest.
5. To reduce the lumbar curvature and place the lumbar vertebrae in closer contact with the table
6. The iliac crests
7. Perpendicular to the midline (midsagittal plane) at the level of the iliac crests (L4) for a lumbosacral examination or $1^1/_2$ inches (3.8 cm) above the iliac crests (L3) for a lumbar examination
8. The bodies, the intervertebral disk spaces, the interpediculate spaces, the laminae, the spinous processes, and the transverse processes
9. From the lower thoracic vertebrae to the sacrum
10. The lateral margin of the psoas muscles
11. An elastic waistband can cause an artifact shadow or distracting soft tissue folds in the image.
12. A. 12th rib
    B. Pedicle
    C. Lamina
    D. Transverse process
    E. Psoas muscle
    F. Intervertebral disk space
    G. Spinous process
    H. Lumbar body
    I. Sacroiliac joint
13. Midcoronal
14. With knees superimposed, flex the patient's hips and knees.
15. Place a radiolucent support under the lower thorax.
16. a

17. b
18. c
19. 5 degrees caudad for males; 8 degrees caudad for females
20. From the lower thoracic vertebrae to the sacrum when using a 30 × 35 cm IR, or from the lower thoracic vertebrae to the coccyx when using a 35 × 43 cm IR.
21. Yes
22. Intervertebral disk spaces should be open.
23. True
24. True
25. False (Close collimation is necessary to reduce the scatter radiation produced within the irradiated area.)
26. A. Body of L2
    B. Intervertebral disk space
    C. Intervertebral foramen
    D. Crest of ilium (iliac crest)
    E. Lumbosacral (L5–S1) interspace
    F. Sacrum
27. c
28. The junction is located in a coronal plane 2 inches (5 cm) posterior from the ASIS and $1\frac{1}{2}$ inches (3.8 cm) inferior to the iliac crest.
29. To the level of $1\frac{1}{2}$ inches (3.8 cm) inferior to the iliac crest
30. b
31. c
32. 5 degrees caudally for males; 8 degrees caudally for females
33. To include the lower one or two lumbar vertebrae and the upper segments of the sacrum
34. A. Body of L4
    B. Spinous process of L4
    C. Body of L5
    D. L5–S1 (lumbosacral) interspace
    E. Sacrum
35. 30 degrees; 50 degrees
36. 30 degrees
37. Right
38. L3
39. c
40. a
41. At a point approximately 2 inches (5 cm) medial to the elevated ASIS and $1\frac{1}{2}$ inches (3.8 cm) above the iliac crest.
42. It indicates that the articular processes are demonstrated.
43. A. Superior articular process
    B. Transverse process
    C. Pedicle
    D. Pars interarticularis
    E. Lamina
    F. Inferior articular process
44. Left
45. From the lower thoracic to the sacrum
46. b
47. a
48. True
49. False (The patient should stop breathing at the end of complete expiration for the exposure.)
50. False (Seeing the "Scottie dog" in the image means that the zygapophyseal joints are demonstrated.)
51. True
52. False (The central ray should always be directed perpendicular to the IR for AP oblique projections.)
53. True

54. A. Pars interarticularis
    B. Transverse process
    C. Zygapophyseal joint
    D. Inferior articular process
    E. Pedicle
    F. Superior articular process
55. The lower limbs may be extended or abduct the thighs to the vertical position
56. Lumbosacral (L5–S1) and sacroiliac joints
57. Lumbosacral
58. At a point approximately $1\frac{1}{2}$ inches (3.8 cm) superior to the pubic symphysis
59. 30 degrees cephalad for males; 35 degrees cephalad for females
60. Stop breathing for the exposure.

Exercise 5: Positioning for the Sacroiliac Joints, the Sacrum, and the Coccyx

1. True
2. True
3. 25; 30
4. 1 inch (2.5 cm) medial to the ASIS of the elevated side
5. To the level of the ASIS
6. Stop breathing for the exposure.
7. Perpendicular
8. 1 inch (2.5 cm) medial to the elevated ASIS
9. The supine position places the sacrum closer to the IR than the prone position does.
10. 15 degrees cephalad
11. A perpendicular central ray will cause the sacrum to appear foreshortened.
12. About 2 inches (5 cm) above the pubic symphysis
13. $3\frac{1}{2}$ inches (9 cm) posterior to the ASIS
14. To the level of the ASIS and $3\frac{1}{2}$ inches (9 cm) posterior
15. The midpoint of the IR should be at the level of the ASIS.
16. Stop breathing for the exposure.
17. Short-scale (high) contrast
18. Perpendicularly
19. A. L5
    B. Sacral promontory
    C. Sacral wing
    D. Sacral foramina
20. b
21. An AP projection (patient supine) places the coccyx closer to the IR than does the PA projection (patient prone).
22. 10 degrees caudad
23. On the midline of the patient at a point about 2 inches (5 cm) superior from the pubic symphysis
24. No (The use of a gonadal shield on a female patient would superimpose the coccyx; close collimation should be used instead.)
25. c
26. c
27. $3\frac{1}{2}$ inches (9 cm)
28. 2 inches (5 cm) inferior to the ASIS
29. Stop breathing for the exposure.
30. True

Exercise 6: Scoliosis Series (the Ferguson Method)

1. a
2. False (The patient should be either standing or sitting upright for both projections.)

3. True

4. False (The second radiograph requires that the patient be standing on a support block.)

5. False (Regardless of the projection, gonadal shielding should be placed between the patient and the x-ray tube.)

6. False (No compression band should be used.)

7. The thoracic and lumbar vertebral columns and about 1 inch (2.5 cm) of the iliac crests should be seen.

8. PA projections significantly reduce the amount of radiation exposure received by the gonadal area compared with AP projections.

9. 60 inches (162 cm)

10. Left

Exercise 7: Identifying Projections of the Vertebral Column

1. AP axial projection, cervical vertebrae
2. Left lateral projection, cervicothoracic region (Twining method)
3. AP projection, thoracic vertebrae
4. Left lateral projection, lumbar vertebrae
5. Left lateral projection, L5–S1 lumbosacral junction
6. Left lateral projection, sacrum
7. Left lateral projection, coccyx
8. AP projection (open mouth), atlas and axis
9. AP projection (Fuchs method), dens
10. Left lateral projection (Grandy method), cervical vertebrae
11. Left lateral projection (hyperflexion), cervical vertebrae
12. Left lateral projection (hyperextension), cervical vertebrae
13. AP axial oblique projection (LPO position), right intervertebral foramina, cervical vertebrae
14. PA axial oblique projection (RAO position), right intervertebral foramina, cervical vertebrae
15. AP projection, lumbar vertebrae
16. AP axial projection, sacrum
17. AP projection, coccyx
18. AP axial projection, lumbosacral junction and sacroiliac joints
19. AP oblique projection (RPO position), right zygapophyseal joints, lumbar vertebrae
20. AP oblique projection (RPO position), left sacroiliac joint

Exercise 8: Evaluating Radiographs of the Vertebral Column

1. The head is tilted back too far, allowing the occipital base to superimpose the dens.

2. The head is not tilted back enough to make the line from the lower edge of the upper incisors to the tip of the mastoid process perpendicular to the IR, thus the upper front teeth superimpose the dens.

3. Not all of the seven cervical vertebrae are demonstrated.

4. a. RPO

   b. The chin should be elevated so that the mandible does not overlap the vertebrae. The intervertebral foramina should be open with those farthest from the IR well demonstrated.

   c. Instruct the patient to elevate the chin higher to ensure that the mandible clears the vertebrae, and ensure that the patient is rotated 45 degrees from the AP body position.

5. Not all intervertebral foramina are clearly demonstrated because an earring superimposes a superior foramina.

6. a. Not all lumbar vertebrae are included. (L1 is not seen in its entirety.)

   b. The patient is rotated, as evidenced by the posterior margins of the vertebral bodies, not superimposed, and the ribs not superimposed posteriorly. The intervertebral disk spaces are not open, probably because the vertebral column was not parallel with the image receptor.

   c. The patient is rotated, as evidenced by the posterior margins of the vertebral bodies not superimposed, and the spinous process is not included within the image.

   d. The patient is rotated, as evidenced by the posterior margins of the vertebral bodies not superimposed and the ribs not superimposed posteriorly, and the anterior portions of L3 and L4 are not included within the image.

7. a. RPO

   b. Right

   c. No (The zygapophyseal joints for L5 are seen, however.)

   d. No (They are too far posterior on the vertebral bodies.)

   e. The patient was rotated too far from the supine position for the upper lumbar region.

8. a. LPO

   b. Left

   c. No

   d. No (They are too far anterior on the vertebral bodies.)

   e. The patient was not rotated far enough from the supine position.

Self-Test: Osteology, Arthrology, and Positioning of the Vertebral Column

1. d	26. d	51. a	76. a
2. d	27. a	52. d	77. c
3. a	28. a	53. c	78. a
4. d	29. c	54. b	79. c
5. c	30. a	55. b	80. c
6. b	31. a	56. a	81. e
7. b	32. d	57. d	82. c
8. b	33. b	58. e	83. b
9. a	34. e	59. a	84. a
10. b	35. a	60. b	85. c
11. b	36. a	61. b	86. a
12. a	37. e	62. d	87. c
13. b	38. a	63. d	88. a
14. b	39. c	64. d	89. b
15. e	40. d	65. b	90. e
16. a	41. c	66. d	91. d
17. e	42. a	67. a	92. e
18. c	43. d	68. c	93. b
19. a	44. c	69. a	94. e
20. a	45. c	70. b	95. d
21. d	46. e	71. b	96. b
22. c	47. d	72. c	97. c
23. b	48. c	73. b	98. a
24. c	49. d	74. d	99. a
25. d	50. b	75. b	100. a

CHAPTER 9 **Bony Thorax**
SECTION 1 **Osteology and Arthrology of the Bony Thorax**

Exercise 1

1. A. 1st rib
   B. 12th rib
   C. 1st thoracic vertebra (T1)
   D. Jugular notch
   E. Manubrium
   F. Sternal angle
   G. Body
   H. Xiphoid process
   I. Costal cartilage
   J. 12th thoracic vertebra (T12)
   K. 1st lumbar vertebra (L1)
2. A. True ribs
   B. False ribs
   C. Floating ribs
   D. Jugular notch
   E. Manubrium
   F. Body
   G. Xiphoid process
3. A. Jugular notch
   B. Sternoclavicular joint
   C. Clavicle
   D. Manubrium
   E. Sternal angle
   F. Body
   G. Xiphoid process
4. A. Thoracic vertebrae
   B. Lumbar vertebrae
   C. True ribs
   D. Costal cartilages
   E. False ribs
   F. Floating ribs
5. A. Head
   B. Tubercle
   C. Neck
   D. Angle
   E. Body
6. A. Sternum
   B. Costal cartilage
   C. Rib
   D. Vertebral body
   E. Head of the rib
   F. Rib tubercle
   G. Transverse process
   H. Costovertebral joint
   I. Costotransverse joint
   J. Spinous process

Exercise 2

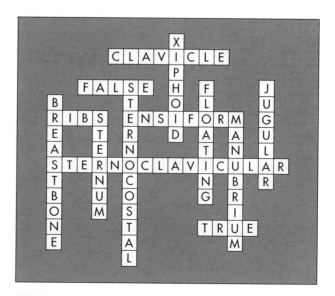

Exercise 3

1. i
2. b
3. h
4. a
5. d
6. k
7. g
8. f
9. e
10. j

Exercise 4

1. Sternum, 1; ribs, 12; thoracic vertebrae, 12
2. To protect the heart and lungs
3. Sternum
4. Manubrium, body, and xiphoid process
5. c
6. b
7. a
8. b
9. b
10. a
11. c
12. b
13. b
14. b
15. c
16. c
17. a
18. The first seven
19. 8, 9, and 10
20. 11 and 12
21. Heads of ribs with thoracic vertebral bodies
22. Transverse processes of thoracic vertebrae
23. Manubrium
24. True
25. False (The thickness, or breadth, of ribs gradually decreases to the 12th rib.)

SECTION 2 **Positioning of the Bony Thorax**

Exercise 1: Positioning for the Sternum

1. c
2. a
3. a
4. b
5. b
6. b
7. a
8. b, c
9. c
10. b
11. b
12. True
13. True
14. False (The right sternoclavicular joint should not superimpose vertebrae.)
15. A. Jugular notch
    B. Sternoclavicular joint
    C. Manubrium
    D. Sternal angle
    E. Body
    F. Xiphoid process
16. d
17. c
18. Posteriorly rotate the patient's shoulders to move the arms behind the patient and lock the patient's fingers together.
19. Extend the arms over the patient's head.
20. Large breasts of female patients should be drawn to the sides and held in place with a wide bandage.
21. Stop breathing after deep inspiration.
22. To obtain more contrast between the posterior surface of the sternum and adjacent structures
23. To keep the long axis of the sternum horizontal with the IR
24. True
25. False (Direct the central ray to the lateral aspect of the midsternum.)
26. False (The patient should suspend respiration after deep inspiration.)
27. True
28. True
29. True
30. A. Manubrium
    B. Sternal angle
    C. Body
    D. Xiphoid process

Exercise 2: Positioning for Sternoclavicular Articulations

1. Spinous process of T3
2. Place the patient's arms along the sides of the patient with the palms facing upward.
3. The patient's head should be rested on the chin for the bilateral examination.
4. The turning of the patient's head toward the affected side causes slight rotation of the vertebral column away from the sternum.
5. Perpendicular to T3
6. c

7. False (Only the sternal [medial] ends of clavicles need to be demonstrated with SC joints.)
8. False (No rotation of the vertebral column is permitted for a bilateral examination; slight rotation of the vertebral column is permitted only when one SC joint is demonstrated.
9. The affected side
10. 10 to 15 degrees
11. T2–T3 (about 3 inches [7.5 cm] distal to the vertebral prominens)
12. a
13. b
14. From the side opposite that being examined toward the midsagittal plane at an angle of 15 degrees
15. a. Perpendicularly
    b. RAO
    c. Right

Exercise 3: Positioning for the Ribs

1. Above; ribs above the diaphragm with slightly better recorded detail for anterior ribs, especially when the SID is 36 inches or less
2. Upright
3. To place the diaphragm to its lowest level and to demonstrate any fluid level within the thorax
4. With its upper edge $1\frac{1}{2}$ inches (3.8 cm) above the shoulders
5. Rest the backs of the patient's hands on the hips and roll the patient's shoulders forward.
6. Rest the head on the chin without any rotation or tilting.
7. Stop breathing after a full inspiration (to force the diaphragm to its lowest level).
8. Perpendicular to the center of the image receptor (the CR should enter the patient at the level of T7).
9. Direct the CR 10 to 15 degrees caudad.
10. The first nine
11. Upright; to aid in placing the diaphragm to its lowest level and to demonstrate fluid levels within the thorax
12. $1\frac{1}{2}$ inches (3.8 cm) above the upper border of the relaxed shoulders
13. To move the scapulae laterally away from the ribs
14. Stop breathing after full inspiration; to depress the diaphragm
15. Perpendicular to the center of the image receptor
16. Posterior (especially if the SID is less than 36 inches)
17. The first 10 posterior
18. a. Upright
    b. Stop breathing after full inspiration.
19. 35 × 43 cm
20. Supine; to place posterior ribs closer to the IR and to help elevate the diaphragm
21. The iliac crests
22. Stop breathing after full expiration; to elevate the diaphragm
23. Perpendicular to the center of the image receptor
24. The lower five (pairs 8 through 12)
25. a. Supine
    b. Stop breathing after expiration
26. True (with emphasis on the axillary portion)
27. True
28. The affected side
29. 45 degrees
30. a. Top border of the IR $1\frac{1}{2}$ inches (3.8 cm) above the shoulder
    b. Lower border of the IR at the level of the iliac crest
31. The location of the affected rib(s) with reference to the diaphragm
32. The first 10
33. The lower 5 (pairs 8 through 12)

34. a. LPO (left PA oblique)
    b. Left, with emphases on the posterior and axillary portions
    c. Left posterior
35. Right
36. RAO
37. Right-side
38. a
39. a. LAO
    b. Right anterior
    c. Left anterior
    d. Stop breathing after full inspiration
40. b, c, d, f, h

Self-Test: Osteology, Arthrology, and Positioning of the Bony Thorax

1. a	14. c	27. d	39. c
2. b	15. b	28. c	40. d
3. a	16. a	29. a	41. b
4. c	17. b	30. a	42. c
5. c	18. b	31. c	43. a
6. b	19. c	32. a	44. c
7. c	20. c	33. b	45. a
8. b	21. c	34. c	46. d
9. d	22. a	35. d	47. d
10. c	23. d	36. b	48. d
11. d	24. a	37. c	49. c
12. a	25. b	38. b	50. c
13. a	26. c		

CHAPTER 10 Thoracic Viscera
SECTION 1 Anatomy of the Chest

Exercise 1

1. A. Mediastinum
   B. Superior aperture
   C. Trachea
   D. Left lung
   E. Heart
   F. Diaphragm
   G. Inferior aperture
2. A. Right lung
   B. Trachea
   C. Left lung
   D. Diaphragm
   E. Heart
3. A. Pleura
   B. Right primary bronchus
   C. Bronchiole
   D. Trachea
   E. Larynx
   F. Left primary bronchus
   G. Terminal bronchiole
   H. Alveolar duct
   I. Alveolus
   J. Alveolar sac
   K. Pleural space
   L. Carina

4. A. Trachea
   B. Superior lobe
   C. Left primary bronchus
   D. Inferior lobe
   E. Carina
   F. Right primary bronchus
   G. Superior lobe
   H. Secondary bronchi
   I. Secondary bronchi
   J. Inferior lobe
   K. Heart
5. A. Apex
   B. Superior lobe
   C. Horizontal fissure
   D. Middle lobe
   E. Inferior lobe
   F. Oblique fissure
   G. Cardiac notch
   H. Hilum
   I. Base

Exercise 2

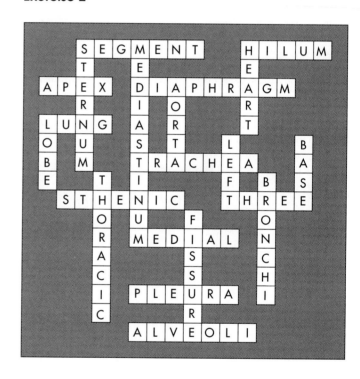

Exercise 3

1. a
2. d
3. a
4. a
5. a
6. a
7. b
8. b
9. a
10. b
11. b
12. a

13. Three; two
14. Right (because of its close proximity to the liver and heart)
15. a. Visceral pleura
    b. Parietal pleura
    c. Pleural cavity

Exercise 4

1. a
2. i
3. l
4. e
5. j
6. b
7. g
8. k
9. h
10. d

SECTION 2 Positioning of the Chest

Exercise 1: PA and Lateral Projections

1. At least 72 inches (180 cm); to reduce magnification of thoracic structures
2. To allow the diaphragm to reach its lowest level and to prevent engorgement of the pulmonary vessels
3. Midsagittal
4. Rest the backs of the hands low on the hips, below the level of the costophrenic angles; this maneuver rotates the scapulae laterally so that they do not superimpose the lungs.
5. c
6. b
7. c
8. b
9. d
10. c
11. Take in a breath and blow it out, then take in another full breath and hold it in. (Suspend respiration after the second full inspiration.) The greatest area of lung structures is demonstrated in full expansion and without strain after the patient suspends breathing on a second inspiration.
12. To demonstrate pneumothorax or to check for a foreign body
13. To prevent elongation of the heart caused by a full inferior movement of the diaphragm
14. a. Fig. 10-8
    b. The costophrenic angles are better visualized in that image.
15. a. Fig. 10-9
    b. More lung area is seen because the lungs in Fig. 10-9 are more expanded than the lungs in Fig. 10-10.
    c. 10
16. a, b, d, e, f, i, j, l
17. A. Air-filled trachea
    B. Lung apex
    C. Clavicle
    D. Scapula
    E. Aortic arch
    F. Bronchopulmonary markings
    G. Heart
    H. Diaphragm
    I. Right costophrenic angle

18. a
19. d
20. Midcoronal
21. Extend the arms directly upward, flex the elbows, and with the forearms resting on the elbows, hold the arms in this position.
22. A patient who is unsteady may use the IV stand for support.
23. $1^1/_2$ to 2 inches (3.8 to 5 cm)
24. Suspend respiration after full inspiration of the second breath.
25. Perpendicular to the midline of the IR, entering the patient on the midcoronal plane at the level of T7
26. False (The midsagittal plane should be parallel with the plane of the image receptor.)
27. True
28. True
29. a, b, c, d, e, f, i, j, l
30. A. Collimated radiation field
    B. Lung apex
    C. Esophagus (air-filled)
    D. Trachea
    E. Sternum
    F. Hilar region
    G. Superimposed posterior ribs
    H. Heart shadow
    I. Diaphragm
    J. Costophrenic angle

Exercise 2: PA Oblique Projections—Right Anterior Oblique (RAO) and Left Anterior Oblique (LAO) Positions

1. The one farther from the image receptor
2. Left
3. $1^1/_2$ to 2 inches (3.8 to 5 cm) above the vertebral prominens
4. 45 degrees
5. The desired structures to be demonstrated (more rotation when the heart is of primary interest)
6. 45 degrees
7. 55 to 60 degrees
8. After the second full inspiration
9. T7
10. Right PA oblique projection (RAO position)
11. True
12. True
13. True
14. a. Fig. 10-17
    b. Fig. 10-16
    c. Fig. 10-17
    d. Fig. 10-16
    e. Fig. 10-17
15. A. Trachea
    B. Esophagus
    C. Right lung
    D. Aorta
    E. Vertebral body
    F. Heart

Exercise 3: AP Oblique Projections—Right Posterior Oblique (RPO) and Left Posterior Oblique (LPO) Positions

1. The one closer to the image receptor
2. Left AP oblique (LPO position)
3. 72 inches (183 cm)
4. a
5. c
6. $1^1/_2$ to 2 inches (3.8 to 5 cm) above the vertebral prominens or about 5 inches (12.7 cm) above the jugular notch
7. Stop breathing after the second full inspiration.
8. 3 inches (7.6 cm) below the jugular notch
9. A. Trachea (air-filled)
   B. Vertebral column
   C. Magnified heart shadow
   D. Diaphragm
   E. Right costophrenic angle
10. a. Left AP oblique projection
    b. LPO position
    c. Left posterior
    d. Left

Exercise 4: The AP Projection

1. 72 inches (183 cm) or 60 inches (150 cm), depending on equipment limitations
2. Midsagittal plane
3. The upper border of the IR should be $1^1/_2$ to 2 inches (3.8 to 5 cm) above the relaxed shoulders.
4. With elbows flexed, pronate the hands and place them on the hips to draw the scapulae laterally.
5. Stop breathing after the second full inspiration.
6. To ensure maximum expansion of the lungs
7. 3 inches (7.6 cm) below the jugular notch
8. a. The heart and great vessels appear somewhat magnified.
   b. The lung fields appear shorter.
   c. The clavicles are projected higher.
   d. The ribs assume a more horizontal appearance.
9. a, e, f, g, h, i
10. A. Horizontal right clavicle
    B. Aortic arch
    C. Heart
    D. Diaphragm
    E. Costophrenic angle

Exercise 5: The AP Axial Projection (Lordotic Position)

1. b
2. With the patient standing and facing the x-ray tube, instruct the patient to move about 1 foot in front of the vertical grid device and lean backward, placing the upper back in contact with the grid device. The elbows should be flexed, and the posterior surface of the hands should be on the hips to better rotate the shoulders forward.
3. Stop breathing after the second full inspiration.
4. On the midsagittal plane, on the midsternum
5. a, c, f, g, h

Exercise 6: Lateral Decubitus Positions

1. To demonstrate air or fluid levels in the thorax
2. False (The patient must be positioned lateral recumbent.)
3. True
4. True
5. True
6. False (To demonstrate a fluid level, place the affected side down.)
7. False (Only the affected side needs to be entirely seen.)
8. d
9. Right
10. To enable free air within the thorax to rise and be better visualized against the lateral border of the ribs instead of overlying the vertebral column (if the affected side were down)
11. To enable the fluid to gravitate and be better visualized against the lateral border of the ribs instead of overlying the vertebral column (if the affected side were up)
12. Stop breathing after the second full inspiration.
13. a. Left
    b. Right
    c. Fluid
14. a. Right
    b. Up
15. a, c, d, e, g

Exercise 7: Ventral and Dorsal Decubitus Positions

1. Supine
2. Prone
3. Horizontally
4. 2 to 3 inches (5 to 7.6 cm)
5. 5 minutes; to allow fluid to settle and air to rise
6. Extend the arms well above the head.
7. Vertically with the top of the IR at the level of the thyroid cartilage
8. After the second full inspiration
9. On the midcoronal plane, approximately 3 to 4 inches (7.6 to 10.2 cm) distal to the jugular notch for the dorsal decubitus, and at T7 for the ventral decubitus
10. a, b, e, f

Exercise 8: Evaluating Radiographs of the Chest

1. The lung fields should be seen from the apices to costophrenic angles, but they are not.
2. a. The ribs posterior to the vertebral column should be superimposed, but those on the image are not.
   b. No shadow of the arm or its soft tissue should overlap the superior lung field, but the soft tissue shadow of the upper arm overlies the upper lung fields.
   c. The IR is positioned too low because the hilum is not seen in the approximate center of the radiograph.
3. a. The patient appears to be rotated, because the distance from the vertebral column to the lateral border of the ribs is not the same on both sides.
   b. Because the patient appears to be slightly rotated into the RPO position, the patient's position needs to be corrected by moving the left shoulder closer to the IR and ensuring that the patient is in the true AP projection position without any rotation.

Self-Test: Anatomy and Positioning of the Chest

1. b	6. c	11. c	16. c	21. c
2. c	7. b	12. d	17. d	22. c
3. d	8. a	13. b	18. c	23. b
4. b	9. b	14. a	19. b	24. a
5. b	10. b	15. d	20. d	25. a

CHAPTER 11 Long Bone Measurement

Review

1. The radiographic procedure whereby the perpendicularly directed central ray passes directly through each joint of a limb to provide accurate measurement of long bones
2. Lower limbs
3. Three
4. Movement by the patient could affect the accuracy of the measurement.
5. Anteroposterior (AP)
6. Under the affected leg and on top of the table
7. Flex the normal knee to the same degree and support both knees on supports of identical size.
8. Both sides should be radiographed.
9. a. Over the superior margin of the head of the humerus
   b. $\frac{1}{2}$ to $\frac{3}{4}$ inch (1.3 to 1.9 cm) below the plane of the humeral epicondyles
   c. Midway between the styloid processes of the radius and ulna
   d. 1 to $1\frac{1}{4}$ inches (2.5 to 3.2 cm) laterodistally at a right angle to the midpoint of an imaginary line extending from the anterior superior iliac spine to the pubic symphysis
   e. Just below the apex of the patella at the level of the depression between the femoral and tibial condyles
   f. Directly below the depression midway between the malleoli
10. The ends of bones are imaged with divergent rays; therefore, some magnification is produced.
11. Use the minimum object-to-image receptor distance (OID) and the maximum source-to-image receptor distance (SID) possible.
12. Because the central ray is perpendicular to and passes through the specified joint for each exposure
13. By subtracting the numerical values projected over the selected joints
14. To the midline of the table between two similar joints
15. In the anatomic position with slight medial rotation
16. Midsagittal
17. At the top of the table so that part of it is included in each of the exposure fields
18. One
19. Examine each limb separately
20. More consistent reproduction of the image and less radiation exposure to the patient

Self-Test: Long Bone Measurement

1. a	6. c
2. b	7. b
3. b	8. b
4. b	9. a
5. d	10. c

CHAPTER 12 Contrast Arthrography

Review

1. Radiography of a joint or joints
2. Magnetic resonance imaging
3. Menisci, ligaments, articular cartilage, and bursae
4. a. Water-soluble, iodinated medium
   b. Gaseous medium
   c. Combination of gaseous and water-soluble, iodinated media
5. Knee
6. True
7. False (A radiologist injects the contrast medium for arthrography.)
8. A radiologist
9. To put pressure against a joint in an attempt to widen the side of the affected joint
10. To permit better distribution of the contrast medium around the meniscus
11. AP projection; AP oblique projection with 20-degree medial rotation; AP oblique projection with 20-degree lateral rotation; lateral; and an intercondyloid fossa projection.
12. Hip dislocation
13. To detect a loose hip prosthesis or to confirm the presence of infection
14. AP projection with internal rotation; AP projection with external rotation; 30-degree AP oblique projection; axillary projection; and tangential projection
15. Computed tomography
16. Computed tomography and magnetic resonance imaging
17. Disk
18. $\frac{1}{2}$ inch (1.3 cm) anterior to the tragus of the ear
19. Tomography
20. Closed, partially open, and fully open

Self-Test: Contrast Arthrography

1. b	6. d
2. d	7. d
3. d	8. b
4. d	9. a
5. b	10. c

CHAPTER 13 Trauma Radiography

Review

1. A sudden, unexpected, dramatic, forceful, or violent event.
2. Level I trauma centers provide the most comprehensive medical and emergency car, whereas Level IV trauma centers provide care for basic injuries and can assess and stabilize patients for transfer to a larger trauma center.
3. 6 feet
4. Cool, clammy skin; excessive sweating; increased drowsiness; loss of consciousness; and patient complains of thirst.
5. Document the alterations for the referring physician and radiologist.
6. Lateral projection, dorsal decubitus position
7. When the entire cervical spine and the interspace between C7 and T1 is not well demonstrated with the lateral projection
8. Permission is granted from the attending physician after review of the lateral projection.

9. When the patient cannot depress the tube-side shoulder
10. To blur rib shadows
11. The attending physician
12. The compound CR angle will cause grid cutoff.
13. At a compound angle of 15 to 20 degrees cephalad and 45 degrees lateromedially
14. Slightly lateral to the midsagittal plane at the level of the thyroid cartilage, and passing through C4
15. Lateral projection, dorsal decubitus position
16. Horizontal and perpendicular to the center of the IR
17. Permission from the attending physician to transfer the patient to the radiographic table
18. Immediately inform the attending physician.
19. To prevent grid cutoff and image distortion
20. To allow any free air to rise and be visualized
21. Internal hemorrhaging and hemorrhagic shock
22. Immediately alert the attending physician.
23. Approximately perpendicular
24. Always include both joints.
25. Do not remove unless directed to do so by the attending physician.

Self-Test: Trauma Radiography

1. d
2. b
3. c
4. a
5. a
6. d
7. d
8. c
9. a
10. c
11. b
12. b
13. d
14. b
15. d
16. c
17. c
18. d
19. c
20. a